Praise for *Ginseng Diggers: A History of Root and Herb Gathering in Appalachia*

"*Ginseng Diggers* is a tour de force in the still-emerging field of US commons history. Manget guides us surefootedly through nineteenth-century Appalachian forests, excavating the intricate ecologies, economies, and cultural contexts medicinal plant gatherers routinely navigated. A worthwhile read for anyone interested in imagining more sustainable futures."—Kathryn Newfont, author of *Blue Ridge Commons* and coeditor of *The Land Speaks*

"Manget provides a fresh environmental context for considering issues crucial to Appalachian history, including the changing forest commons and the vagaries of capitalism in small communities. This is a must-read for anyone interested in ecology, economics, and the enduring legacy of the Appalachian 'sang digger.'"—Timothy Silver, author of *Mount Mitchell and the Black Mountains* and coauthor of *An Environmental History of the Civil War*

"Manget's impressive research in merchant records, correspondence, diaries, and local newspapers provides a fascinating glimpse at the evolution of ginseng culture in Appalachia and its connection to the national economy and society. A major addition to our understanding of land use, the role of the commons, and capitalism in the mountains."—Ronald D Eller, Distinguished Professor Emeritus at the University of Kentucky and author of *Uneven Ground*

"*Ginseng Diggers* provides crucial new insights into Appalachian subsistence practices. Manget opens up a whole new world of root and herb gathering, the business surrounding it, and the commons practices that made it possible. A must-read for scholars of Appalachia and anyone interested in the region's culture and history."—Daniel S. Pierce, author of *Tar Heel Lightnin'*

"Manget's study joins a number of books in recent years that challenge reductive narratives about Appalachia's cultural and economic history. *Ginseng Diggers* belongs in any library of books devoted to this necessary course correction."—*Chapter 16*

"*Ginseng Diggers* demonstrates that people find small avenues for persistence, just as ginseng and other threatened plants somehow do themselves. . . . Manget's book, centered on a humble (but medically efficacious) plant, is a fine Appalachian history."—T. R. C. Hutton, *Journal of Southern History*

"The impressive and extensive use of primary and secondary sources, documented with copious endnotes (some of which read like brief essays on their own), is tempered by Manget's engaging gift of storytelling. . . . A great read for anyone interested in the history, culture, and ecology of the Appalachian region."—Betty J. Belanus, Smithsonian Center for Folklife and Cultural Heritage

"A powerful account. . . . In a region historically plagued by extractive industry, new interpretations of capitalism may be exactly what is needed. For that, *Ginseng Diggers* is an impressive step forward."—Riccardo D'Amato, *Register of the Kentucky Historical Society*

"Manget puts a new focus on Appalachian and American history through the lens of 'commons commodities' (herbs and plants that through customary use belong to the gatherers and not to the landowners). He shows how these herbs, bolstered by early America's Jacksonian democracy and religious individualism, helped revolutionize American medicine. Furthermore, he describes how these 'commodities' enabled the formation of supply chains from the gatherers all the way to the metropolis and beyond and permitted the region to survive and contribute to the war efforts in the Civil War and World War I."—Dykeman C. Stokely, founder of Wakestone Books

"A model of the kind of Appalachian history the world needs now. . . . By building up a better understanding of how various individuals made use of the commons, *Ginseng Diggers* illustrates how mountain people played a central role in the development of botanical medicine—a story that extends far beyond the mountains and one that continues to have an impact on contemporary Appalachia."—Jeffrey A. Keith, professor of global studies at Warren Wilson College

"*Ginseng Diggers* begins to illustrate how the interconnection between East Asian markets and Appalachian medicinal remedies influences the perception of Appalachia, intimately addressing topics on gender roles, class relations, forest use, and commons management. . . . It's written so well that you'd think this unmatched understanding of ginseng was simple knowledge, but it's the first of its kind. It's relevant, original, globally thinking, and it's simply Appalachian."—Loyal Jones Appalachian Center at Berea College

GINSENG DIGGERS

GINSENG DIGGERS

A History of Root and Herb
Gathering in Appalachia

Luke Manget

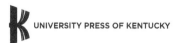
UNIVERSITY PRESS OF KENTUCKY

Editorial and Sales Offices: The University Press of Kentucky
663 South Limestone Street, Lexington, Kentucky 40508-4008
www.kentuckypress.com

Cataloging-in-Publication data available from the Library of Congress

ISBN 978-0-8131-8381-7 (hardcover)
ISBN 978-0-8131-8382-4 (pdf)
ISBN 978-0-8131-8383-1 (epub)
ISBN 978-1-9859-0180-3 (paperback)

This book is printed on acid-free paper meeting
the requirements of the American National Standard
for Permanence in Paper for Printed Library Materials.

Manufactured in the United States of America.

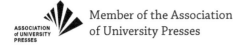

Member of the Association
of University Presses

To my grandmother, Orbenia Greer Stewart Burges,
who grew up digging roots and gathering herbs
in the mountains of eastern Kentucky
and who first stimulated my interest
in the botanical drug trade.

Contents

Introduction

From "Roots and Herbs" to "Crude Botanical Drugs"

> In locating her laboratories in different parts of the world, nature selected, as one of them, a vast wilderness in the mountainous region which one day was to be the southeastern United States. Here, in what is now southern Virginia and North Carolina, there gradually developed through the ages a wonderful flora, influenced by the tropics on one side and the bracing climate to the northward, of which perhaps some six hundred or more species have had medicinal application. Out of this Blue Ridge section of the Southern Appalachian System now comes 75 per cent of North America's contribution to the drug supplies of the world.
> —Henry C. Fuller, *The Story of Drugs*, 1922

HENRY WEBB SCANNED THE GROUND FOR PLANTS AMONG THE forested mountainsides surrounding the picturesque hamlet of Valle Crucis on the Watauga River. It was 1873 and, as in every other spring, the forest floor of this spot in northwestern North Carolina was decorated in a colorful carpet of wildflowers and herbaceous plants. Trilliums, trout lilies, Solomon's seal, blue cohosh, black cohosh, and dozens of other plants grew in the shade of Fraser magnolias, chestnuts, striped maples, sugar maples, beech, buckeye, and basswood trees. Webb may not have known every species of mountain flora, but he knew the ones that brought good prices at Henry Taylor's store down in the valley. The ultimate prize was ginseng, but it was becoming harder to find, so he settled for the lower-valued mayapple, bloodroot, angelica, and jack-in-the-pulpit, which everyone referred to as Indian turnip.[1] Webb referred to them collectively as "roots and herbs," and he could certainly use the bartering power these plants offered. Like everybody else's life in the Watauga Valley, Webb's had been severely disrupted by the war-torn 1860s. In 1870, pushing sixty years old, he had moved residences at least three times during the previous decade, married a wife half his age, had a son, and moved again to Valle Crucis, where he found work as a farm laborer. However, his wages alone did not provide his family with any measure of comfort. So he dug the roots of the medicinal plants that abounded in the mountains. From 1873 to 1876, he used $23.50 worth of roots to buy corn, sugar, tobacco, fishhooks, leather, and other necessities.[2] It may not have been much, but it was all the store purchases he made from Taylor during that time.

At his store in Valle Crucis, Henry Taylor collected a variety of roots and herbs from customers like Webb. He had done so for more than two decades. At least once every fall, "Uncle Henry," as he was affectionately called by the people of the valley, loaded up a wagon with his peculiar produce and hauled it down the mountain to sell. Before the war, he took his roots to a store near Wilkesboro owned by Calvin Cowles, exchanging them for goods that he hauled back up the mountain to sell in his own store. After the war, he started taking his roots and herbs to George W. F. Harper in the Piedmont town of Lenoir. Although it was not his entire source of revenue, the trade in native medicinal plants helped Taylor weather the post–Civil War depression when cash was scarce. In 1883, he opened a new store with a new partner, W. W. Mast, operating it until he died in 1899. In 1913, Mast purchased Taylor's interest, and the store became known as Mast General Store. There are now ten Mast General Stores scattered around the southern mountains.

George W. F. Harper, a veteran of the Confederate Fifty-Eighth North Carolina Infantry, returned from the Civil War to revive his father's store in Lenoir. Domestic demand for roots and herbs had grown since the war, and Harper eyed profits in purchasing roots and herbs from storekeepers like Taylor and selling them to wholesalers in New York, Boston, St. Louis, and Cincinnati who would, in turn, sell them to druggists, patent medicine makers, and pharmaceutical manufacturers. The roots and herbs that Harper and his competitors obtained from rural Appalachians eventually made their way into drugstores, physicians' offices, traveling medicine shows, and ultimately human bodies across the United States. As these roots, leaves, berries, flowers, barks, and seeds were abstracted from their mountain environment and entered the webs of exchange that scattered them to distant markets, they became known as "crude botanical drugs," or sometimes just "crude botanicals."

Harper found an eager buyer for his crude botanicals in Boston wholesaler Gardner S. Cheney. A mason in Boston before the war, Cheney had enlisted in a Massachusetts artillery company five days after President Lincoln's call for troops on 15 April 1861, and crossed Burnside's Bridge at Antietam. After the war, he jumped with both feet into the wholesale drug trade, forging a partnership with a former Harvard Shaker named Elisha Myrick to form Cheney and Myrick. Despite their divergent allegiances during the war, Cheney and the ex-Confederate Harper found common cause in the botanical drug trade. From 1867 to 1869, Cheney purchased nearly $10,000 worth of crude botanicals from Harper, far more than any other buyer. In the summer of 1869, the two spent a week botanizing and trout fishing in the Watauga Valley.[3]

Webb, Taylor, Harper, and Cheney formed one of many supply chains established in the wake of the Civil War that would turn the Southern Appalachian bioregion into the United States' largest supplier of medicinal plants to global markets. Stimulated by the Civil War and its aftermath, the pharmaceutical industry in the United States entered a period of rapid expansion and consolidation, and demand for crude botanicals skyrocketed. Consequently, between 1865 and 1900, root digging and herb gathering became a general occupation in some mountain communities. One observer claimed that more than forty thousand people gathered roots and herbs for one wholesale herb dealer in Western North Carolina alone during the height of the botanical drug boom in the 1880s.[4] By the turn of the twentieth century, according to one US Department of Agriculture estimate, the region supplied some three-quarters of all the native medicinal plants sold commercially in the United States.[5] Unmatched before or since, this botanical drug boom left a lasting impression on Appalachian communities.

On a basic level, this is a story about humans, plants, and mountains. While scholars have long known that Appalachian people engaged in root digging and herb gathering, this is the first monograph dedicated to the topic.[6] This book digs into the roots (pun intended) of the unique relationship between the Appalachian region and the global trade in medicinal plants to explain how and why the region became so integral to the trade. Re-creating the ecologies of root digging and herb gathering, it explores how the trade functioned on the ground, how that experience changed over time, and how the burgeoning commercial relationship influenced the region's land use, social relations, culture, economy, and ecology. While the trade involved hundreds of different kinds of plants, this book focuses primarily on a select handful of the most commonly traded, including mayapple (*Podophyllum peltatum*), bloodroot (*Sanguinaria canadensis*), wild ginger (*Asarum canadense*), lobelia (*Lobelia inflata*), and pink lady's slipper (*Cypripedium acaule*). The star of the book, however, is American ginseng (*Panax quinquefolium*). Ginseng was one of the first Appalachian herbs traded on a global scale, and it remained the most lucrative and sought-after throughout the nineteenth and twentieth centuries. Indeed, any understanding of the botanical drug trade in Appalachia must begin and end with ginseng. This book does just that.

On another level, this is a story of capitalism through the lens of a commodity.[7] By exploring the supply-chain dynamics of this trade, from the global context down to the local, this book presents a view of capitalism from the bottom up. And it is a different view than offered by most commodity studies. One significant characteristic that distinguished Appalachian roots and herbs from many other commodities was that they were not entirely privatized. Even as they stimulated the development of the early pharmaceutical industry, and even as elsewhere in the United States farmers had begun to supply botanical drug markets with plants cultivated on private farms, Appalachian roots and herbs were not raised in gardens prior to the twentieth century. Due to ecological, economic, and cultural factors, they remained what I call "commons commodities"—commodities harvested from the commons.

Never firmly codified in American law, the commons was a socially constructed institution that comprised overlapping use rights that governed access to unimproved interstitial spaces between improved areas of the landscape.[8] These rights—a feature of many rural areas in nineteenth-century America—were established by custom through both explicit and tacit negotiations among residents of a community. In many Appalachian communities, local custom dictated that the forested mountainsides were open to virtually all members of the district to obtain game, fish, livestock forage, firewood, honey, berries, fruits, greens, maple syrup, feathers, and medicinal plants, among many other resources. In effect, these resources comprised a species of property widely acknowledged as belonging to the harvester or gatherer rather than the landowner. Council Main, who grew up in the 1930s and 1940s in the Pottertown (now Tamarack) community of Watauga County, not too far from where Henry Webb harvested roots in the 1870s, explained the commons to an interviewer in 2005: "Back when I was little, you used to go anywhere and get [roots], and nobody would say nothing to you. That was the way of life, you know. If I found something on your land, I could get it. Or if they found it on ours, they could get it. You didn't have these 'no trespassing' signs. . . . The tops of the mountains were just for everybody."[9] These resources were often consumed at home, but enough extralocal markets existed for them that they could also provide commons users with access to the broader consumer economy. The commons custom made the postwar botanical drug boom possible at the same time that the botanical drug boom reinforced the commons custom in the mountains.

The concept of commons commodities can enhance our understanding of both capitalism and commodification in intriguing ways. Scholars who have examined the history of single commodities tend to reinforce a similar narrative: about how commodification fueled the development of industry and science, enclosed the commons, strengthened private property regimes, restructured ecological communities, and led to the accumulation of capital and the exploitation of labor. Commodification, in short, created and reinforced systems of inequality.[10] The story of roots and herbs, however, does not conform to this standard narrative. In the late nineteenth century, root diggers became an important part of the supply chains of some of the earliest and largest pharmaceutical companies, and yet they were remarkably free to engage with the market on their own terms. In this case, the market did not supplant the commons. It reinforced it. In her insightful study of the Matsutake mushroom pickers of the Pacific Northwest, anthropologist Anna Tsing has found a similar anomaly. Both the mushroom pickers and Appalachian root diggers operated within the framework of capitalism. That is, both were (are) mobilized by global markets and contributed to the concentration of capital that defines capitalism. However, the forces that brought these products to market did not lead to the rationalization of

5

labor and nature. They resisted the conditions of the plantation. They refused to be scaled up. They have their own story. Tsing calls this "salvage capitalism" and defines it as a system in which "lead firms amass capital without controlling the conditions under which commodities are produced."[11] As Tsing contends, the concept of salvage capitalism can broaden our perspective regarding alternative forms of capitalism. Indeed, if we pay closer attention to the peculiarities of individual markets and the human and nonhuman communities that supplied crude botanicals, we can see another way in which Appalachian communities structured their relationships with global economic systems. And it stokes the imagination.

This story also broadens our understanding of one of the oldest and richest veins of Appalachian scholarship: the transition to capitalism in the nineteenth century.[12] This discussion grew out of the War on Poverty in the 1960s as part of a national debate regarding the origins of the region's poverty. Talking back to those who blamed Appalachian people themselves for their poverty, scholars such as Harry Caudill and Ron Eller began to argue that Appalachia's poverty could be traced instead to the uneven or exploitative ways in which the region was incorporated into the capitalist economy. While scholars have disagreed over when the transformation began and the role that mountain people themselves played in it, most agree that the transformation from subsistence farming to industrial wage work at the end of the nineteenth century was chaotic and destabilizing, creating inequality, dependency, and poverty.[13] The story of the root and herb trade serves as a reminder that the specific impacts of the region's capitalist incorporation depended on the ecology of a particular commodity's production. Indeed, the production of medicinal plants for the pharmaceutical industry had very different impacts on human and nonhuman communities than the production of coal, timber, tobacco, or virtually any other extractive or agricultural product. This story also suggests that we must pay attention to the enclosure of the commons as a key causal factor in the region's transition to capitalism. Scholars have identified demographic pressures, adverse federal policies, depressed agricultural markets, and exploitative land-purchasing practices as the most important reasons why mountain communities transitioned away from agrarian independence. However, Steven Stoll has recently brought much-needed attention to the role of commons enclosure in undermining the ecological base of subsistence communities.[14] The story of the rise and decline of the root and herb trade illuminates one way in which commons enclosure contributed to the erosion of this agrarian world and accelerated the shift toward the wage-earning economy.

This book benefits from increased attention to the history of commons and common rights over the past twenty years. A lively debate regarding fence laws in the late nineteenth-century South has enriched our understanding of the southern livestock range as one iteration of common rights.[15] And historians examining localized contexts elsewhere have found evidence of such commons in the early republican Low Country, in the Great Dismal Swamp region in the mid-nineteenth century, in the Georgia Upcountry in the late nineteenth century, and among New Yorkers around Adirondack Park in the late nineteenth century.[16] Although they look at different types of resources, these scholars all identify a similar commitment to popular access to certain undeveloped resources. Stephen Aron refers to "rights-in-the-woods," suggesting that these were a powerful cultural force in late eighteenth-century Kentucky.[17] Christine Keiner has also found such rights among Chesapeake watermen's claims to oyster beds in the early twentieth century.[18] Appalachian scholars have long known of the existence of this informal system of use rights, but Kathryn Newfont's *Blue Ridge Commons,* which itself took a page from folklorist Mary Hufford's work, applied the term *commons* and demonstrated that it could be a valuable analytical lens to explore the region's history of land use.[19] Indeed, Newfont's scholarship, in many ways, laid the groundwork for this book.

A full history of such commons is difficult to uncover. It requires exploring that hard to reach space between the letter of the law and its enforcement, between the hegemonic system of private property and the informal systems that governed daily use. And it requires tight focus on local contexts and careful reading of primary sources. Often, commons users did not articulate their ideas unless they were threatened with enclosure. There were always tensions between those who wanted to limit access to the commons and those who wanted right of entry to it, and that tension bubbles up into the historical record from time to time. Little by little, scholars are piecing together the history of the American commons, revealing that it was much more widespread and powerful than once imagined.

Because it features some of the most significant commons commodities, the root and herb trade can provide a rare window into how the commons functioned and the purposes it served. Four broad claims, woven throughout the pages that follow, reveal insights into the history of Appalachia and the commons. First, the commons served as *both* an important social safety net for the landless and land poor in times of distress and as a preferred mode of production. Many root diggers were small farmers who relied on roots and herbs to supplement their farm production. Some were young, just starting out as independent producers, and needed the extra source of bartering power to purchase goods or pay their taxes. Some were devastated by the economic impacts of the Civil War and used roots and herbs to avoid the poorhouse and feed their families. Yet the commons was not solely an avenue of last resort. For others, it was an alternative to both the agricultural and industrial economy, a financial means of supporting a life dependent on hunting, fishing, and gathering. Cherokee Indians relied heavily on selling ginseng and other roots as a way to maintain their traditional land-use practices. Some Euro-Americans also preferred digging roots to hoeing corn or working for wages, and they engaged in this activity specifically to resist the pull into these types of labor. Thus, whereas some mountain people fell back on the commons during hard economic times, they also pursued it as preferred alternative to prevailing modes of production. These dynamics changed over time and were frequently in tension with one another.

Second, the commons was not a static institution. It was a historical institution, subject to change over time as markets evolved and use rights were negotiated and renegotiated. One of the changes detailed in this book is the shifting class dynamics of the commons over the course of the nineteenth century. Whereas root digging and herb gathering had been mostly a part-time activity of small farmers prior to the Civil War, it became more often a full-time occupation after the war. As the mountain economy struggled, and markets for more plants opened, men and women specialized in hunting roots and herbs, putting different pressures on the commons and creating different tensions within communities. Due to these changes, the Appalachian gathering commons underwent a significant renegotiation in the late nineteenth and early twentieth centuries. Scholars have given some attention to the closing of the open range and the game and fish laws passed in the late nineteenth century, but the enclosure of the medicinal plant commons has received virtually none. This enclosure took place at different times in different communities, and it unfolded in a variety of forms. Rooted in tensions within communities that emerged during and after the Civil War, pitting landowners and part-time commons users against full-time diggers, this enclosure movement blossomed with a wave of state laws that strengthened landowners' rights to the wild-growing plants on their property. Focused primarily on ginseng and other lucrative roots, this movement often manifested itself in the literal enclosure of plants within fences, but it took other forms as well. The loss of markets for some specific plants in the mid-twentieth century indirectly aided the enclosure movement and effectively ended much of the root digging and herb gathering in Appalachia.

Third, as medicinal plant populations declined, some diggers adapted by adjusting their habits and values, thus ensuring that the struggle for conservation would play out across time and space at a grassroots level. Thus, this book provides something of a corrective to the (in) famous claim of biologist Garrett Hardin. In his 1968 essay in the journal *Science,* "The Tragedy of the Commons," Hardin offered a grim assessment of the fate of nature in a commons. "Picture a pasture open to all," he wrote. Each herdsman in this hypothetical pasture, acting in his own self-interest, would gradually increase the size of his herd, thereby consuming more of a particular resource (in this case grass) until it collapsed. Hardin was making the Malthusian point that the pressures of population growth on the resource base has no technical solution and therefore requires a reorientation of Americans' laissez-faire culture. However, the message that has resonated with academics ever since was his assumptions about the commons. Those resources are destined for collapse, he implied, because users lack necessary incentives to conserve them. "Ruin is the destination towards which all men rush, each pursuing his own interest in a society that believes in the freedom of the commons," he wrote. "Freedom in a commons brings ruin to all."[20]

Hardin's work has stimulated tremendous interest in property regimes and resource use, and academics and resource managers remain deeply divided over his thesis. Philosophical conservatives saw this warning as an argument for privatization, whereas liberals and many conservation biologists used it to champion greater state management of common resources. Moreover, critics challenge Hardin's basic thesis by asserting that his open-access pasture was a rhetorical invention, not an actual commons. Thus it did not account for contingencies such as market forces or the ability of commons users to mobilize cultural forces to mitigate overuse. Scholars have shown that rural peoples around the world have developed viable commons systems that effectively conserve resources.[21] Economist Elinor Ostrom won a Nobel Prize in economics in 2009 for her work on human behavior and common-pool resources in which she points out the many alternative systems that exist for limiting commons harvests without relying on either privatization or state management. She argues that models explaining the inevitable collapse of commons resources do not take enough consideration of local context.[22]

Indeed, local context matters. This book suggests that a more complicated set of factors contributed to the eventual decline of the root and herb commons. Not all root diggers were always motivated by maximizing profits, and not all carelessly exploited their resource. While it is difficult for the historian to tell if there was ever a time when the gathering commons was effectively managed on a local level for sustainable yields, it is safe to say that some tried to adjust their practices to adapt to declining populations of roots and herbs. This history suggests that the cultural forces of exploitation and conservation were constantly in tension with one another, and they interacted with other factors, such as population growth, class dynamics, and market demands, to shape the way the commons changed over time. In short, this book injects historical contingency into the discussion of commons use.

The fourth theme highlights how the commons in general and root digging in particular informed popular perceptions of mountain people. While scholars have thoroughly deconstructed Appalachian stereotypes—from moonshiners and "hillbillies" to feudists and Unionists—root diggers have not yet received any scholarly attention. From the 1860s through the 1910s, newspaper reporters, magazine writers, missionaries, and novelists created a distinct mythology surrounding the root diggers and herb gatherers of Appalachia. They were most often called "sang diggers," or "sangers," epithets based on the colloquial term for ginseng, "sang." Despite the fact that they were enmeshed in the supply chains of one of the most significant growth industries of the last 150 years, in the hands of these writers, they became the most backward of all mountaineers, totally isolated from the main social, cultural, political, and economic currents sweeping the nation. The commons and mountaineers' relationship to it thus formed an important component of the broader hillbilly stereotype that continues to inform popular perceptions of the region.[23]

These four themes unfold here in a roughly chronological narrative that begins in the 1710s when American ginseng was first commodified. Chapter 1 explores the evolution of the ginseng market in China and how ecological and political factors led to the discovery of ginseng in Canada in 1716. It also focuses on how the first ginseng boom of the 1750s shaped the experiences of both Native Americans and Euro-American settlers along the borders of Iroquoia. Chapter 2 follows the ginseng boom into the Ohio Valley and the mountains of West Virginia and Kentucky, where it facilitated the Euro-American settlement of the region in the late eighteenth and early nineteenth centuries. Over the course of the antebellum era, ginseng was incorporated into rural communities' seasonal subsistence patterns, which depended on both the forest and the farm. By the 1850s, it had surpassed skins and furs as the most commonly traded forest product.

Chapter 3 shifts the focus away from ginseng and examines the creation of markets for a wide variety of other Appalachian plants. Sectarian challenges to medical orthodoxy and the rise of patent medicine and pharmaceutical manufacturing in the 1840s and 1850s stimulated demand for indigenous plants to be made into medicines. Calvin Cowles of Wilkesboro, North Carolina, was one of the first to link Appalachian plants to these burgeoning markets, and by the outbreak of the Civil War, he had established a trade network that stretched from country stores on the Blue Ridge to manufacturers in the midwestern and northeastern United States as well as in Europe. Chapter 4 charts the emergence of Southern Appalachia as the nation's premier botanical drug–exporting region and the role the Civil War played in stimulating it. The decades following the war witnessed the rise of some of the largest wholesale botanical drug dealers in the nation, if not the world, and most of them were located around the southern mountains.

The next two chapters bring the focus to the forests of Appalachia to detail the local dynamics of the post–Civil War root and herb boom.

Chapter 5 makes the case that the economic depression that settled on the region after the war made root digging and herb gathering an attractive alternative to the agricultural economy, and many people fell back on the forests to make ends meet. In the process, roots and herbs shaped class and gender dynamics across the landscape and led to the rapid depletion of ginseng populations. Chapter 6 explores the social tensions that the postwar root and herb boom engendered and the many efforts undertaken by local landowners and commons users to conserve that most illustrious of all roots, ginseng. Beginning in the 1870s, the commons system that supported the gathering of medicinal plants underwent a significant renegotiation as landowners worked to curb common rights, a process that continues today.

This book's final chapter explores the growth of the sang-digger myth, the role it played in shaping outside perceptions of Appalachia, and the functions it served for a rapidly modernizing nation. Another form of literary exploitation, the myth originated inside Appalachian communities by mountain elites who wanted to distance themselves from their more rural neighbors. Writers, journalists, and missionaries took it to a national audience, for whom it served as a commentary on civilization and savagery and the proper relationship between nature and culture. The stereotypes achieved the same purpose for mountain life as the enclosure movements. They undermined a way of life that depended on the farm and forest commons by further delegitimizing the commons in the eyes of the national community.

These deeply held prejudices both within and outside Appalachia have contributed to an overall dearth of reliable historical sources on the region's root diggers and herb gatherers. The commerce in roots and herbs was not consistently documented by any government agency or trade association until the second half of the twentieth century. While export data can provide some loose parameters for the trade dating back to the 1790s, they are not reliable for re-creating the scale and extent of the trade in any given locale. Moreover, nineteenth-century economic boosters were not interested in discussing the trade as an important industry going forward. In the rare instance in which they promoted ginseng, for example, as a potentially lucrative commodity, they almost always championed privatization as the path forward. The commons played no role in regional boosterism. It was something to be overcome, to be enclosed and privatized, so that the region's economic future could be realized. Foraging was too closely associated with "savagery." Local historians writing in the nineteenth and early twentieth centuries touted their counties' railroads, factories, banks, and other measures of capitalist "progress." They rarely mentioned roots and herbs. Those writers and journalists who did describe the region's root diggers were more interested in feeding mountaineer stereotypes. For the mountain "elite," root digging was an aspect of mountain life to be ridiculed or ignored.

Telling this story, therefore, requires overcoming this bias in the historical record. It involves creative use of an eclectic collection of sources culled from the holdings of state and university libraries, local history museums, and country stores in five states. It includes diaries, correspondence, newspapers, and census records as well as ecological and anthropological studies. This story relies most heavily on business records from mountain merchants, Piedmont wholesalers, northern pharmaceutical manufacturers, and patent medicine makers. In total, I examined some sixty-five store ledgers and daybooks that document the business carried on at roughly thirty-four different establishments. Geographically, they range within Appalachia from northern West Virginia to southwestern North Carolina and outside the region from New York and Philadelphia to Boston. Temporally, they range from the late eighteenth century through the early twentieth century. The availability of these sources has imposed some limitations. Some time periods and geographic areas are more fully represented than others. For example, ledgers from East Tennessee and eastern Kentucky are decidedly lacking, and there are far more ledgers available from the late nineteenth century than the early nineteenth century. Nevertheless, as the first comprehensive history of the botanical drug trade, this book breaks new ground where furrows did not exist.

In the interest of full disclosure, I come from a family of root diggers and herb gatherers. My grandmother and her siblings grew up digging sang, mayapple, and bloodroot in the forests of Pike County, Kentucky. Their grandfather (my great-great-grandfather), John U. Greer, learned to hunt sang in those mountains from his father in the 1870s and later taught his son and grandchildren how to find it. After Consolidation Coal Company opened up the Elkhorn Coal Fields in the 1910s and built the company town of Jenkins, Greer refused to work in the mines like his sons and continued to dig ginseng in the mountains. By all accounts, it was one of his favorite things to do.

I saw my first ginseng plant in July 1996 on a mountainside along Beefhide Creek near the border of Pike and Letcher Counties. I was fifteen years old and visiting Kentucky for our biennial family reunion when my cousin Paul Randy Osborne pointed it out behind the barn on my family's property. On a hike, I might have walked right past it, but Paul Randy had been watching that plant all season, waiting for it to produce berries so he could dig it and sell it to the dealer in Jenkins. Despite having hiked through countless forests in the mountains near my home in North Georgia and Western North Carolina, I had never seen this elusive plant outside of a field guide. Some years later, Paul Randy told me with bitterness that he had built up his patch of ginseng over several years only to have his plants dug up and stolen. Surprisingly, the thief did not hide his deeds. When Paul Randy confronted him, he admitted, "I just couldn't help myself. It was such a pretty patch of sang." It was yet another episode in the struggle over the ginseng commons.

I did not grow up digging roots, but thanks to the stories I heard from my grandmother and the rest of my family, I took to hunting roots in historical archives as a graduate student. In telling this story, I aim to shine light on family history as well as regional and American history.

1 The Journey of Ewing's Roots

American Ginseng and the China Trade

IT MAY HAVE BEEN GROWING AMONG THE OLD-GROWTH CHESTNUTS ON the side of Little Mountain. Or perhaps it had matured under the butternut trees on the banks of Turkey Creek. Somewhere near the brand-new hamlet of Union in the western Virginia backcountry in October 1783, a Scots-Irish settler named William Ewing spotted a small plant among the deep green understory. He saw the cluster of bright red berries perched atop a peduncle that protruded from the center of the twenty-inch-high herb. He counted the leaves: four. His heart beat a little faster. It probably had a large root. If he could find a few more like this, he could buy a knife, a pair of spectacles, a pound of gunpowder, a bushel of salt, or maybe a pint of rum.[1]

The Iroquois called it *garangtoging,* or "child's thigh."[2] The Cherokee named it *atali-guli,* "the mountain climber," and sometimes *Yunwi Usdi,* "the little man."[3] William Byrd of Virginia referred to it as the "plant of life," and the Tartars, living in the northern Chinese province of Tartar, called it *Orhota,* or "queen of the plants."[4] Linnaean taxonomists would later label it *Panax quinquefolium.* Ewing knew it as "sang," a shortening of the word *ginseng,* which was itself derived from the Mandarin *jen-shen.*"[5] Indeed, it was a world-famous plant.

Ewing had only one month to gather the plant before it disappeared for the season. A deciduous perennial, ginseng can grow for dozens if not hundreds of years, but its top—that is, everything but the root and rhizome—dies back every year after the first frost. He likely knew that it

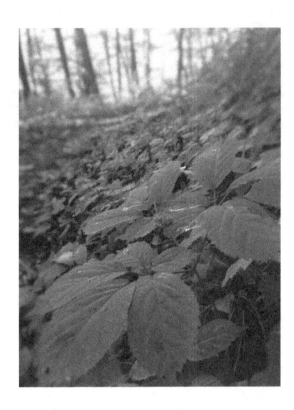

American ginseng (*Panax quinquefolium*). (Photo by Daniel Manget.)

grew in cool deciduous forests, and although it could be found in the Piedmont, it seemed to prefer what one mid-eighteenth-century observer called "the hills that lie far from the sea."[6] As early as the 1730s, colonists recognized the tendency of the plant to grow on the "north sides of mountains and very high hills, that are shaded with trees."[7] Seeds are typically dispersed by gravity and rain runoff, most ending up less than a few feet from their mother plant.[8] Thus, Ewing was unlikely to encounter ginseng on a short jaunt, but when he did find one plant, there were probably hundreds more nearby. It was like treasure hunting.

Ewing uprooted the full ginseng plant from the earth, cut the leaves and stem off, and placed the gnarly root in a small sack, where this singular specimen joined hundreds of its kinsmen. His 186 pounds of roots were taken to James Alexander's trading post in Union, where they were exchanged for, among other things, one pound of gunpowder, a hat, a pint of rum, and two saddles. At the end of the season, as the weather turned bitterly cold, Alexander would have loaded Ewing's roots up with thou-

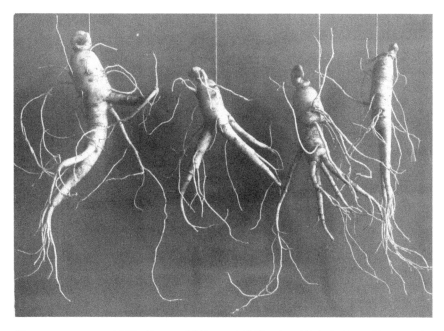

Ginseng roots, ca. 1902. (State of Missouri Collection, P0018, State Historical Society of Missouri.)

sands of other ginseng roots and hauled them in a covered wagon to Staunton in the Shenandoah Valley. At Staunton, there is a good chance that they were purchased for close to 4 shillings per pound by Dr. Robert Johnston, who had procured large amounts of ginseng there in the summer and fall of 1783. If they had ended up in Johnson's hands, they would have been taken to Philadelphia, then up the coast to New York where they, along with some fifty-seven thousand pounds of other ginseng roots dug from the Virginia and Pennsylvania backcountry, were loaded on the *Empress of China* bound for the Far East. These roots would prove crucial in opening trade relations between the United States and China.[9]

The trade that brought Ewing's roots from western Virginia to the Far East was made possible by a worldwide market built by cultural developments, social and political struggles, and ecological relationships that unfolded on a spatio-temporal scale that was both global and evolutionary. Originating in northern China, the market for ginseng was extended deep into the backcountry of Southern Appalachia over a period of centuries by emperors and missionaries, colonists and Native Americans, wealthy merchants and itinerant storekeepers. This market transformed the plant from an inconspicuous herbaceous perennial into a lucrative commodity for mass consumption.

Nature, Culture, and Ginseng in East Asia and Eastern North America

The market that provided Ewing with his store-bought goods was made possible by ecological forces 300 million years in the making. The ancestor of American ginseng, the first in the *Panax* genus, likely originated in the mountains of northeastern China sometime well before the Pleistocene glaciation.[10] At that time, mixed mesophytic (medium moisture) forests blanketed most of the Northern Hemisphere, and the environments of China and North America had similar climates and terrain. Over ensuing ages, the plant, along with other Asian flora and fauna, migrated into North America. Scholars disagree on exactly how and when it got there, but most biogeographers believe that through the very gradual process of seed dispersal, it crossed the Bering land bridge that connected the two continents beginning around 10 million years ago.[11] As glaciers covered much of the Northern Hemisphere during the Pleistocene, ginseng's range fragmented and the plant underwent a process called vicariance. Cut off from its ancestral populations, it developed new characteristics in North America and became genetically distinct, forming a new species, *Panax quinquefolium*. By the time the glaciers retreated around eleven thousand years ago, most of the world's *Panax* populations were limited to eastern North America and eastern Asia.[12] The species' Asian homeland was primarily between the thirty-ninth and forty-seventh parallel in the thick forests that covered rugged mountains in northern China—the so-called Tartary region—and the Korean Peninsula. American ginseng grew in eastern North America across a wide geographical range that formed something of an inverted triangle. It grew as far north as southern Canada, stretching from Minnesota and Ontario in the west to Nova Scotia in the east, and as far south as North Georgia, with small populations in the Ozarks of Missouri and Arkansas. Ginseng was not the only plant to find refuge among the eastern mountains from global environmental forces. Indeed, the regions share some 120 genera of flowering plants, most of which likely made similar journeys. The existence of genetically similar species in two geographically different regions of the world is a phenomenon biogeographers call disjunction, and the East Asia–eastern North American connection is one of the most striking examples of disjunction in the world.[13]

Over the ensuing millennia, ginseng became woven into the cultural fabric of Asian and North American peoples, often in remarkably similar ways. Many writers on ginseng claim that the Chinese incorporated the plant into their medical systems as early as 2600 BC when a man named Shen Nung penned the first Chinese medical text, the *Pen Ts'ao Ching*.[14] Its value was in the role it played in a system of medicine grounded in a cosmology of balance.[15] Influenced by both Confucian and Taoist thought, the Chinese believed that the universe was infused with a vital life force called *Qi* that operated according to the polarizing yet complementary forces of *yin* and *yang*. The human body, like the rest of nature, was a temporary assemblage of Qi that was kept in balance by the interplay of yin (femininity, darkness, earth, and passivity) and yang (masculinity, lightness, heaven, and activity). This balance could be affected by the presence or absence of certain sensory experiences, elements, or emotions, or the relative activity of certain organs (or viscera), specifically the kidney, spleen, pancreas, liver, heart, and lungs.[16]

By the end of the first millennium AD, the Chinese had integrated Taoist herbal therapies into Confucian theories on health, developing a pharmacology that ascribed specific uses to ginseng and other plants according to the yin-yang system of correspondence. According to the *Pen Ts'ao Ching*, ginseng was used for "repairing the five viscera, harmonizing energies, strengthening the soul, allaying fear, removing toxic substances, brightening the eyes, opening the heart, and improving thought. Continuous use will invigorate the body and prolong life." In short, ginseng could help strengthen the yang in order to restore balance, which can partly explain why the root became known as an aphrodisiac. It was, as physician Stephen Fulder states, the most important herb in a "pharmacology of harmony."[17] By the time of the Ming Dynasty (1368–1644), ginseng had become one of the most widely prescribed herbs in Chinese medicine.[18]

Although ginseng had been an article of trade among Asian kingdoms since at least the Han Dynasty (202 BC–AD 220), evidence suggests that by the early eighteenth century, overharvesting had become a significant problem. Because harvesting the root kills the entire plant, and because it takes at least eight years, preferably ten to fifteen, for the plant to reach harvestable size from seed, ginseng was particularly susceptible to overharvesting.[19] But the decline of ginseng accelerated as it assumed a significant commercial role in imperial politics during the seventeenth century. The founders of the Qing Dynasty (1644–1911), which overthrew the Ming Dynasty (1368–1644) in midcentury, were ethnic Manchus from the ginseng-growing regions of Tartary (now Manchuria). The monopolization of the ginseng trade formed the financial base of their power both before and after their overthrow of Ming rulers.[20] With Manchus in control of the empire, Qing emperor Kangxi moved to protect their homeland from encroachments by ethnic Han Chinese, including the protection of their ginseng from Han poachers. When the French Jesuit priest Pierre Jartoux visited the Manchu region on a surveying expedition in 1709, he noted that the local Tartars had erected a fence of wooden stakes around their mountainous ginseng strongholds and patrolled it with armed guards. This was no effort at conservation but rather an ethnically motivated attempt to monopolize the exploitation of the plant. To control the harvest, Kangxi ordered ten thousand Tartars, under Mandarin overseers, to comb the mountains and forests and pluck every ginseng plant they found, each person to give the emperor two ounces of the best root.[21] Each digger in this "army of herbalists," wrote Jartoux, carried only a small shovel and a sack of millet and braved the weather, as well as wild animal attacks, for six months out of every year. "These poor people suffer a great deal in this Expedition."[22] Despite these precautions taken by the Qing emperor, thousands of Han Chinese risked their freedom and their lives every year to cross into the ginseng region and harvest the plant for sale.

Habitat loss also played a role in ginseng's decline in East Asia. Because the plant requires the rich humus and heavy shade found in cool deciduous forests, deforestation for agricultural purposes had deleterious effects on ginseng populations. As Jartoux observed, ginseng grew best in heavily forested mountainous areas; it "is not to be met with in Plains, Vallies, Marshes, the bottoms of Rivulets, or in Places too much exposed and open."[23] By the late seventeenth and early eighteenth centuries, agricultural expansion had begun to take its toll north of Beijing. Enormous population growth in China proper forced millions of migrants north, and agricultural estates spread into the once heavily forested Tartary, destroying ginseng's habitat along the way.[24]

The scarcity of Asian ginseng populations resulting from overharvesting and agricultural expansion raised its value. The plant, always associated with a realm beyond human habitation, was so rare and hard to find that, as Jartoux commented, only the nobility could afford to purchase it. Chinese consumers were desperate for more sources of ginseng.

Native American peoples in North America also incorporated the plant into their systems of medicine.[25] The wave of ethnographies conducted in the late nineteenth and early twentieth centuries suggest that ginseng was prized by many tribes, but no tribe held it in higher esteem than the Cherokee. Frans Olbrecht, who studied Cherokee ethnobotany in the 1920s, observed that ginseng was "one of the most important plants in the Cherokee medical botany. . . . There is no other plant that is treated with so much respect by the laity as well as by the medicine men."[26] Like the Chinese, the Cherokee used it as a "love medicine" as well as to treat pain in the chest, chills, fever, headache, cramps, and "female troubles."[27] Evidence suggests that the Cherokee realized the medical virtues of the plant long before the emergence of a global market.[28] David Cozzo, an ethnobotanist with the Eastern Band of Cherokee Indians in Western North Carolina, has pointed out the cultural saliency of the root in the tribe. The etymology of the term for it, a'tali'guli, meaning "It climbs the mountain," also suggests that its use long predated the arrival of Europeans.[29] Furthermore, it was one of the most commonly occurring plants in Cherokee medicine and religious ceremonies from an early date, and we know from the trader James Adair's account of the 1760s that the "Indians use it on religious occasions."[30]

Native Americans, like the Chinese, used ginseng as part of an expansive system of medicine that embraced not only therapeutic practices but also systems of knowledge and power that reaffirmed their position in nature. Although views varied considerably across cultures, Native Americans generally conceptualized the earth as a living being and their relationship to it as one of mutual respect and reciprocity.[31] They believed that the world, in historian Annie Booth's words, "exists as an intricate balance of parts, and it was important that humans recognized this balance and strove to maintain and stay within it."[32] The Cherokee concept of to'hi exhibited fascinating similarities with the Taoist concept of Qi. In their analysis of the concept, Heidi Altman and Cherokee linguist Thomas Belt argue that to'hi referred to the "normal state of the Cherokee universe." It was "smoothly flowing, evenly and moderately paced, fluid, and peaceful." In order to maintain to'hi, "humans must observe a system of natural laws instilled through oral tradition."[33] Unethical actions among humans or between humans and the rest of nature could disrupt this flow of energy, which would bring on illness and disease.

According to Cherokee mythology, there was a time when humans, animals, and plants all coexisted in harmony, but as human populations increased, they began to kill off more animals. The vengeful animals resolved to introduce diseases that would destroy the humans, but the plants, who remained friends of the humans, agreed to provide them with all the antidotes to disease.[34] Cherokee people thus maintained a relationship with an estimated eight hundred different species of plants, and they believed that every plant possessed healing properties, even though they might not know what those properties were.[35] They developed a complex classification system that grew organically out of the uses to which they put these plants, and they concocted elaborate formulas that often contained more than ten different types of plants.[36] James Mooney, the Smithsonian ethnographer who spent his career studying the Cherokee and other native tribes in the late nineteenth century, observed that due to the especially "luxuriant flora" of their homeland, the "vegetable kingdom . . . holds a far more important place in the mythology and ceremonial of the [Cherokee] than it does among the Indians of the treeless plains and arid sage deserts of the West."[37] Appalachian floral diversity and Cherokee cosmology exerted an unmistakable influence on each other. Indeed, this ethnobotanical knowledge, gleaned from centuries of interaction with the region's flora, would play a large role in stimulating the botanical drug industry in Southern Appalachia.

While all plants were important or potentially important to the Cherokee, ginseng played an outsized role in sustaining tohi, which earned it a high degree of respect and reverence. In addition to treating specific ailments, the Cherokee used it in a number of religious ceremonies aimed at ensuring continued harmony between humans and the universe. In the 1840s, missionary Daniel Butrick mentioned its use as one of seven articles of purification in the elaborate Green Corn Dance and the Great New Moon Feast.[38] The Cherokee held that all life was sacred, and ginseng was no exception. James Mooney observed that ginseng, referred to as the "Great Man" in the sacred formulas, was, as the most important of the "plant gods," treated with utmost respect. One formula dictated that when hunting ginseng, a medicine man should pass by the first three plants then approach the fourth by circling it counterclockwise one to four times while reciting a prayer. After assuring the mountain that "he comes only to take a small piece of flesh [ginseng] from its side," he would dig up the root and place a small bead into the hole in the ground as payment.[39]

Despite the ecological implications of this concept of medicine, Native American peoples struggled to live up to their ideals in the face of economic pressure. As numerous scholars have shown, Cherokee and other Native American peoples contributed to destructive ecological trends, including the deerskin trade beginning in the seventeenth century. When the cultural values that had worked to mitigate the overharvesting of ginseng came into dramatic conflict with the commercial values of a growing market culture, ginseng would lose.

Commodification and the Failures of Colonial Science

At the time of Jartoux's expedition to the Manchu region in 1709, a trade in ginseng did not exist in North America. However, Jartoux's visit set into motion a series of events that stimulated the first of several backcountry ginseng booms in a different hemisphere. Because of his training as a mathematician, Jartoux was chosen by the emperor to accompany the Jesuit cartographer Jean-Baptiste Régis on surveying expeditions to the empire's northeastern border. In July, in a small village less than a dozen miles from the Korean border, a local Manchu climbed a nearby mountain and brought back to the expedition party four ginseng plants in a basket. Eager to sketch this unfamiliar plant and send a detailed description back to France, Jartoux attempted to learn as much as he could. He wrote the procurator general of missions in Paris, "No Body can imagine that the Chinese and Tartars would set so high a Value upon this Root. . . . The most eminent Physicians in China have writ whole Volumes upon the Virtues and Qualities of this Plant and make it an ingredient in almost all Remedies. I am persuaded that it would prove an excellent

Medicine in the Hands of any European who understands Pharmacy."[40] Displaying a prescient understanding of the East Asian–eastern North American disjunction, he speculated that "if it is to be found in any other country in the world, it may be particularly in Canada, where the forests and mountains, according to the relation of those that have lived there, very much resemble these here."[41] His report, which was translated and published in the *Philosophical Transactions of the Royal Society of London* in 1713, was met with great curiosity in scientific circles around the Atlantic and touched off a widespread search for the plant in North America.[42]

In Canada, another Jesuit priest, Joseph-François Lafitau, who lived among the Iroquois in Sault-Saint Louis, induced local Iroquois to help him find ginseng based on Jartoux's description. After three months of searching in 1716, an Iroquois woman found it growing by a nearby house. One of Lafitau's Mohawk informants recognized it immediately as one of their "ordinary remedies."[43] When he published his findings several years later, his report was widely circulated and drew intense interest from the merchants of Montreal and Quebec. Although Lafitau himself was interested in ginseng more for the support it provided for his theory of a common human history than for its potential commercial value, his discovery soon touched off a commercial frenzy in Canada. The late 1740s and 1750s seem to have been its peak. When Peter Kalm, a Swedish student of Carl Linnaeus, visited Canada in 1748, he observed that the ginseng trade was "very brisk. . . . All the merchants at Quebec and Montreal received orders from their correspondents in France to send over a quantity of ginseng."[44] He noted that most of the roots were dug by Native Americans who "travelled about the country in order to collect as much as they could and sell it to the merchants at Montreal."[45] In 1752, merchants in New France sent 34,580 pounds to the French port at La Rochelle, thence to travel on to China.[46] By the mid-eighteenth century, the forests around Montreal were suffering from overharvesting and habitat destruction. "By all accounts [ginseng plants] grew in abundance round Montreal," wrote Kalm, "but at present there is not a single plant of it to be found, so effectually have they been rooted out."[47] Consequently, ginseng harvesting began to spread south.

The Iroquois played a role in expanding knowledge of and involvement in the ginseng trade throughout their territory, which stretched roughly from the area south of Montreal to northwestern Pennsylvania.

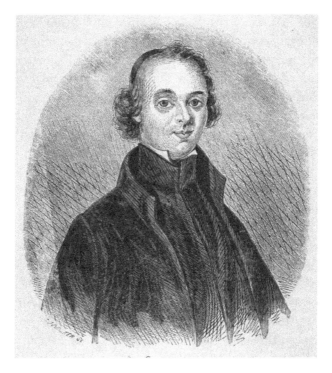

Joseph-François Lafitau, a Jesuit missionary in Quebec who first discovered that a ginseng species resembling the Chinese plant grew in North America. (Joseph-François Lafitau, *Mémoire présenté à Son Altesse Royale Mgr. le duc d'Orléans, régent de France:Concernant la précieuse plante du gin-seng de Tartarie découverte en Amérique* (Orleans: Philipe, 1858).

Kalm reported that the Montreal trade "obliged the Indians this summer to go far within the English boundaries to search for the root."[48] A French engineer and surveyor confirmed in 1752 that "all the sauvages had left to trade in New England, or were collecting geinseing; all the cabins were closed."[49] That same year, Moravian missionary J. Martin Mack observed around one hundred Oneida and Cayuga digging the roots in New York's Mohawk Valley.[50] Indeed, sources are clear that Native Americans were heavily engaged in the trade and likely did the bulk of the harvesting.

Not to be outdone by the French, the English soon evinced a strong interest in discovering more ginseng within their borders. Following the appearance of Jartoux's description in its own publication in 1713, members of the Royal Society of London stimulated a search for the plant as part of a broader campaign to develop a Western commerce in the plant. William Byrd, a Virginia planter and one of the few colonial members of the Royal Society, was instrumental in its discovery in Virginia in 1729 and its promotion to the Royal Society. He carried some with him on his journey to survey the dividing line between Virginia and North Carolina in 1728. "I us'd to chew a Root of Ginseng as I walked along," he wrote. "This kept up my Spirits, and made me trip away as nimbly in my half Jack-Boots as younger men cou'd in their Shoes."[51] He evidently procured this root from somewhere other than Virginia, for he would later credit Robert Beverley for its discovery in that colony the following year.

During a 1729 expedition to the Shenandoah Valley of Virginia, Beverley, the son of the author of *History and Present State of Virginia* (1705), carried along a copy of Jartoux's Royal Society article and found a plant growing on a north-facing slope in the Blue Ridge Mountains that resembled Jartoux's plant. He took a specimen back to Byrd at Westover.[52] Convinced that this plant was the exact same as Jartoux's, Byrd traveled to the Blue Ridge the following year to find some of the plants for himself. Over the next few years, believing in the medical virtues of the plant, he sent specimens to his friends in the Royal Society, including John Perceval, Earl of Egmont, and Charles Boyle, Earl of Orrey. He told Hans Sloane, the Royal Society president and the king's physician, that "the earth has never produced any vegetable so friendly to man as ginseng."[53] He also sent a root to Prime Minister Robert Walpole, who apparently did not use it.[54]

Byrd's news of discovery in Virginia intrigued the Royal Society, including the Quaker botanist Peter Collinson, who in 1737 asked Byrd to procure him a specimen. Byrd's response was not promising. "The ginseng grows only on [our mountains], and consequently not easily to be got by us, who live at [150 miles'] distance."[55] Collinson then implored his other American botanist friend, John Bartram, to consult with Byrd and attempt his own search for the plant. "I mightily want it," he told him.[56] The following year, Bartram found it growing in Western Pennsylvania, the news of which was heralded by Benjamin Franklin's *Pennsylvania Gazette*.[57] Bartram soon shipped Collinson a live specimen of ginseng, which he successfully transplanted to his garden, proclaiming it the first cultivated in England.[58]

Over the next six decades, botanists in both Europe and North America continued to try to cultivate American ginseng in their gardens. A few seem to have been successful. In addition to Collinson, another Quaker botanist, John Fothergill, claimed to have raised at least one plant at his garden in Upton, England, from a specimen sent by Bartram in 1769.[59] If they could unlock the botanical secrets that would enable the plant to be cultivated, these botanists continually asserted, they could develop a thriving industry for both home consumption and Chinese trade. "I am well assured it will prove a very profitable commodity to China," Collinson told Bartram.[60] The publication of Jean-Baptiste Du Halde's *The General History of China* in 1735, which listed some seventy-seven ginseng recipes used by the Chinese to treat various illnesses, stoked vigorous discussion among European physicians and businessmen of the medical and commercial value of the plant.[61] It seemed as though a ginseng industry would soon develop as European demand for the root would rise, as had happened with other medicinal plants obtained from the colonies, specifically cinchona.[62] If ginseng could be made a plantation crop, the trade could be controlled by wealthy planters like Byrd, who could apply slave and other forms of labor to its profitable cultivation.

However, despite half a century of experiments in cultivation by the most talented botanists and gardeners in Europe and despite continued interest from the most influential scientists of the age, ginseng culture failed to thrive in either the colonies or Europe. Byrd gave up trying to cultivate it and seemed resigned to the fact. "I have sowed seeds of it, but it never came up," he told Charles Boyle. "Providence I sopose has ordered it thus, lest so great a blessing should be too common."[63] Cultivation experiments had still not paid off by 1786, when Joseph Banks, successor to Sloane as president of the Royal Society, asked Humphry Marshall to send him a few hundred pounds of the root so that he could perform some experiments in cultivation that "may become of importance both to your country and mine."[64] To help him find the plant, Marshall, a Pennsylvania plant collector and cousin to John Bartram, enlisted his nephew, the botanist Moses Marshall, who was obliged to travel "two hundred miles to the westward, through a dismal mountainous part of our country" to procure the root. Moses Marshall hired another man at $1 a day to help him dig, and the two men spent twenty days camping and tromping around the mountains before they acquired the requested weight.[65]

That this event occurred at all indicates that the secrets of successful ginseng cultivation had not been unlocked. Banks, perhaps the most well-connected man in botany, was nevertheless required to order specimens to be gathered in the wilds of Pennsylvania at great expense. Thus, the ecology of ginseng operated to defy the wishes of the most powerful men in the Atlantic world. This circle of transatlantic botanists maintained a small trade in ginseng seeds and nursery stock, but commerce in the plant would continue to be driven by China, and the vast majority of the work of ginseng harvesting for the China market would be performed not by forced laborers on plantations but by Native Americans and Euro-American settlers in the backcountry of North America. The process of commodification avoided privatization; ginseng remained a commons commodity.

Ginseng and the Opening of the US-China Trade

While the ginseng trade flourished on the borders of Iroquoia in the 1740s and 1750s, it seems to have had a negligible impact on the southern colonies prior to the American Revolution.[66] Despite Byrd's role in colonial science, he was unwilling to engage Native Americans to gather the wild root for him, as Lafitau had done in Canada, and he was unwilling to promote the trade among white settlers. Perhaps with an eye toward controlling labor, he did not advocate gathering the plant in the wild.[67] Further south, Indian trader James Adair, writing in the 1770s, suggested that merchants in the southern backcountry were unwilling to engage in the trade with Native Americans. He observed that the plant was "very plenty on the fertile parts of the Cheerake mountains," but he lamented that "it is a great loss to a valuable branch of trade, that our people neither gather it in a proper season, nor can cure it."[68] Apparently, merchants would not take it. However, he did report that some inhabitants of the upper Yadkin valley in North Carolina, near the western edge of Euro-American settlement where Daniel Boone lived, had begun digging the root from the mountains and hauling it two hundred miles to

Charleston themselves, but they seem to have been atypical. By 1766, an economic report showed that only one bag of ginseng had been brought out of the upper reaches of the James River the previous year.[69] The earliest trading post records to have survived from the Greenbrier River valley (now West Virginia) reveal that only ninety pounds of ginseng were traded from 1771 to 1773.[70] Thus, while southern colonists were familiar with the trade, there is hardly any evidence to suggest that western Virginia or the Carolinas produced any sizeable quantity of ginseng prior to the 1780s.

The lack of trade in the southern colonies can be partly attributed to a collapse of Chinese demand in the mid-eighteenth century just as the trade in Canada and the northern colonies was picking up. Nearly every observer commented on this, but they do not agree on exactly what caused it. Kalm claimed that it was due to oversupply, whereas others attributed it to successive shipments of poorly prepared or adulterated roots.[71] The bottom dropped out of the ginseng market in the 1760s and 1770s, which slowed the trade in the North and hindered its development in the South.

During the American Revolution, the ginseng trade seems to have virtually halted, as Americans could not spare ships, but almost before the ink had dried on the Treaty of Paris in 1783, the ginseng trade began to blossom into a social, economic, and ecological force in the southern backcountry. US control over the trans-Appalachian west brought renewed popular interest in ginseng as a potential article of commerce as settlers began to pour across the Proclamation Line of 1763 looking for valuable forest products. During his tour of the newly independent American colonies that same year, German traveler and physician Johann Schoepf ran into a man leading two horses loaded with five hundred pounds of ginseng roots in the mountains of Western Pennsylvania. The man declared that during the war, virtually no roots had been harvested, and he hoped to cash in on the new bounty.[72] At the same time, eastern merchants were looking for ways to secure quality tea, open trade relations with China, and help establish American economic independence from the British. American trade with China prior to the Revolution had been limited and restricted by both the Chinese themselves and British mercantilist policies. When the Qing emperor Kangxi finally began opening up China to increased foreign trade at the end of the seventeenth century, British mercantilist policies prevented American colonists from directly engaging in the China trade. All exports of ginseng and any other goods going to China had to pass through Britain and be loaded onto ships belonging to the East India Company, thus precluding any accumulation of profits by American merchants.[73] With US independence, merchants and financiers up and down the Eastern Seaboard were eager to open up direct trade with the Celestial Empire.[74]

Ginseng as a commodity had significant benefits to financiers eager to establish trade relationships with the Far East. First and foremost, the Chinese seemed to want a lot of it. Despite the few decades of low demand since the 1750s, the Chinese were rumored to continue to significantly desire it. Second, it grew wild in the backcountry and many inhabitants were knowledgeable veterans of the trade in Iroquoia, so it was readily available for an immediate trade expedition. Third, it was a commodity to which European traders had very little access, as the plant did not grow in Europe. The US monopoly on the root provided the new country with an advantage and thus a way to break into the Chinese market that had previously been dominated by the British and the Dutch.[75]

In August 1783, Boston financier Daniel Parker informed the Philadelphia concern Messrs. Turnbull, Marmie, & Co., "We are in want of 10,000 lb. Ginseng" and requested the company "to procure that Quantity if to be had at your Market."[76] Realizing it had precious little time to fulfill the order before ginseng died back for the winter, the company hired Robert Johnston, a thirty-three-year-old Pennsylvania physician, and fronted him $1,000 to travel the backcountry to procure the root. He quickly began a race against time. Within a week, Johnston arrived at Fort Pitt but found very little root. "After a most tiresome Journey across the Frontier of Pennsylvania," he wrote to Turnbull and Marmie, "I have not been able to procure more than 400 weight of Ginseng." Yet he sounded a word of optimism. "Tomorrow I set out for Stantown [Staunton] and Augusta, where I am informed large Quantities of Ginseng has been sent from the Frontier parts of this State [Virginia]."[77] His intelligence was accurate. Ginseng was flowing into the Shenandoah Valley from the mountains of western Virginia and Pennsylvania. Unfortunately for Johnston, the people who were digging it were reluctant to take bank notes or even gold for the root. Instead, they wanted goods, so

Johnston, unable to haul wagonloads of goods across country, resolved to purchase the roots from various storekeepers and country merchants who themselves bartered with the diggers. On his first jaunt, Johnston procured some fourteen thousand pounds of "the best Ginseng which I have seen" and made arrangements with other storekeepers to ship further roots to Baltimore.[78] By the end of December 1783, he had succeeded in accumulating an astounding fifty-seven thousand pounds of ginseng root from the mountains of Virginia and Pennsylvania.[79]

On a cold winter day in February 1784, the *Empress of China,* laden mostly with ginseng and Spanish silver, weighed anchor in the icy waters of the Hudson River and set sail for the Far East. The ambitions and hopes of the young nation sailed with it.[80] The voyage was long and rough. The *Empress of China* followed the western coast of Africa down to the Cape of Good Hope and turned east, crossing the Indian Ocean in June and continuing north through the East Indies. On 28 August 1784, the ship arrived in Canton, where it remained for four months while the ship's merchants negotiated the sale of its cargo. The final destination of the ginseng from the mountains of western Virginia cannot be determined from available evidence. Perhaps the roots were consumed by men and women in Canton. More than likely they exchanged hands a few more times as they made their way into the Chinese interior, where they would have been gradually sliced up and boiled into tea. Meanwhile, in December, weighed down with seven hundred chests of black tea, one hundred chests of green tea, and thousands of pieces of porcelain ware, the *Empress of China* set sail on its return voyage. In April 1785 it arrived safely in New York, some fourteen months after it left.

The return of the *Empress* from her maiden voyage to Canton in the spring of 1785 brought high hopes for the future of ginseng and for American economic independence. In order to secure "permanent advantage to this rising empire," one observer quipped, "it is only necessary to encourage the cultivation and proper curing of ginseng, to prevent its exportation to any other country than China, and that in our own vessels."[81] "The inhabitants of America must have tea," wrote Samuel Shaw, the chief merchant on board the *Empress* and first American consul to China. "It must be pleasing to an American to know that . . . the otherwise useless produce of its mountains and forests will, in a considerable degree, supply him with this elegant luxury."[82] Ginseng, predicted one observer from South Carolina, "may become to us, that is, the backcountry, very valuable articles of commerce."[83]

The commodification of ginseng was a process that unfolded over several centuries, beginning in Asia and eventually extending into North America due to a botanical twist of fate that occurred in the Tertiary Period. As we have seen, the difficulty in cultivating the plant determined that wild harvesting remained the key feature of the trade throughout the seventeenth and eighteenth centuries. This fact had far-reaching social and cultural implications. Its high market value and the desire of indigenous peoples to access that market worked to overwhelm any cultural adaptations that these societies may have developed to limit the overharvesting of the plant. Consequently, the plant began a slow decline, and the centers of extraction shifted from northern China to French Canada to, eventually, the British colonies. By the 1780s, the centers of extraction had moved further southwest into Pennsylvania and Virginia. "In these mountains the plant is still common," confirmed one observer of western Virginia in 1783, "but in the lower parts it has pretty well disappeared."[84] Thus, the Southern Appalachian region, still a sparsely settled backcountry in the postrevolutionary period, was poised for its first large-scale ginseng boom.

2 | Appalachia's First Ginseng Boom and the Evolution of Commons Culture

IN THE SUMMER OF 1789, JOHN MAY LOADED FIVE TONS OF CONSUMER goods onto flatboats in the Monongahela River some fifty miles upstream of Pittsburgh. An agent for the Ohio Company and former colonel in the Massachusetts militia, May hoped to sell plow points, knives, gunpowder, and an array of other goods to settlers around emerging commercial hubs along the Ohio River, including Marietta and Wheeling.[1] The Ohio River valley was open for business in the late 1780s. The British restrictions on settlement across the Appalachians were nullified by the Treaty of Paris, inviting a wave of settlers to settle on land that several Indian tribes still claimed in the valley. Merchants like May hoped to cash in on the fledgling commercial economy, but instead they found an economy very much dependent on ginseng.

At the town of Marietta, May found a bustling economy with ten traders hawking their wares, whereas the year before there had been only one. Ginseng seemed to have facilitated much of the boom. Referring to the merchants' dependence on the plant, he called it "their darling Gensang" and claimed that a sudden depreciation of ginseng prices threatened to derail the burgeoning economy.[2] Marietta is "filled with merchants who cannot dispose of their goods, as the dealing medium of exchange ginseng has utterly depreciated," May wrote in his diary. "It seems to be a prevailing opinion that two thirds of the traders referred to will be ruined by this summer's business."[3] May initially refused to accept ginseng as payment due to the uncertainty of the market that year and the difficulty in handling the roots. "Ginseng is worse than nothing," he wrote in his diary on 3 July 1789.[4] However, May quickly found he could not avoid it. Having failed to unload much of his stock by the time he reached Wheeling, he realized that "if we would do anything, we must take deer skins, furs, and ginseng in exchange for goods."[5] After spending a few weeks in Wheeling and Marietta, he headed inland across the mountains of Virginia. Along the way, he collected fourteen hundred pounds of skins and furs and twenty-eight hundred pounds of ginseng. He claimed he could have had a thousand more pounds of the root but a frost and heavy rain killed the plant tops in early October, thus shortening the season by nearly a month. After drying the roots in the sun, he packed them up in large bags and sent them on wagons some 250 miles over the mountains to Baltimore.[6] May had hoped that the commercial economy of the region had evolved to the point at which cash purchases would sustain his business, but instead he had to rely on bartering the products of the forest.

May's diary gives us a fascinating glimpse into the role that ginseng played in the economic and cultural transformation of the Ohio Valley and Central Appalachia around the turn of the nineteenth century. The earliest white inhabitants of the valley had come to the region in the 1750s and 1760s to hunt, fish, and generally live off what eighteenth-century Virginia writer Robert Beverley called the "spontaneous productions of that country."[7] These men held fluid notions of property and believed that unimproved forests, streams, and other crucial resources—regardless of ownership—should be treated as semi-public property. While they were certainly not opposed to private landownership, they struck a balance between private property and public necessity, creating a system of what historian Stephen Aron calls "rights-in-the-woods."[8] These patterns of behavior, infused with customs stretching back to Europe, helped create commons across the landscape.[9] Ginseng fit neatly into this world of commons. It provided early white inhabitants much-needed purchasing power to build their new lives, buy land and implements, pay taxes and fines, and start businesses. It was the "only species of colonial produce in Kentucky," French botanist François Michaux remarked during his journey to the region in 1802, "that will bear the expense of carriage by land from that state to Philadelphia."[10] Despite a rocky start that saw ginseng prices fluctuate wildly, the root eventually became one of the leading mediums of exchange in a frontier region that lacked hard cash and reliable transportation systems. It was one of the pillars of the economy.

By the opening decades of the nineteenth century, however, the world of the hunter was rapidly giving way to the world of the farmer, the merchant, and the lawyer, and the culture began to change with it. This transformation was gradual, beginning in the most heavily populated and commercialized areas along the river courses. As the Monongahela, Ohio, and Mississippi Rivers became commercial highways for emerging cash crops such as hemp, corn, cotton, and whiskey, new landowners began to assert greater control over the resources on their land, and by the opening of the nineteenth century, the rights-in-the-woods were giving way to a new legal culture with a more stringent view of property. Property rights were more readily invoked, trespassing prosecuted, and commons enclosed.[11] The persistence of the ginseng trade illustrates how this transformation unfolded across time and space. Indeed, ginseng helped usher in this commercial transition in some areas, but it did not wholly succumb to the new property regime—at least not yet. Like deerskins, beaver furs, wild bird feathers, and other roots, barks, and herbs, it was a product of both worlds. It was a tradable commodity created by global markets. It helped grease the wheels of commercial development in an area that struggled for traction. Yet it was also a commons resource, available to hunters and farmers alike, according to widely accepted use rights. The fact that the ginseng trade not only continued to thrive but expanded in scope and scale suggests that common rights-in-the-woods did not disappear in the 1790s. Rather, they persisted and evolved even as the social, ecological, and economic dynamics changed around them.

Hunting, Surveying, and Digging

Most ginseng harvesters in western Virginia and Kentucky during the boom times of the 1790s were hunters who knew the forests well, had little or no agricultural business to attend, and could afford to spend days on end in the woods in September and October. "The hunters collect it incidentally in their wanderings," remarked Johann Schoepf in 1784.[12]

Around 1800, one anonymous diarist (possibly the Virginia planter John Preston) hired some sixteen hunters to join his party of surveyors in the Coal River basin in (West) Virginia.[13] Their job was to provide food for the surveyors and to dig ginseng. Upon crossing the "high and rough ridge and mountain" between the New River and the Coal River, they discovered "plenty of root" and constructed a camp next to a small branch to serve as a base for a few days of gathering.[14] Some hunters with the knowledge and skill to find and harvest the plant became specialists whose services were much in demand by merchants. May relied for most of his roots on a "Dutchman from Kentucky" and spent weeks courting his business. "I have bin playing out my best Cards to the Dutch man— have kept his skin full, and prevented his having any correspondence with the many packers who Came here to Carrey Loads, least he should Send off his Sang [to another party]," he wrote in his diary.[15] May's preoccupation with this Dutchman suggests that knowledge of how to find and harvest the root empowered knowledgeable hunters to dictate the terms of their labor.

Some early ginseng hunters also purchased roots from others, becoming middlemen in the long chain that would take the product to China. Perhaps the most famous ginseng digger in history was Daniel Boone, whose experience in the trade shows the perils and promises of dealing in the root. In 1787, two years after he had moved his family to Maysville at the mouth of Limestone Creek, Kentucky, and three years after he had become nationally famous by way of John Filson's biography, fifty-three-year-old Boone got caught up in ginseng fever. According to his son Nathan, he and his father frequently dug ginseng "out among the hills" near the Ohio River. He also hired "several hands" to dig for him and purchased more ginseng from other diggers. For two seasons, he collected ginseng in this way and stored it in a warehouse before hauling it by keelboat up the Ohio. At the very least he stood to make a few thousand dollars, but disaster struck: the boat capsized and the roots were soaked. Boone dried them out, poled them up to Redstone, Pennsylvania, loaded them onto packhorses, and hauled them to Philadelphia. Because of water damage, however, he received only half their usual market value.[16]

Surveyors themselves often found that digging ginseng along their routes could turn their expeditions into more profitable ventures. In July

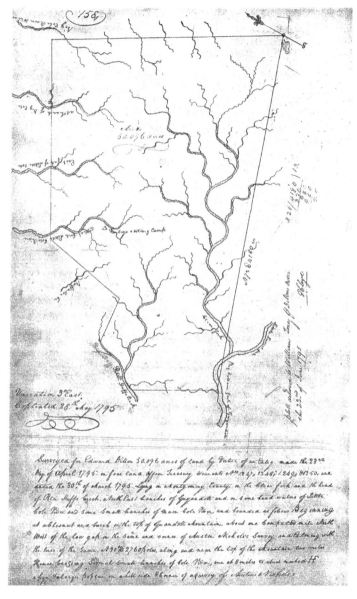

 A plat of the Coal River basin, 1795. Note "Farley's Rooting Camp" in the middle of the page. (Coal River Folklife Project collection [AFC 1999/008], American Folklife Center, Library of Congress.)

1786, the Confederation Congress appointed John Mathews, a twenty-one-year-old Massachusetts man, to survey the lands in what is now southeastern Ohio, recently ceded by Wyandotte and Delaware peoples.[17] In September, Mathews and four others in his surveying party took advantage of a lull in their duties, camped on the headwaters of Short Creek, and found ginseng growing "in great abundance." They spent five days wandering the nearby forests digging roots. Demonstrating a detailed knowledge of digging practices, Mathews claimed that the best diggers could dig more than forty pounds a day, a considerable sum that could have earned him upwards of £20 worth of goods at the nearest mercantile.[18] Even as they engaged in the symbolic enclosure of the commons by delineating property boundaries and thus hastening the transformation of the Ohio Valley, surveyors nevertheless asserted a right to ginseng.

Unlike their participation in the earlier ginseng boom in Canada and New York, Native Americans did not engage in the early trade on the Virginia frontier. As Euro-American settlers flowed into the Ohio Valley in the 1780s and 1790s, forcing ever greater land cessions from native tribes, the relationship between white Americans and Indians was at its nadir. Ginseng digging by white settlers often exacerbated the problem, as Native Americans exacted reprisals on those they found on their territory. Shortly after his digging expedition in 1786, Mathews heard that another party of men "out after ginseng" was attacked by Indians. Three were killed and another taken prisoner, which led him to remark, "I feel very happy that I have reached my old quarters and will give them liberty to take my scalp if they catch me after ginseng again this year."[19] Similarly, May filled his diary with anxious speculation about Indian attacks. He estimated that they had killed some fifty men and women during the summer of 1789, reinforcing his suspicion that "there will be an Indian war."[20] Thus, on the Virginia frontier in the 1780s and 1790s, ginseng harvesting was conducted exclusively by white Americans under the cloud of frontier violence. Such findings support the claim recently put forward by Allan Greer, Virginia Anderson, and others that the clash between native peoples and Euro-Americans was not only an abstract contest between a system based on communal, usufruct property rights and one based on absolute, individual property rights: white frontiersmen and Native Americans initially experienced the conflict as a fight over the commons. They fought over who could hunt, fish, run livestock, and dig ginseng and where they could engage in these activities.[21]

As surveyors designed towns and drew property borders, and as new human communities situated themselves on the Appalachian landscape, ginseng played a crucial role as a medium of exchange and quickly became woven into the fabric of community life. New settlers used the proceeds of the root to pay taxes; they traded it for land, horses, and tools; and they relied on it to sustain the civil and legal functions of their communities. According to court records from Greenbrier County in 1785, for example, John O'Neal, the loser in a lawsuit, was ordered to pay the plaintiff twenty-two pounds of ginseng. That same year, one John Smith weighed sixty-nine pounds of ginseng due to John Brown in Augusta County, presumably a reference to a verification of payment in a judgment.[22]

The store records of James Alexander in the Greenbrier River valley reveal just how dependent frontier communities were on ginseng in the 1780s and 1790s. One of the first Euro-American settlers in what is now Monroe County, West Virginia, twenty-two-year-old Alexander built a farm in 1774 near a prominent intersection of two Indian paths on the eastern slope of the Alleghenies and a short jaunt from the Wilderness Road. He also operated a small trading post following the Revolution.[23] From 1783 to 1785, Alexander conducted 87 percent of his sales in ginseng, trading for roughly six thousand pounds, worth £643. Around 47 percent of Alexander's customers used ginseng to pay for their entire purchases for those two years, while most of the remainder used some combination of ginseng, saltpeter, and cash. In the fall, they would bring their ginseng in sacks and open a line of credit that they would use through the winter, spring, and summer to purchase plow points, scythes, knives, gunpowder, and dozens of other goods.[24]

Virtually all early settlers found ginseng an easy means of extracting some quick wealth while they busied themselves with the tasks of improvement. Alexander's customers, most of whom were Scots-Irish, included many prominent landholders. Dozens received original land patents from 1783 to 1794 and became owners of some of the choicest property along the river bottoms. William Blanton, for example, purchased 400 acres along Turkey Creek from the Greenbrier Company in 1783 and, the same year, traded 225 pounds of ginseng for a variety of merchandise. Blanton had been appointed constable in 1773 and later purchased a lot from Alexander in the new town of Union. William Ewing, mentioned in chapter 1, also received a Greenbrier patent, his for 170 acres. A majority of Alexander's customers, including Blanton and Ewing, cast votes for electors in the presidential election of 1800, which means they met the property and residency requirements of Virginia.[25] Alexander became a large landholder as a result of his ginseng venture, donating 26 acres in 1806 to construct the town of Union, which would become the county seat of Monroe.[26] Thus, Alexander's store records indicate that people of all levels of wealth, from squatters to sizeable landowners, participated in the ginseng economy in the early years of resettlement.

Indeed, ginseng helped shape fortunes across the Ohio Valley landscape, enabling some merchants who were willing to engage in the trade to accumulate wealth. Andrew Beirne, a twenty-four-year-old itinerant merchant with little property and a stock of goods, arrived in Monroe County in 1795 and immediately set to work trading goods for ginseng.[27] According to what locals told Anne Royall, who toured the Virginia backcountry in 1826, Beirne often went door to door taking people's roots in exchange for goods.[28] Beirne decided to stay in the county; a few years later, he moved to Union and constructed a store, where he faced stiff competition from another able merchant, Hugh Caperton. Determined to prevail over his commercial rival, Beirne expanded his operations and opened several other stores in the county, where he accepted ginseng and other produce for goods. Within a few years, Beirne had acquired seventy-two parcels of land, presumably in exchange for nonpayment of store debts, becoming the largest landowner and slaveholder in the county.[29] Ginseng greatly assisted Beirne's rise from itinerant merchant to slaveholder, and Beirne helped spread the trade into the more inaccessible parts of the county.

The Rise of Ginseng Manufacturing

Beginning in the late 1790s, aspiring businessmen imported into the Ohio Valley the knowledge and techniques to better cure ginseng roots, what many referred to as "ginseng manufacturing." In the 1780s, the vast majority of the ginseng handled by merchants was prepared for market by drying it in the sun, but in the 1790s, a few merchants began acquiring knowledge of how to prepare the roots in the way the Chinese preferred: a process of steaming and drying called clarification. This process had been vaguely described by Jartoux in 1713, but it was not until the 1790s that merchants began to perfect it. While in Kentucky in 1802, Michaux noted that "several persons begin even to employ the means made use of by the Chinese to make the root transparent."[30] In order to perform it on a large scale, they erected "factories" and hired laborers to help carry out the work. The spread of ginseng factories in the Ohio Valley and North Carolina may help explain why ginseng exports, after averaging under 30,000 pounds annually through most of the 1790s, jumped to 281,000 pounds per year from 1798 to 1807.[31]

Typically, such facilities consisted of two rooms, one for steaming and the other for drying, under the same roof with a door between them. They contained no windows and featured carefully planned ventilation systems. The clarifying process began outside, where laborers, usually from three to five boys or men, washed the roots, scraped them gently with the back of a knife, and polished them, first with a shoe brush and then with a toothbrush. The roots were then brought into the steaming room, where they were placed near the top of an iron kettle at least eighteen inches in diameter on a coarse linen cloth suspended above boiling water. After about an hour of steaming, once the roots turned a translucent "whitish" color, they were wrapped up in the linen and plunged into cold water for a few minutes until cool. Then they were transferred to the drying room and laid out on a clapboard to dry. A furnace gently warmed the air "somewhat more than heat of sun on warm summer day." The process, which took the better part of a day, rendered the roots "a beautiful amber color."[32] Although little is known about why the Chinese preferred their ginseng prepared in this way, modern scientific studies have demonstrated that in this process the root undergoes a chemical transformation, rearranging the ratios of various ginsenosides, the active compound in the root. However, due to the complex phytochemistry of the plant and the relative lack of clinical studies, scientists do not know how that affects ginseng's medical efficacy.[33]

Knowledge of the clarification process was a closely guarded secret. Upon giving his instructions for the construction of a ginseng factory to John Preston, the Tennessee politician John Rhea made it clear that Preston "will not make it known to any . . . without my consent" and instructed him to take care to keep the contents of the factory "well guarded from public inspection," including the gaze of his laborers.[34] This secrecy was a business strategy. According to Michaux, Kentuckians paid those with the desired knowledge $400 for instructions on how to clarify roots.[35] It was apparently worth it, as clarified roots sold for $6 or $7 per pound on the coast, more than ten times what simple dried ginseng fetched.[36]

Merchants therefore realized that with a little investment, they could add enormous value to their roots and increase their profits by making their commodity more attractive to their Chinese customers. Robert Wellford, a prominent Fredericksburg physician who had once counted George Washington as a patient, constructed what was likely the first ginseng factory, in Scott County, Virginia. Leaving his medical business behind in October 1801, he headed west on the Wilderness Road to Powell Mountain, Virginia. He may have obtained the knowledge of clarification from John Preston, who was Wellford's patient and had accompanied him on part of his journey. By the time Wellford arrived, the laborers he had hired under the direction of his partner, a Dr. Carter, had constructed three cabins and were busy processing roots. Wellford purchased roots from locals with goods hauled in from Virginia.[37]

The frontier ginseng boom came to Western North Carolina a little later than to the Ohio Valley. As discussed in chapter 1, ginseng was not an economic factor on the southern frontier prior to the American Revolution. By the 1780s and 1790s, the Cherokee had begun to dabble in it, but the extent of this trade is unclear. A 1790 report from Indian traders in the Piedmont region of North Georgia informed Congress that "ginseng abounds in that country, but is not yet gathered in any considerable quantities."[38] Yet in his 1802 book, *View of South Carolina,* John Drayton remarked, "Ginseng has been so much sought by the Cherokee Indians for trade, that at this time, it is by no means so plenty, as it used formerly to be in this state."[39] Evidently, the trade among Native Americans was only getting started in the 1790s, but it escalated quickly. Virginia merchants began looking south, believing that the southern reaches of the Appalachians still contained virgin ginseng patches waiting for the "sang hoe." Perhaps reflecting this optimism, Michaux noted in 1802 that the plant "grows chiefly in the mountain regions of the Alleghenies, and is by far more abundant as the chain of these mountains incline south west."[40]

American settlers pouring into Western North Carolina found it plentiful, and itinerant merchants discovered it to be a very useful medium of exchange with the early settlers there.

James Patton helped expand the trade into Western North Carolina. Born in Ireland in 1756, Patton fled high rents and oppressive landlords, arriving in Philadelphia in 1783, from where he immediately set out for the backcountry. He undoubtedly developed experience with ginseng as he worked various jobs in Western Pennsylvania, and within a few years, he headed south along the Great Valley and entered the world of frontier commerce in Western North Carolina. According to an autobiographical letter he left for his children, Patton spent the early 1790s traveling around the mountains purchasing ginseng, furs, beeswax, and snakeroot. He remained in each location for a week or two, having sent word ahead announcing his imminent arrival to give the inhabitants time to gather these products. He was so successful at this business that he eventually hired a partner, Andrew Erwin, purchased land in several states, and opened an inn and store in Wilkesboro, North Carolina, on the Yadkin River.[41] Itinerant merchants like Patton and Beirne relied on ginseng to sustain their businesses in the early years of settlement, and they provided a market for settlers to engage the commercial economy.

Ginseng manufacturing began in Western North Carolina with the arrival of Isaac Heylin from the Ohio Valley. An able physician and active member of the Philadelphia medical community, Heylin traveled in the 1790s to China, where he likely learned about the clarification process, for upon returning to the United States, he set off for the Ohio River valley to use his new knowledge on the ginseng frontier.[42] Near the upper reaches of Limestone Creek, upstream from where Daniel Boone was doing business, Heylin spent around $1,000 to build a ginseng factory, making him one of the first to clarify ginseng in Kentucky. He must have done well, for in 1802, he hauled four thousand pounds of clarified root on two wagonloads to Limestone Creek, where the product was put on a keelboat for Pittsburgh. If Michaux's estimates are accurate, Heylin stood to make as much as $24,000 on the shipment. He soon grew dissatisfied with the trade in the Ohio River valley, however—perhaps due to the root's increasing scarcity—because when the explorer and land speculator George Hunter passed through Kentucky later that year, Heylin offered to sell him his business for $2,000. Hunter told him he'd think about it.[43] Although Hunter's journal makes no mention of whether he accepted the offer, Heylin probably found a buyer somewhere, as he was soon investing time and money in ginseng clarification in Western North Carolina.

Over the next three decades, Heylin induced several prominent merchants in Western North Carolina to build factories and sell their ginseng to him. He must have established connections with James Patton and his partner Andrew Erwin in Wilkesboro, for when Erwin, who was married to Patton's sister, had his third child in 1807, he named him Isaac Heylin Erwin.[44] In 1808 the noted botanist John Lyon mentioned passing through "Patton & Erwines ginseng works" near Scott's Creek in Haywood County, which suggests Heylin may have taught them the art of clarification.[45] Lyon's reference is the earliest indication of a ginseng factory in Western North Carolina, and sources are sparse for the next two decades. Sometime in the late 1820s, Heylin convinced two young Buncombe County citizens, Nimrod S. Jarrett and Bacchus J. Smith, to move further west to Jonathan's Creek and operate a ginseng factory.[46] A few years later, Smith joined John McElroy at another of Heylin's factories along the Caney River in Yancey County, where in 1837 they produced some twenty-five thousand pounds of clarified roots from eighty-six thousand pounds of green roots.[47] In 1851, Mary Kite stayed a night with the owner of one of these factories near Jefferson in Ashe County—this was likely Bacchus Smith, who had recently come from the Caney River to open a new branch—and claimed that he "had as much as ten thousand pounds gathered."[48] These were the pioneers of ginseng manufacturing in Western North Carolina, and Heylin was the driving force behind them.

The impact of the frontier boom on ginseng populations in Central and Southern Appalachia was noticeable. When the boom commenced in the mid-1780s, diggers found virtually untouched patches of ginseng that consisted of hundreds, even thousands, of individual plants. The slow-growing nature of the plant and challenges to seed germination dictate that patches also grow very slowly. Although long-term studies of wild ginseng populations are surprisingly lacking, short-term studies have suggested that for a patch to increase from a handful of individual plants to over one thousand could take hundreds of years.[49] In the late eighteenth century, there were many virgin patches of such a size. Both

John Mathews and Johann Schoepf, two men familiar with the practice in the mid-1780s, asserted that one experienced digger could harvest between forty and sixty pounds in one day, a remarkable amount that would never again be matched.[50] Mathews, measuring their age by counting the growth rings on the rhizome, claimed that even the medium-sized roots he dug were twenty or thirty years old. Just two decades later, François Michaux, who visited the Ohio Valley in 1802, claimed that "a man cannot pull up above eight or nine pounds of fresh roots per day."[51] Michaux himself was able to collect half an ounce, "which was a great deal, considering the difficulty there is in procuring them."[52] One observer, referring to Pennsylvania in the 1780s, declared that "ginseng is either dug up for sale, or rooted up by the hogs so much, that it begins to grow scarce in the inhabited parts, especially where the people are any ways thick settled; and seems likely to be entirely demolished amongst the inhabitants in a few years."[53] Even if all observers were exaggerating slightly, these kinds of reports suggest that overharvesting began to take its toll in much of the plant's range within two decades of the boom.

Aside from such anecdotal evidence, assessing the impacts of the Ohio Valley ginseng boom from existing traditional sources is a difficult task, but ecology can help. When determining the impact of harvests on ginseng populations across wide geographic areas, ecologists take into account three factors as they relate to a hypothetical ginseng patch: (1) the likelihood that harvesters will find a particular patch, (2) how much of the patch they harvest, and (3) other mitigating factors such as the number of seeds they successfully replant.[54] The first factor was typically a function of geography. It depended on the range covered by diggers and the location of the patches. The second and third factors, however, were largely functions of culture. When diggers approached a patch of ginseng, they brought with them certain cultural principles that determined how much of that patch they harvested and whether they took measures to replenish it. If they harvested an entire patch and took no further measures to replant seeds, it may have taken decades for the patch to regain what ecologists call a minimum viable population size, which may be as few as two hundred plants—or perhaps the patch might never recover.[55]

Of course, each individual entered the forest with his or her own complex web of cultural values and attitudes, and sources that could help us reconstruct them are difficult to come by. What seems clear is that harvesters during the initial boom period had little incentive to conserve the plant. First, they were mobile, often lacking long-term land tenure. Without the legal means of ensuring multigenerational tenure, one strong incentive for long-term stewardship was lacking. Second, with the exception of their coveted use rights, hunters generally eschewed social rules, both statutory and informal. Indeed, many of them, like Daniel Boone, were attracted to a life in the woods because of the freedom it offered and did not readily submit to limits on that freedom. As Johann Schoepf observed in 1783, "They shun everything which appears to demand of them law and order, dread anything that breathes constraint. . . . Their object is merely wild, altogether natural freedom, and hunting is what pleases them."[56] Hunters' track record with other game species suggests that they placed little value on conservation. They hunted buffalo and elk to extirpation in the Ohio Valley, and they significantly reduced the numbers of bear, deer, beaver, and any other animal whose hides could be marketed. The occasional call for game conservation always went unheeded, leading Stephen Aron to conclude, "About the only ceiling that pioneer hunters observed was that set by the supply of powder and bullets."[57] When these hunters approached a patch of ginseng, therefore, all indications suggest that they typically dug the entire patch.

Moreover, evidence suggests that harvesters took no measures to replant ginseng seeds. In order to replant seeds, one must harvest only in the late fall, typically after mid-September when the plants begin to produce seeds. François Michaux remarked in 1802 that unlike the Chinese, who began digging in the autumn, Americans "begin gathering ginseng in the spring, and end at the decline of autumn."[58] John May's diary further suggests that people did not wait until the autumn to harvest. When he arrived in Marietta in June, he noted that several other merchants were already taking ginseng. He was bombarded by potential customers who brought undried, "green" ginseng to trade.[59] James Alexander purchased green ginseng throughout the summer and fall. By not waiting until the plant went to seed, harvesters contributed to the rapid depletion of the plant near the Ohio River. Following the initial "smash and grab," ginseng populations retreated deeper into the more inaccessible places, mostly located in the mountains. Here, patches still existed that had never seen harvesting pressure.

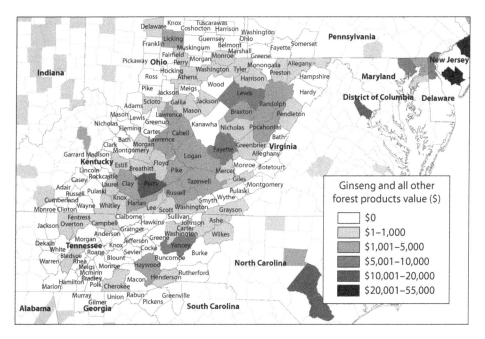

Ginseng production by county, 1840. (Map by author; data from: US Census Office, *Compendium of the Enumeration of the Inhabitants of the United States* [Washington, DC: Thomas Allen, 1841].)

The Evolution of a Commons Culture

By 1840, the dynamics of the ginseng trade were changing in the Appalachian region. As part of the 1840 census, federal enumerators recorded the only county-level statistics of ginseng production from the nineteenth century, shedding rare light on the changing economics and geography of ginseng digging. Based on a survey of local merchants in every county, the census revealed that while upstate New York still produced large quantities of ginseng (as much as $140,000 worth that year), North Carolina ($46,000), (West) Virginia ($35,000), and Kentucky ($35,000) were the clear leaders south of New York.[60] The vast majority of ginseng from these states came from the least accessible and least populated sections of Central Appalachia. A map of this data reveals two clusters of ginseng extraction: the mountainous headwaters of the Tug Fork of the Big Sandy River and further east in the high ridges of Fayette, Pocahontas, Randolph, and Greenbrier.[61] Whereas ginseng was found throughout much of the Ohio Valley in the eighteenth century, the geography of ginseng harvesting was moving further into the mountains.

The 1840 census reveals that the ginseng trade thrived in areas distant from major transportation routes where the agricultural economy was least developed. Perhaps not surprisingly, western Virginia's counties that produced significant quantities of ginseng in 1840 (more than $1,000 worth) on average produced some 13 percent fewer cattle, 14 percent less corn, and 70 percent less wheat than counties that did not export ginseng. This has much to do with the fact that major ginseng-producing counties contained, on average, 40 percent fewer people than counties that did not produce ginseng.[62] Thus, there was a strong inverse correlation between population, economic development, and ginseng production.

A closer look at Randolph County, (West) Virginia, one of the most prolific ginseng-producing counties in the 1840s, provides a useful glimpse into the changing social and economic roles the plant played during the late antebellum period. As the seventh most productive ginseng county in the state, reaching at least $2,000 that year in sales, Randolph County displayed a developing agricultural economy that was still very much dependent on the forest.[63] From 1790 to 1840, the population of Randolph grew from 951 to 6,200, and cattle, corn, swine, and wheat emerged as the county's leading commodities. It was not a prolific producer of these farm commodities in 1840, but it was near average among western Virginia counties.[64] Incorporated in 1790 on the east bank of the Tygart River, Beverly grew steadily as the commercial hub of the county, expanding as agricultural development proceeded. Wagon roads crisscrossed the Tygart Valley, ascending the mountains along all the major tributary creeks. By 1850, Beverly boasted a population of roughly 200, including two wagonmakers, three saddlers, two lawyers, two carpenters, two blacksmiths, and four proprietors of country stores.[65] The eastern and southern ends of the county remained more sparsely populated and heavily forested. Randolph had one of the lowest population densities in western Virginia in 1850: nine persons per square mile. Beneath the façade of agricultural development, Randolph suffered from unequal land distribution. Tenancy was a persistent problem. Nearly half (49 percent) of all households owned no real estate in 1850, while the average real estate value for those who did own their farms was $2,000. A legacy of the land engrossment during the frontier phase, 44 percent of the total real estate value reported to the census in 1860 was owned by fewer than fifty individuals.[66]

Ely Butcher, whose parents had moved to Randolph County in the 1790s from Eastern Virginia, was a commercial and civic leader in Beverly. Sometime around 1840, he opened a store twelve miles southwest in the small and more rural community of Huttonsville on the upper reaches of the Tygart River, placing his fourteen-year-old son, Ely Baxter, in charge of the establishment.[67] The records of this store, which span the years 1841 to 1857 (with a few years missing), are among the most comprehensive from the Ridge and Valley region in the antebellum era. Analysis of one calendar year, from the spring of 1840 to the spring of 1841, reveals that some 64 percent of Butcher's revenues came from cash transactions, and 10 percent came from bartering for farm products such as bacon, corn, and wheat. The remainder (26 percent) came from bartering products from the forest commons, including ginseng (9 percent), skins and furs (4 percent), maple sugar (4 percent), and chestnuts (3 percent).[68] More than a quarter of the economy that funneled through Butcher's store came from the commons.

Butcher's records provide some quantitative evidence to support what anecdotal sources suggest: that ginseng was the cornerstone of the commons economy. Local historian John Sutton, who grew up in antebellum Braxton County in what would become West Virginia, later claimed that "the value of wild ginseng has been many times greater in a commercial sense to the inhabitants of central West Virginia than all the magnificent timber that has stood as stately sentinels in the forest for a thousand years. Ginseng was the greatest source of income the common people had for a half century after the settlement of the country."[69] Gathering $10 worth of roots might take five days, he pointed out, whereas it took a three-year-old steer or ten large walnut trees to bring in the same amount. Ginseng was simply easier to obtain without investments in land or other overhead costs.[70] Thus, the commons was a vital part of the local economy, and ginseng was the most crucial. In this regard, Butcher's community seems to have been fairly typical of ginseng-producing Appalachian counties. By 1840, according to the census, ginseng had replaced skins and furs in Appalachian states as the most valuable forest product. In Kentucky, the hunters' paradise of Daniel Boone's generation, rural residents now traded nearly twice as much ginseng as skins and furs.[71]

Ginseng served important social and economic functions for local communities, providing something of a social safety net for land-poor farmers. Of Butcher's 305 customers, more than one-third, or 105 of them, paid him in ginseng. Most of these customers were clustered in the same general area in the mountains west of Huttonsville. Of those 105 customers who could be identified in census returns (40), some 45 percent owned no land, and 92 percent owned less than $2,000 worth of real estate. The vast majority of Butcher's ginseng customers were young heads of household, twenty to thirty years old, with either no children or very young children and who owned less than $500 worth of land, if they owned any at all. Both Isaac Dodrell and James Ware, for example, were twenty, landless, and newly married when they first appear in Butcher's records, and they both relied heavily on the forest commons to build their new adult lives. Every fall, Dodrell brought in a load of ginseng to pay for most of his store purchases, which averaged roughly $5 per year. Ware, similarly, brought in roots, maple sugar, and venison as well as corn and one calf. Lewis Cowgar covered a $103 bill over a period of five years with $36 in ginseng, $24 in skins, $12 in fish, $4 in beeswax, and the rest in cash, wool, and "merchandise." In 1841, Daniel Wamsley, a thirty-three-year-old tenant farmer with a wife and two young children, paid most of an $18 bill with $16 worth of ginseng. Thus, the pattern was clear: the county's small and landless farmers, especially those living in the highland areas in the Tygart Valley headwaters, used the root to procure supplies when their farm could not produce the surplus needed to purchase them. These land-poor farmers created lives for themselves that integrated the forests into their seasonal agrarian routines, and ginseng was the pillar of their forest economy.

While the county's smallholders leaned heavily on the forest commons to access the national economy, landowners of sizeable wealth still participated in the trade. Some 8 percent of Butcher's ginseng customers owned more than $2,000 in real estate, a sum that placed them in the top wealthiest quarter of landowners. John Sutton later recalled, "A great many of the best citizens and successful businessmen of central West Virginia bought their school books and made their first pocket change by digging the greatest of all the herbs known."[72] One of them was James B. Hamilton. Born in 1830 and raised on a large farm in Fayette County, West Virginia, Hamilton was, by 1858, a successful farmer, surveyor, and active member of the Ansted community. His diary from that year indicates that from late August through September, he hunted ginseng almost daily in the hills along the New River near its confluence with the Gauley. On good days, he dug as much as $1.37 worth of roots. During the rest of the year, he surveyed roads, worked in the fields, tended livestock, participated in the annual muster, worked the polls on Election Day, and attended church meetings.[73] By 1860, ginseng and this assortment of other income streams helped him accumulate $6,000 worth of real estate and $1,000 worth of personal property, making him one of the wealthiest landowners in the community.[74] The development of a cash-based agricultural economy had provided landowners with more options for accessing the market than they had in the 1780s. Nevertheless, the ginseng economy that operated alongside still served a wide swath of western Virginia society.

Several of Butcher's customers who owned large farms may have participated in the trade less out of economic necessity than from tradition. The family of Jesse Wamsley, who owned $6,000 worth of land, for example, brought in regular loads of roots every fall. The load that Jesse's son and three daughters traded every September was almost always the first of the store's ginseng transactions for the year, after which they disappeared from the ledgers. This suggests that digging ginseng had become something of an annual Wamsley family tradition rather than an effort to fulfill economic needs. An older son, twenty-two-year-old Samuel, who had recently moved from the homeplace to his own farm, fell back on that tradition. Although he owned $5,000 in real estate in 1850, he used the root to make ends meet, paying 22 percent of his $57 bill with it. Similarly, landowner Henry Vandevender brought his four daughters to the store to trade their roots. They used ginseng to cover all their purchases from 1841 to 1847, which ranged from $3 to $27 per year and consisted primarily of nonessential things like candy, toys, and dolls.[75] Thus, the local landowning elite participated in the ginseng hunt, but their hunt was more for recreation and luxuries, less for subsistence.

Even as ginseng's economic importance to the region continued throughout the antebellum era, the process of commodification remained incomplete due to economic, ecological, and cultural factors. There is no evidence that anyone cultivated the plant in private gardens, which raises the question: why not? Ecology played a role, but it cannot fully answer the question, as it was possible—as it is today—to cultivate the plant. As discussed in chapter 1, William Byrd could not raise ginseng, but that was because he tried to do it on the Virginia peninsula where the climate was too warm. One North Carolina newspaper reported in 1860, "Attempts have been made to propagate it by seed, but so far have failed, though an experienced Ginseng dealer informs us that he has no doubt it can be done by adhering to the habits of the plant as to location."[76] This ginseng dealer was correct, and rural Appalachians did know the habits of the plant. Over the first half of the nineteenth century, hunting ginseng became deeply woven into the fabric of rural life throughout the southern mountains. Inhabitants of the area came to know it intimately: its seasonal cycle, its ecology, where it grew, what it grew next to, and how it interacted with climate and soil. Since at least the 1890s, ginseng has been successfully cultivated across the United States, demonstrating that its growing conditions could have been replicated by diligent efforts in the mid-nineteenth century. The answer then, it seems, involves a more complex set of factors.

First, because ginseng takes several years to mature to harvestable size, many lacked the land tenure that would allow for such delayed returns. From 1763 to 1776, land companies such as the Transylvania, Greenbrier, Loyal, and Ohio acquired titles to roughly 5 million acres of Indian lands in the trans-Appalachian region, and those settlers who had moved into the region to build homesteads found themselves unable to secure title to their land without purchasing power. Many of them took up residence as squatters on land purchased by absentee owners and faced near-constant threats to their tenure. John Mathews ran into ten white families squatting on federal lands along Muskingam Creek who were in the midst of a protracted struggle with federal troops who sought to remove them.[77] The 1802 diary of land speculator George Hunter is full of references to finding people living on lands to which he claimed a patent.[78] As late as 1810, absentee owners held title to some 93 percent of the land in what is now West Virginia, and these patterns continued through the antebellum era, ensuring that some communities suffered from high rates of tenancy.[79] Perhaps tenant farmers did not want to invest money and time into improving land that was not their own with such delayed returns as ginseng offered.

A second reason has more to do with the culture that developed around the commons. There were enough landowners who could have pioneered ginseng cultivation, but by the 1850s, accepted patterns of land use had become established in rural communities. The rights-in-the-woods that predominated among early hunters due to the necessities of survival had evolved into common rights to certain naturally occurring resources. Rural Americans in general and Appalachians in particular adhered to something of a Lockean conception of property: they believed the ownership of land resulted from the mixing of labor with it. Therefore, if a plant grew wild and was not the result of any human labor, it was not owned by anyone and could thus be harvested and used by anyone. Custom dictated that ginseng was the property of the harvester, rather than the landowner, and this proved difficult to reform.[80] After all, the social relationships within mountain communities were very much influenced by the relationships between humans and the land. Accessing the property of others to hunt, fish, and forage—and, conversely, allowing others access to one's own property—was an integral part of membership in a community. "To do so unneighborly a thing" as restricting access or fencing off one's property, as one observer put it, "would be to make undying enemies."[81] In other words, even if landowners wanted to assert more ownership over the ginseng plants on their property, they were unlikely to convince their neighbors to acknowledge their exclusive right to it. Perhaps they were unwilling to challenge convention in that way.[82]

There is also ample evidence to suggest that Appalachian people simply preferred the freedom of harvesting the plant from the forest commons to the financial profitability of cultivating it, and they could find enough in the wild to bolster their security and independence. Much like hunting and fishing, digging ginseng blurred the line between leisure and labor. Many rural residents developed an intense fondness for wandering the hills in search of the plant. "A day of sanging had all the fun of gambling with no risk of losing any of your own nickels," one West Virginian later remembered of the antebellum era. "It was similar to an Easter egg hunt with higher stakes for the adults."[83] Some pursued ginseng out of necessity, and others because they enjoyed it, but for most rural folk, it was a false dichotomy. They hunted the root because they needed the money *and* because they enjoyed it. Author Anne Royall, who grew up in Monroe County, (West) Virginia, in the 1810s before moving to the East Coast, wrote that people in the remote mountain communities of Greenbrier, Monroe, Randolph, Pocahontas, Giles, and Tazewell Counties preferred a life dependent on the commons. Their employments consist in "farming, raising cattle, making whiskey (and drinking it), hunting, and digging sang."[84] In his social history of Appalachia during the late antebellum era, John Sherwood Lewis has argued that the people who settled in the remote sections of West Virginia did so not because they saw commercial potential in these areas, but rather because they desired different economic structures that balanced freedom and stability. Displaced by economic developments associated with the market revolution elsewhere in the United States, they moved to these isolated areas because, like the hunters before them, they wanted to live off the "spontaneous productions of nature." The forest commons provided access to a wealth of resources that they could not, or would not, produce on a farm.[85] They did not live independent of markets, and they did not oppose markets per se, but they preferred a different relationship to the land than the ambitious agriculturalist, one that blended light farm work with the work of hunting, fishing, and foraging.

Across Appalachia, ginseng digging provided mountaineers with a shared experience that reinforced a sense of community. While diggers were particularly secretive about where they found ginseng, they were more than willing to show off their large roots at the country store and spin tales about the ones that got away. According to one observer, "Wonderful sang patches found in the mountains and lost again, although carefully sought, form the staple of many of the simple legends of these parts."[86] As a node of commerce and a meeting place, the ginseng factory also served some important social functions. Allen T. Davidson, who grew up in Haywood County, North Carolina, in the 1820s, remembered seeing "the great companies of mountaineers coming along the mountain passes . . . with pack horses and oxen going to the 'factory' as we called it. It was a great rendezvous for the people where all the then sports of the day were engaged in, such as pitching quoits, running foot races, shooting matches, wrestling, and sometimes, a good fist and skull fight. But the curse and indignation of the neighborhood rested on the man who attempted, as we called it, 'to interfere in the fight, or double-team, or use a weapon.'"[87] Davidson's colorful portrait of the ginseng rendezvous suggests that the shared experience of ginseng digging and trading, based on equal access to the forest commons, helped strengthen relationships among some sparsely settled farmers.

Ginseng also played an important cultural role in some Native American communities. Some Indians preferred the work of harvesting ginseng to farming and often used it to resist acculturation efforts by missionaries, including the imposition of European-style agriculture. Scholars have tended to characterize Indians' engagement in the ginseng trade as a form of acculturation, as another node of dependency that pulled them away from their traditional patterns of life and into the orbit of white society.[88] However, as we have seen, not all commodities are created equal, and while ginseng did grant native communities access to the Atlantic consumer economy on which they had grown increasingly dependent, it also helped them reduce their dependency on the modern agroecological complex built around individual, private farms. From the eighteenth century, Native Americans used the ginseng market in ways that inspired resistance to other acculturation efforts. For example, the Iroquois depended on the plant to defy the wishes of colonial authorities who sought to coerce Indian labor for farm work. Peter Kalm noted that the Indians around Montreal were "so much taken up with this business [digging ginseng] that the French farmers were not able during that time to hire a single Indian, as they commonly do to help them in the harvest."[89] In a private letter in 1752, the Reverend Jonathan Edwards noted the blossoming of the trade around Albany, New York, lamenting that it has "occasioned our Indians of all sorts, young and old, to spend abundance of time in the woods, and sometimes to a great distance, in the neglect of public worship and their husbandry, and also in going to Albany to sell their roots, which proves worse to them than going into the woods, where they are always much in the way of temptation and darkness."[90] Thus, ginseng enabled the Iroquois to circumvent the colonial labor system, avoid coerced worship, and maintain a way of life built around the forests.

In southwestern North Carolina during the antebellum era, the Cherokee similarly utilized ginseng to maintain a more traditional relationship to the land dependent on the forest commons. In 1839, Waynesville native William Holland Thomas opened a store in Cherokee County near Fort Butler in the southwestern tip of North Carolina. One of the stockades constructed two years earlier by the US Army to facilitate the removal of the Cherokee from their homes, Fort Butler became the locus around which newly arriving white settlers created the town of Murphy. Thomas, a white man who also owned two other stores in neighboring Haywood County, sold goods to both white settlers and the few hundred Cherokee whom he had helped remain in the mountains. He had traded in ginseng as a clerk for Felix Walker in 1818 and then again in Qualla Town as a teenage storeowner in the early 1820s, but in 1839, he encouraged the Cherokee to bring in the root, and he jumped into the trade with both feet. Placing much hope in ginseng, he ordered his clerks to give it "closer attention than any business you have ever had charge of" and cautioned that it "has more responsibility attached to it" than any other article.[91] In addition to ginseng, he took in other commons commodities for barter, especially skins and furs, chestnuts, and pinkroot, which was sold throughout the Southeast to treat intestinal worms.[92] While his correspondence does not indicate how much money he stood to make on ginseng, the two counties in which he owned stores produced nearly $2,000 worth in 1840, according to the census.[93]

Thomas's records reveal that virtually all the ginseng he purchased came from the Cherokee. According to his store ledgers from 1839 to 1850, Thomas's white customers used cash, bank notes, labor, or some form of farm produce to purchase their goods, whereas the Cherokee relied heavily on ginseng, chestnuts, deerskins, and pinkroot.[94] Thomas's correspondence with his store managers indicates that the bulk of his ginseng came from Shoal Creek, a remote area in western Cherokee County near Wacheesee Town and Turtle Town, where a cluster of Cherokee families had resisted the removal orders and remained. Such findings suggest that race played a key role in determining commons use in antebellum Cherokee County. Interestingly, Thomas's white customers were just as likely to purchase chestnuts and pinkroot as the Cherokee were to sell it.[95] Three other area store ledgers have survived from the late 1830s and early 1840s: Jesse Siler's store just across the Cherokee County line in Macon County, William Walker's store on the Valley River, and A. R. S. Hunter's store near Fort Butler. These stores served a clientele that was virtually all white. None of them dealt in ginseng.[96]

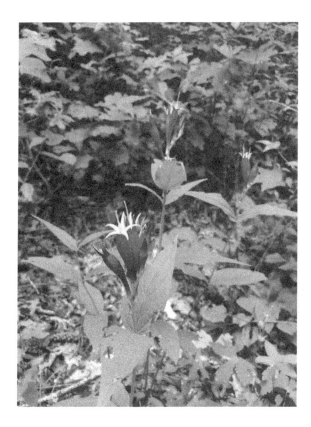

Pinkroot (*Spigelia marylandica*). (Photo by author.)

Reasons for this racial divide remain unclear. Thomas would certainly have taken ginseng from white customers. Nowhere in his voluminous correspondence with his store managers did he indicate that he wanted ginseng from the Cherokee only.[97] His white customers simply did not supply ginseng as the Cherokee did. Perhaps there was a social stigma associated with the forest economy, a phenomenon further explored in chapter 7. Or perhaps simple economics was at work. Thomas's white customers were relatively well positioned for an income that depended on the sale of farm commodities. The earliest wave of whites to move into the area following Cherokee removal settled on former Cherokee farms on the rich bottomland along the Valley and Hiwassee Rivers. They had little knowledge of local flora and fauna, but they knew how to grow crops, often with the help of enslaved people. Within two years of removal, the county boasted agricultural production that rivaled its longer-resettled neighbors Macon and Haywood Counties. By 1860, Cherokee was one of the fastest growing counties in Western North Carolina. Its inhabitants owned more slaves and slaughtered more livestock than any other western county outside of Buncombe.[98]

The region's Cherokee, on the other hand, had the economic incentive, ecological knowledge, and cultural proclivities to harvest ginseng. Even prior to the arrival of the US Army, they were among the Cherokee Nation's poorest members, if poverty can be measured by a lack of slaves and a lack of merchantable agricultural commodities. While many Cherokee in the North Georgia Piedmont owned large plantations and were among the wealthiest individuals in the region, white or Indian, those in the North Carolina mountains tended to cling to a more traditional lifestyle.[99] They raised a little corn and owned small farms, but they drew more heavily on the forests for their subsistence. During the years following removal, the lives of those Cherokee who resisted removal were so disrupted that many faced starvation. According to Thomas's store clerk in Qualla Town, "There came from the towns of Alarka, Nantahalla, Stekoah, and Cheoah, a good many poor and destitute Indians who stated they had been deprived of all their means of support during the emigration."[100] Thomas obliged by lending them corn. Ginseng not only supplied them with a readily available means of support; it also provided a way to reconcile their traditional forest-based lifestyle with the need to access the consumer economy, much like the case of the Iroquois a century earlier. Therefore, it seems likely that the Cherokee, due to their tenuous economic position and their cultural proclivities, not to mention their knowledge of how to find it, harvested the bulk of the ginseng from far southwestern North Carolina in the antebellum era.

The Evolving Ecology of Ginseng Digging

By the outbreak of the Civil War, the human-ginseng relationship seems to have evolved beyond the initial smash-and-grab phase of the frontier boom. There is some evidence that ginseng began to grow scarce even in the remote parts of Southern Appalachia. Ely Butcher's records show a gradual decline through the 1850s, from 500 pounds in 1849 to 129 pounds in 1851 and 86 pounds by 1857.[101] Observers elsewhere noticed a gradual disappearance as well. Henry Colton remarked in 1859 that, in Yancey County, North Carolina, "the day had been when anybody could gather six or eight pounds, but now it took a right smart hand to get that much."[102]

Evidence suggests that as the root became scarce, mountain people began to adjust their practices to boost ginseng populations. Some began more conscientiously tending the commons, replanting seeds where they found ginseng growing. Recalling his youth in mid-nineteenth-century Appalachian Ohio, for example, one physician recalled that he would "plant the seeds of ginseng in the woods as I would dig the roots, think-ing that they would not grow outside their own environment or natural habitation. . . . I just planted them and left them to 'work out their own salvation.' . . . After a few years, I began to see the result of my work; I found little bunches of ginseng throughout the woods which convinced me that my labor had not been in vain."[103] He did not describe what he was doing as cultivating. Rather, he was replenishing the roots he took from the commons. Sources that could reveal how typical these practices were in the 1840s are nonexistent, but it is not unreasonable to assume that the people who saw ginseng as a vital resource for their future took measures to ensure the long-term health of the plant, including replant-ing seeds.

In order to successfully mitigate overharvesting through seed replanting, diggers would first have to wait until the plant produced seeds, typically in September or October. Butcher's records indicate that mountain communities did indeed begin to limit their harvests to the fall season over a decade prior to states passing laws mandating the same ginseng season (beginning in the late 1860s). The first of September seems to have been the unofficial start of the ginseng season at Butcher's store in the 1840s and 1850s. By paying attention to whether Butcher noted that the ginseng was traded as "green" (undried) or dried in his ledger, the historian can approximate when the ginseng was harvested. Throughout the month of September, Butcher accepted only the green root, which indicates it was recently harvested. Starting in October and continuing, in a few cases, into the winter, he took dried root. He took virtually no green and very little dry ginseng out of season. Indeed, the only time green ginseng appears in his books out of season, he apparently felt the need to justify it, scribbling a note in the margin explaining that the customer "had to pay for boy's boat."[104] Thus, in this case, the exception may prove the rule: an unofficial, locally sanctioned ginseng season had developed since the area's initial settlement. Whereas James Alexander purchased ginseng throughout the summer and fall in the 1780s, Butcher's customers waited until the plant went to seed.

The fact that locals adhered to a season does not in itself prove that a conservation ethic was widespread among rural communities. The refusal of merchants to take ginseng before September could have been an attempt to appeal to Chinese tastes. They realized that in the fall, the plant acquires "its full degree of maturity and perfection," which is one reason the Chinese harvested it only at that time of year.[105] Experts today assert that the young roots can double or triple their size during each of their first few growing seasons, and mature roots expand roughly 20 percent through the course of a year.[106] Waiting until September to purchase ginseng gave these traders added assurance that they were getting the best possible root for shipment. Market forces, in this case, worked in the plant's favor.

That harvesters and storekeepers observed a particular season reveals a few significant aspects of the antebellum ginseng trade. First, it suggests that competition among merchants for the ginseng trade was not as fierce as it would later become. Indeed, Butcher was likely one of the only merchants in western Randolph County buying ginseng and could, thus, enforce this season simply by refusing to take it at any other time without worrying about losing customers. Second, the social and economic conditions were such that people could afford to wait until the fall to harvest. Utilizing an economy balanced between the farm and the forest, diggers likely had other means of obtaining store credit throughout the year. In other words, they were not desperate. Third, the fact that this season existed in Butcher's records indicates that one of the most important components of ginseng conservation was present in antebellum forests: trust. For someone to willingly forego harvesting a lucrative commodity in, say, the summer, that person must be able to trust that no one else will harvest that plant until the right time. Apparently, in western Randolph County, there existed enough trust to ensure that people waited until the fall to harvest, thus giving the plants a fighting chance to reproduce. These dynamics would change, however, following the Civil War, as we will see in chapter 6.

The frontier economy in Central and Southern Appalachia depended heavily on the Chinese demand for ginseng and the transpacific trade network that it helped establish. As the ginseng boom spread from Canada and New York into the Ohio Valley, the plant served as a widespread medium of exchange that enabled early merchants to sustain their businesses, hunters to access the consumer economy, and new residents to purchase necessities. As economies diversified, the geography of ginseng digging moved further into the mountains of Central and Southern Appalachia, where it was incorporated into the seasonal routines of rural communities and played an important social and economic role. The initial smash-and-grab phase of the frontier boom eventually gave way to a more complex human-ginseng relationship in which individuals and communities worked collectively to mitigate overharvesting. Nature in the form of agroecological challenges and culture continued to interact to shape the process of ginseng's commodification. Instead of becoming a privately cultivated cash crop, it remained a commons commodity. While they could have cultivated ginseng in large gardens, rural residents insisted that it—like all other naturally growing plants—remain the property of the harvester rather than the landowner. This fact reinforced a general commitment to common rights-in-the-woods and an egalitarian economic structure that formed the basis of community. Still, this commons system faced increasing pressures as population grew and forests were cleared for livestock and agriculture. Meanwhile in the mid-nineteenth century, changing medical practices and improved transportation opened new markets for a variety of other roots and herbs.

3

Marketing the Mountain Commons

Calvin J. Cowles and the Origins of the Botanical Drug Trade

IN SEPTEMBER 1850, CALVIN J. COWLES, A MERCHANT FROM WILKES County, North Carolina, said good-bye to his wife and two young sons and headed north with his brother Josiah leading a wagon with a peculiar cargo. Inside the bales of burlap piled high behind the twenty-nine-year-old merchant were seeds from lobelia plants, bark from elm trees, and the roots of wild ginger, lady's slipper, bloodroot, mayapple, and several more plants. He hoped to sell them to businessmen in the North to eventually be made into tinctures, extracts, ointments, and patent medicines. After a long journey through Virginia, he stopped at Washington City, where he met President Millard Fillmore, and pushed on to Philadelphia, where he visited the grave of Benjamin Franklin. He continued north, spending some time shopping in New York City. All along his route he could find only a few buyers for his roots and herbs. "I see I shall have to go to New Lebanon to sell out," he informed his wife, Martha, in November. New Lebanon, New York, a small town some thirty miles east of Albany on the western slope of the Berkshire Mountains, was an emerging center of the manufacturing of botanical medicines. There, he sold the rest of his cargo and began the long journey home. "I think I have made a good trip," he told his wife. "Our prospects for the future are bright enough for substantial good."[1] Indeed they were.

Cowles took a risk when he traveled north in 1850. He had already purchased these roots and herbs from local diggers and country storekeepers with goods, and now he had to sell them for a good price or else suffer a loss on the venture. Country merchants like Cowles had experience trading in roots and herbs on a local level, supplying nearby physicians with plants harvested from the surrounding fields and forests. But Cowles had larger ambitions, and with this trip he hoped to tap into the emerging national markets for medicinal plants that changing medical practices, new pharmaceutical manufacturing technologies, and transportation improvements had only recently made possible. It was not an easy beginning, but with the help of his roots and herbs, Cowles eventually met with some financial success and became a prominent Republican politician in North Carolina politics after the Civil War. Cowles had an unmistakable impact on the root and herb trade in the late nineteenth century. By demonstrating that buying and selling roots and herbs to pharmaceutical manufacturers could be profitable, he established a model that subsequent merchants would emulate. Indeed, Cowles's 1850 trip north was a turning point that paved the way for Southern Appalachia to become the nation's most prolific supplier of "crude botanical drugs."

A New Kind of Merchant

Born in Hamptonville, North Carolina, in 1821, Calvin J. Cowles grew up in a world of developing trade and commerce. His father, Josiah Cowles, had moved from his native Connecticut in 1815 to peddle Yankee wares among Cherokee and Creek Indians and backcountry settlers in exchange for skins and furs before settling down and opening a shop in Surry County, North Carolina. The elder Cowles embraced the changes brought by the market revolution and sought to profit by them. He pushed for internal improvements, opposed the putative backward policies of Andrew Jackson, and became a prominent Whig in Surry County. Largely self-educated, Calvin developed a nose for business. He grew up in and around his father's store in Hamptonville and worked there as a clerk from his teenage years into his early twenties. His mother died young, and when his father remarried, his new wife brought three children into the marriage, including the young Martha Duvall. Cowles fell in love with her, and the two married in 1844. Within two years, they had a son, Arthur Duvall. Six more children eventually followed.[2]

In 1846, eager to make his own name in business, Cowles moved with his wife and infant son twenty miles west to Wilkes County, North

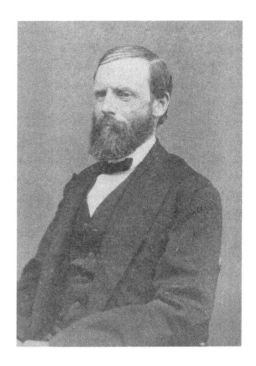

Calvin J. Cowles, Wilkesboro, North Carolina, merchant, in 1867. (Courtesy of W. L. Eury Appalachian Collection, Special Collections, Belk Library, Appalachian State University, Boone, NC.)

Carolina, and settled in Elkville where Elk Creek empties into the Yadkin River. There he constructed a store and began operating in partnership with his father under the name J. and C. J. Cowles. In many ways, Elkville in the 1840s was a remote outpost for a commercial enterprise. Located some seven miles from the crossroads of Wilkesboro along a local wagon road, it was a small cluster of farms at the foot of the imposing Blue Ridge escarpment, which quickly rose to over six thousand feet within a few miles from the Yadkin Valley. Beyond the ridge lay Ashe, Yancey, and Watauga County (created in 1850), which included some of the most sparsely populated sections of the state. But Wilkes County was also a community on the make. Wilkesboro, the county seat, was connected to larger commercial centers like Greensboro, Statesville, and Morganton by major thoroughfares, and within a few years, Greensboro would boast a railroad that linked the city to Raleigh, Wilmington, and beyond. Cowles was aware that greater commercial involvement was in store for northwestern North Carolina, and he wanted to be a part of it.

Cowles was ready to barter for his business, and he began, like many other merchants in the area, trading for ginseng, furs, skins, bird feathers, and a variety of other farm and forest goods. Thus, in an area lacking cash, Cowles, like other storekeepers, was compelled to engage in a variety of markets. Not only did he have to purchase wholesale goods at a price from which he could profit, but he also had to find buyers for the produce for which he bartered in order to realize the full value of his sales. Under the watchful eye of his father, he struggled through the first few years in business, but around 1848, he decided to branch out from ginseng and deal in other forest commodities. He purchased chestnuts from customers and sold them in Greensboro and Raleigh, where they were likely boiled or roasted and eaten. He bought wormseed, or Jerusalem oak (*Chenopodium anthelminticum*), used as a vermifuge to treat worms in children, and the seeds of lobelia (*Lobelia inflata*), used as a purgative for stomach troubles. He also traded in Seneca snakeroot and pinkroot, used to treat fevers and worms, respectively.

Initially, the markets he tapped were local. North Carolina doctors and druggists sporadically purchased from him a few pounds of a handful of different plants. His earliest business records reveal that he sold snakeroot to a Dr. Carter in Hamptonville and pinkroot and lobelia seeds to another local doctor, Alva Spears.[3] Although documentation is rare, it appears that this kind of local trade was not uncommon in the opening decades of the nineteenth century. According to family lore, David Worth, who would become a leading citizen of adjacent Ashe County, first came to the mountains in the 1830s to purchase roots and herbs for a family druggist in Greensboro.[4] However, the demand for native medicinal plants was limited prior to the 1840s. Most physicians relied heavily upon imported drugs from Europe, and most lay practitioners—those healers with no formal training in a medical school—harvested the plants themselves.

This local trade was not extensive and produced little income for Cowles. His father, despite occasionally relaying orders through his correspondence, was not enthusiastic about Cowles's move toward the botanical trade and urged caution. "I am not without my misgivings," he wrote to his son in 1849. "The market is liable to become over marked, the article to fluctuate very much in price. . . . You may be destined to labor too hard often on the same article if not in the same action."[5] The elder Cowles's advice was prescient, as the early years of piecemeal trade with local doctors were indeed precarious and unprofitable. What the elder Cowles did not realize was that vast new markets were beginning to open for the plants of Western North Carolina. Ever the visionary entrepreneur, the younger Cowles paid close attention to national market trends, constantly on the lookout for potential profits. By the 1840s, market trends, spurred by changes in medical ideology and practice, pharmaceutical manufacturing, and transportation improvements, promised to open profitable horizons.

The Rise of Botanical Medicine

Cowles was certainly aware that during his lifetime, the demand for native medicinal plants was on the rise nationwide. This was largely the result of challenges to the medical profession by lay practitioners and patients, mostly in the western and rural areas. At the turn of the nineteenth century, medicine in the United States was at a significant crossroads. Would Americans continue to embrace Old World therapeutics based on theories of illness and disease that dated back to Galen and the ancient Greeks, or would they move toward a new system that drew on empirical observations and utilized a pharmacopoeia with more native American plants?[6] Would the speculative rationalism of Europe or an American-flavored empiricism dominate American medicine? This was more than an academic debate. Rather, it was fueled by and embedded in a culture clash emblematic of the Age of Jackson, and it would have significant ramifications for the forests of Southern Appalachia.

In the late eighteenth century, professional physicians trained in a university setting tended to be wealthy elites who jealously guarded their prerogatives against pretenders and quacks. After the University of Pennsylvania established its medical school in 1765, the number of medical schools in America grew, but the fount of most medical knowledge circulating in the United States was the University of Edinburgh, Scotland. There, would-be physicians like Benjamin Rush and Benjamin Smith Barton were versed in the ancient theories of Hippocrates, Galen, Dioscorides, and other Greco-Roman physicians dating back to the first century AD. Although the veracity of ancient humoral theory had been undermined by various discoveries over preceding centuries, it still formed the basis for medical practice into the nineteenth. According to humoral theory, the body's health was determined by the balance of four fluids, or "humors": blood, phlegm, black bile, and yellow bile. Illness was the result of imbalances of these humors, and balance could be restored by building up or removing fluids. Physicians employed a number of techniques to balance the humors, including bloodletting, puking, purging, cupping, and sweating. Despite the important advances in medical science in the eighteenth century, particularly in the field of anatomy and in practices such as inoculation, Galen's basic ideas still influenced the way physicians viewed the causes of disease and the methods they used to treat them.[7]

While ancient theories based on speculative rationalism continued to exert influence over Western medicine, therapeutics had undergone something of a revolution. Plants are the oldest method of therapy used by Westerners, and they dominated therapeutics from the time of Galen (AD 129–216) through the sixteenth century, but as a result of a therapeutic revolution spurred by the sixteenth-century German physician Paracelsus, physicians in Europe began using increasing amounts of mineral-based medicines, such as mercury, antimony, sulphur, and lead. While they also had an impressive botanical materia medica at their command, minerals quickly became the most prescribed drugs in their practices. American physicians trained in Europe transferred this practice to the New World. By the 1790s, frustrated by the lack of success in treating diseases, they prescribed greater, or "heroic," doses of various forms of mercury, including calomel, blue mass, and corrosive sublimate as well as other chemical compounds like camphor, tartar emetic, and arsenic. They also continued to rely on some plant products, such as quinine, ipecac, and calamus, but virtually none of these were native to North America and had to be imported from Europe or other European colonies.[8] Frustrated by the floral ignorance of Virginia doctors, planter William Byrd lamented that "they are not acquainted enough with Plants or other parts of Natural History, to do any Service to the World."[9]

The eighteenth-century countryside was generally devoid of trained physicians and remained disconnected from the medical theories espoused in Edinburgh. Although the number of university-trained physicians was growing, it was still virtually impossible to find one outside of urban areas around the turn of the nineteenth century. Medical historian John Haller estimates that there were fewer than four hundred trained physicians in the United States at the time of the American Revolution, and probably only half of those had earned a medical degree from a university.[10] Lacking access to physicians, rural patients sought help elsewhere. The rural landscape, especially in the South and West, was replete with folk healers, midwives, and self-taught "doctors" who placed less faith in ancient theories and more on empirically derived medical knowledge. They were less interested in how these treatments fit into theories of illness than how effective they were at treating specific ailments. Patients, many of whom lacked faith in or knowledge of medical theories, embraced them.[11]

Many were impressed by Native Americans' abilities to heal people.[12] During his explorations in North Carolina in 1709, John Lawson observed that "an Indian hath been often found to heal an English-man of a Malady . . . , which the ablest of our English Pretenders in America . . . have deserted the Patient as incurable."[13] The Indian trader James Adair, who lived among the southeastern tribes for thirty years in the mid-eighteenth century, admitted that he preferred Cherokee healers to Western-trained doctors in some cases. The Cherokee "have a great knowledge of specific virtues in simples; applying herbs and plants, on the most dangerous occasions, and seldom, if ever, fail to effect a thorough cure, from the natural bush. . . . For my own part, I would prefer an old Indian before any surgeon whatsoever, in curing green wounds by bullets, arrows, &c., both for the certainty, ease, and speediness of cure."[14]

Little by little, this Native American knowledge brought some native plants into general use. Virginia's Dr. John Tennet, who emigrated from England in 1625, learned that the Seneca Indians successfully used an inconspicuous native plant to treat respiratory ailments, including tuberculosis. He introduced the plant as Seneca snakeroot (*Polygala senega*) to friends and colleagues. Sir William Johnson, the British agent to northern Indians in the mid-eighteenth century, reportedly discovered the uses of *Lobelia syphilitica* from the Iroquois, who used it to treat syphilis. And the Charleston, South Carolina, botanist Alexander Garden claimed to have learned from the Cherokee that the plant pinkroot (*Spigelia marylandica*) was an effective vermifuge.[15] Garden shipped a box of pinkroot to his New York colleague Cadwallader Colden. In their studies of North American botany, naturalists such as Colden, Peter Kalm, and John Bartram preserved Indian uses of several plants in mid-eighteenth-century publications.[16] In 1772, Samuel Stearns, a Massachusetts physician, wrote *The American Herbal*, the first book dedicated to the medicinal uses of American plants. These authors relied heavily on Native American ethnobotanical knowledge, and this knowledge often came to them secondhand from the "country people."[17] However, general knowledge of American medical botany remained limited.

From the late eighteenth through the mid-nineteenth century, American physicians became much more aware of their ignorance of native medicinal plants and sought to rectify it. A number of historical events combined to create this new awareness. First, the American Revolution demonstrated the liabilities of relying so much on medicines imported from Europe. Cut off from their traditional sources of medicines, many practitioners realized that more knowledge of native plants and a more dependable domestic supply of medicines were needed.[18] Second, the wave of nationalism that swept across the United States following the Revolution awakened a spirit of scientific inquiry into the natural products of the country. Naturalists like Thomas Jefferson, realizing that much of what Americans knew about their native plants came from foreign sources, undertook a campaign of more systematic study to remedy this deficiency.[19] Third, the American medical establishment became more open to botanical remedies because their patients demanded them. Frustration with regular physicians' inability to confront serious illness and disease (in many cases making it worse) led many Americans to what Haller has called a "crisis of faith" in their physicians.[20] Many patients, as well as some physicians, came to believe that, with its continued reliance on bloodletting, purging, and mercury treatment, American medicine had lost its ability to cure, which severely eroded the relationship between regular physicians and their patients. Everyone was desperate for new therapies.

In a lecture to medical students at the University of Pennsylvania in 1789, Benjamin Rush urged them to search the "untrodden fields and forests of the United States," emphasizing that "the Seneka and Virginia snake-roots, the Carolina pink root, the spice wood, the sassafrass, the butternut, the thoroughwort, the poke, and the stramonium are but a small part of the medicinal productions of America." He continued: "Who knows but it may be reserved for the American to furnish the world, from her productions, with cures from some of those diseases which now elude the power of medicine? Who knows but that, at the foot of the Alleghany mountain, there blooms a flower, that is an infallible cure for the epilepsy? Perhaps on the Monongahela, or the Potowmac, there may grow a root that shall supply, by its tonic powers, the invigorating effects of the savage or military life in the cure of consumptions?"[21] Pointing to the west as the way forward for American medicine, Rush proposed that the botanical diversity in the Appalachian region was an untapped and potentially valuable source of medicines, an idea that future druggists and physicians would reiterate and act upon. In 1798, Benjamin Smith Barton, professor of medical botany at the University of Pennsylvania, took a leap forward with the publication of his *Collections for an Essay towards a Materia Medica of the United States,* in which he laid out some of the more promising vegetable remedies in use in America. In 1818, two influential works appeared that greatly stimulated the study of the United States' indigenous medicines: William P. C. Barton's *Vegetable Materia Medica* and Jacob Bigelow's *American Medical Botany.* These works drew heavily on Native American uses of plants, subjecting them to chemical analysis and scientific scrutiny, thus giving them an air of respectability that physicians could endorse.

Of all the American botanists around the turn of the nineteenth century who branched out into medicine, none was more colorful or influential than Constantine Rafinesque. The Turkish-born, French-reared polymath first moved to the United States in 1802 at age nineteen and began a career of intense study of the natural world. Despite coming from a mercantile family, Rafinesque quickly earned a reputation as one of the greatest—if perhaps the most controversial—scientific minds in a young nation teeming with patriotic students of nature. Ever the sharp-tongued critic, he published hundreds of articles and books in geology, history, zoology, geography, philosophy, and botany. In 1819, he was appointed professor of natural history at Transylvania University in Lexington, Kentucky, where he served until 1826. Late in his life, he turned his perceptive mind to the study of medical botany and, in 1828, published *Medical Flora of the United States,* which remains one of the most comprehensive books on the subject published in the nineteenth century. Based on extensive observations of Native American uses of medicinal plants as well as the folk practices of "country people," *Medical Flora* became a handbook of sorts for an emerging generation of botanically inclined physicians.[22]

In 1820, a group of practicing and academic doctors and professional pharmacists, dominated by men from the northeastern United States, met in Washington City to create *The Pharmacopoeia of the United States of America,* which listed all the drugs commonly used in standard practice. They divided the contents into two lists: "Materia Medica" included the most commonly prescribed drugs, and the "Secondary List" included the less common. Of the 220 medical preparations in the "Materia Medica," only 31 were from plants indigenous to the United States. Nearly 70 preparations on the list were made from foreign plants. However, the "Secondary List" was dominated by indigenous plants. All but 11 of the 87 preparations on this list were indigenous to the United States.[23] Thus, although native plants remained secondary to minerals and foreign plants in the estimation of the nation's medical establishment, they had clearly bettered their reputation over the preceding thirty years.

Two trends in American culture combined to greatly increase the popular demand for botanical therapies, which ultimately pushed the medical establishment in a more botanically friendly direction: the flourishing of democratic sentiment and nationalism typically associated with the Jacksonian era and the revival of religious enthusiasm known as the Second Great Awakening. Both of these helped fuel the emergence of what scholars have called America's first botanico-medical movement.

The so-called Age of the Common Man featured an intense skepticism of anything that reeked of elitism and privilege, and many people directed their ire at regular doctors. "Has it not occurred even to physicians of the learned order, that every man may and ought, at a proper age and to a certain extent, to become his own physician?" quipped J. W. Cooper in his *The Experienced Botanist; or, Indian Physician* (1840).[24] No one harnessed this anti-intellectual sentiment better than Samuel Thomson. The son of an evangelical father born and raised in rural New England, Thomson grew acquainted with plant medicine through a widow named Benton whom his family employed as a healer. After spending years experimenting with herbal remedies and utilizing such methods as the steam bath, he developed a system of medical treatment that relied heavily on steaming, purging, and botanical remedies. He obtained a patent for his system in 1813, and he employed agents to travel the country selling the rights to use his remedies and formulas. He initiated a public relations onslaught against the "poison" of regular medicine, telling people they could "be their own physician" and imploring them to pay attention to "those medicines that grow in our own country, which God of nature has prepared for the benefit of mankind."[25] By the 1840s, at the height of his popularity, he had sold some one hundred thousand patents, and an estimated 3 million people were using his system, including half the population of Ohio.[26] His personal charisma, abrasiveness, and marketing prowess forced American doctors to reckon with botanical medicine.

Thomson's successes invigorated many disillusioned healers and encouraged imitators; by the 1840s, a wide variety of physicians and lay healers were operating under the title of botanic practitioners, including physio-medicals and Neo-Thomsonians. The most important of these post-Thomsonian groups called themselves Eclectics. They believed strongly in the efficacy of indigenous medicinal plants, but they did not go so far as to claim that "every man could be his own physician." Committed to medical science, they helped organize several medical colleges in the 1830s and 1840s to train a new generation of physicians to rely on indigenous plants in conjunction with other proven therapeutics.[27] Although by then the botanico-medical movement had degenerated into factional infighting and internal squabbles, the growth of the movement signaled a historic shift in therapeutics.

With the outpouring of religious enthusiasm brought about by the Second Great Awakening, many Americans came to see the use of native vegetable remedies as something akin to a religious exercise. After all, they were God's medicines, not man's. Mormons, Shakers, Disciples of Christ, and other sects developed a commitment to botanical medicine.[28] As the stern, vengeful God of the eighteenth century gave way to the more benevolent, merciful God of the nineteenth, more Americans embraced the ancient idea that he had endowed the land around them with vegetable remedies for all their ailments. John C. Gunn, author of the eminently popular *Gunn's Domestic Medicine* (1830) and a resident of East Tennessee, harnessed more effectively than most the religious sentiments of Jacksonian democracy and the Second Great Awakening. Referring to pious Americans as "God's patients," he declared, "Piety towards God should characterize every one who has any thing to do with the administering of medicine. . . . God, in the infinitude of his mercy, has stored our mountains, fields, and meadows, with simples for healing our diseases, and for furnishing us with medicines of our own, without the use of foreign articles."[29] He likened the discovery of these medicines to the processes by which religion was revealed to believers. Gunn's pitch was tremendously popular. By the time *Gunn's Domestic Medicine* ceased publication in 1924, it had gone through 234 editions and had been translated into German.[30]

In addition to Gunn's work, dozens of immensely popular self-help medical guides, including Samuel Thomson's *New Guide to Health* (1827), Morris Mattson's *The American Vegetable Practice* (1841), and Peter Good's *Family Flora* (1854), were published between 1820 and 1860. With titles like *The Indian Doctor's Dispensatory* (1813), *The Experienced Botanist; or, Indian Physician* (1840), and *The Cherokee Doctor* (1849), some displayed continued reverence for Native American medical wisdom. Playing up themes associated with Jacksonian democracy and the Second Great Awakening, they insisted that average Americans could take control of their own health and introduced them to native plants with hopeful—and in some cases unrealistic—promises of their medicinal value. Indeed, these medical guides helped lift botanical medicine to unprecedented popularity among the general public. While regular physicians, now referred to as allopathic physicians, were still reluctant to embrace botanical medicine, American consumers successfully pushed medical therapy in a botanically friendly direction. The cures to ailments, they asserted, were not to be found in a chemist's laboratory or in universities but rather in God's nature, in the fields and forests of the American countryside.

Patent medicine makers worked to further these trends and profited from them. They assured customers that they did not have to rely on physicians to manage their own health. All they had to do was purchase Carpenter's Vermifuge or Bristol's Sarsaparilla or Bull's Cherry Pectorals or any number of the thousands of patented medicines that graced the shelves of drugstores.[31] Many of them extolled the virtues of so-called vegetable remedies. Advertisements for McLean's Strengthening Cordial and Blood Purifier assured potential buyers that it was "nature's own remedy, curing disease by natural laws."[32] William Swain's Panacea was one of the most popular medicines. Swain claimed that his remedy consisted of only vegetable ingredients, specifically sarsaparilla and oil of wintergreen, although it was later revealed that there was a secret ingredient: the mercurial corrosive sublimate.[33] The medical establishment ridiculed many of these patent drugmakers for obscuring their ingredients and making absurd claims about their products' efficacy. Yet the popularity of these products attests to the fact that Americans wanted botanical drugs.[34]

Drawing on the knowledge of Native Americans and "country people," botanic practitioners and domestic medical guides succeeded in expanding the use of a handful of indigenous plants in American medical practice. Lobelia (*Lobelia inflata*) became something of a panacea to followers of Samuel Thomson, who claimed to have discovered the medicinal properties of the plant himself when he was a child. While many regular physicians relied on drugs such as tartar emetic, a derivative of antimony, and ipecac, a South American shrub, to produce vomiting, Thomson believed that native *Lobelia inflata* could produce emesis without the harsh side effects, and he used it to treat virtually every ailment he encountered. "It is the most important article made use of in my system," he wrote in his *New Guide to Health*.[35] Thomson is generally credited with introducing it into common use.[36]

Two other important herbs promoted by botanic practitioners that made their way into common use were mayapple (*Podophyllum peltatum*) and bloodroot (*Sanguinaria canadensis*). Mayapple, a perennial herb that grows throughout eastern North American forests, was well known to rural people. Rafinesque declared that "many use it frequently in the country."[37] By the 1820s, botanic practitioners were championing it as an excellent cathartic, or laxative, that could replace jalap, an imported Mexican plant then commonly used by both regular and unconventional physicians. Not only could it be obtained significantly more cheaply than jalap; many claimed that it was much gentler, inducing catharsis without the stomach pain that typically accompanied jalap. By the late 1840s, many Eclectic physicians began prescribing mayapple root instead of mercurials, specifically calomel, in treating bilious complaints, earning it a reputation as the "Eclectic calomel."[38]

Bloodroot, a perennial herb that grows chiefly in the Appalachian Mountains, was the subject of vigorous debate among all kinds of medical circles beginning in the 1820s, when physicians began using its root to treat a wide variety of ailments, from jaundice and croup to bronchitis, pertussis, typhoid fever, influenza, and pneumonia. Eclectics considered it a "very active agent . . . , capable of exercising a powerful influence on the system."[39] In his *Medical Flora,* Rafinesque hailed it as "one of the most valuable medical articles of our country."[40] One of the plants whose reputation extended well beyond botanical doctors, bloodroot attracted the attention of Yale professors William Tully and Eli Ives, who conducted numerous experiments with the plant in the 1820s and promoted its use in treating diseases of the lungs and the liver.[41]

Interestingly, despite enthusiasm for the plant in the seventeenth and eighteenth centuries among people like William Byrd, ginseng was not among those plants that enjoyed widespread use during the botanico-medical movement of the nineteenth century. John C. Gunn dismissed it as "nothing more than . . . a pleasant bitter," and John King as a "mild tonic and stimulant."[42] In his highly influential *American Medical Botany,* Jacob Bigelow, a student of Benjamin Smith Barton at the University of Pennsylvania, declared that "its virtues do not appear, by any means, to justify the high estimation of it by the Chinese."[43] However, Constantine Rafinesque performed many studies on ginseng and concluded that "this article appears . . . to deserve further attention, instead of total neglect." While evidence suggests that some rural people self-medicated with ginseng, and there were some medical thinkers who were not ready to dismiss ginseng so readily, it was not used widely in the United States.[44]

There are a few reasons why ginseng use did not catch on in the United States. The first is the sheer profitability of the root. To the rural mountain people who knew how to find the plant, ginseng was worth much more as a tradable commodity than as a medicine. Second, ginseng lacked the properties that most botanics looked for in a medicinal plant. They wanted action. Plants like mayapple, bloodroot, lobelia, and hellebore produced powerful reactions such as vomiting and diarrhea which, according to common medical thought, indicated that the medicine was working to bring the body back into balance. Botanic medicine, no less than regular medicine, remained under the sway of humoral theory. Ginseng produced none of these reactions. "It is not a very active substance," Bigelow observed. "A whole root may be eaten without inconvenience."[45] Third, members of all medical circles—from botanics to regulars—maintained a prejudice against Chinese practices that may have precluded a

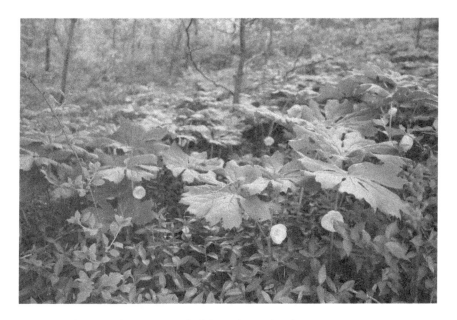

Mayapple (*Podophyllum peltatum*). (Photo by author.)

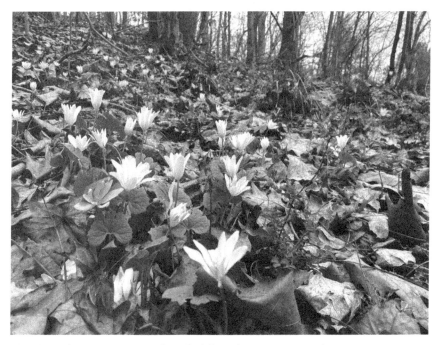

Bloodroot (*Sanguinaria canadensis*). (Photo by Tom Manget.)

thorough consideration of the Chinese panacea. In his *Vegetable Materia Medica* (1818), medical botanist William P. C. Barton sneered that "the numerous beneficial effects ascribed to it by the Chinese" were attributable "to the imagination of a people remarkable for their prejudices, civil, moral, and religious."[46] Gunn agreed: "These people are remarkable for their superstitious prejudices."[47] Thus, it appears that while nineteenth-century Americans could embrace the empirical medical wisdom of Native Americans, trusting Chinese wisdom was a step too far. Until the twentieth century, ginseng remained almost entirely an export product with little domestic use.

The Origins of Botanical Pharmaceutical Manufacturing

The popular rise of botanical medicines in the first half of the nineteenth century stimulated the emergence of manufacturing firms to supply ready-made tinctures, powders, ointments, syrups, extracts, salves, teas, and other botanical preparations to retail druggists and physicians. Prior to the 1840s, those few physicians who prescribed native plants obtained them directly from the fields and forests, although a limited trade in Seneca snakeroot, pinkroot, sarsaparilla, sassafras, and a few other plants did exist. By the 1840s, however, a network of wholesale and retail druggists and manufacturers had emerged to fulfill the demands of the growing number of botanic practitioners. Specifically, the rise of Eclecticism in the 1830s was a significant catalyst for the expansion of botanical pharmacy. Through the 1840s and 1850s, the botanical pharmaceutical industry expanded rapidly, creating opportunities for businessmen like Calvin J. Cowles to profit from the collection and supply of a wide variety of what those in the business increasingly called "crude vegetable drugs"—that is, raw, unprocessed medicinal plants.[48]

New Lebanon, New York, Cowles's destination in 1850, emerged as the center of botanical drug manufacturing due largely to the efforts of the United Society of Believers in Christ's Second Appearing, better known as Shakers. The Shakers had been believers in botanical medicine since they first began forming communities in the 1780s and 1790s. The Shakers established eleven communities across the northeastern and midwestern United States, each with its own physic garden to serve its own medical needs. By the early 1820s, the Shakers had all but aban-

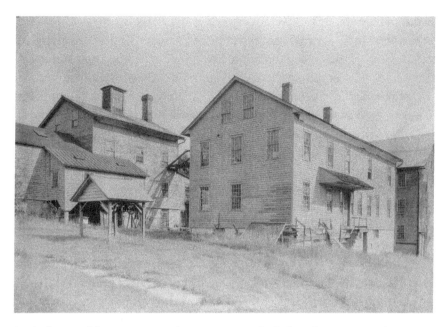

Herb shop and factory, New Lebanon, New York. (Edward Deming Andrews Shaker Collection, Winterthur Museum, Garden, and Archives, Winterthur, DE.)

doned their original sectarian aims of total self-sufficiency and complete withdrawal from "the world" and engaged in the wholesale botanical drug business, among other commercial endeavors.[49] Under the leadership of the medical botanist Garret K. Lawrence, the gardens at New Lebanon grew to become the most elaborate and comprehensive of the Shaker physic gardens. Around 1821, Lawrence began harvesting, processing, and distributing herbs throughout New York and New England.[50]

Within six years, Shaker communities at Harvard (Massachusetts), Union Village (Ohio), and Watervliet (New York), had also entered the trade. Dividing up territory, New Lebanon Shakers sold medicines to druggists and physicians across New York, from New Lebanon to New York City.[51] Harvard Shakers, with Elisha Myrick in charge of the herb department, sold medicines to druggists and physicians across Massachusetts, from Boston to Worcester to Lowell.[52] Most of their early products were fresh and dried herbs, roots, seeds, flowers, and other plant parts, but they also prepared a small assortment of oils and extracts. One of the more popular in the 1820s was Syrup of Liverwort, used to treat liver complaints, coughs, and respiratory ailments. The productivity of the Shakers' gardens, the quality of their products, and their botanical knowledge quickly gained a national reputation. Constantine Rafinesque visited the gardens at New Lebanon in 1827 and 1828, proclaiming them to be the "best medical gardens in the United States" in his *Medical Flora*.[53]

The Shakers had an unmistakable influence on another New Lebanon drugmaker, Tilden & Co. From its beginnings in the 1830s, this Shaker rival would grow to become one of the largest botanical concerns in the nation.[54] The early success of the Shakers convinced Elam Tilden and his sons Henry A. and Moses Y. to abandon their sheep-farming business and enter crude-drug production. In the 1840s, Tilden constructed an herb garden and invested in heavy machinery to manufacture medicines; by 1855, the firm produced twenty thousand pounds of extracts a year.[55] Tilden was the first to use a vacuum evaporator to produce extracts, which enabled the company to distill plants into concentrated form faster and without exposure to the atmosphere, resulting in an ostensibly purer extract. *The American Journal of Pharmacy* declared Tilden's laboratory "the source of the best medicinal extracts prepared in vacuo."[56]

The Shakers followed suit, invested in a vacuum evaporator, and began distributing concentrated remedies throughout the Northeast.[57] Shaker account books reveal that, despite their rivalry, the two firms regularly purchased herbs from each other through the 1850s, presumably to fill orders. This suggests that despite their commercial rivalry, cooperation was important to their survival and growth. They expanded together through cooperation to make New Lebanon a center for the production of botanical products in the Northeast.[58]

Aside from the Shakers and Tilden & Co., most entrepreneurs who entered the botanical drug-manufacturing business during this time were retail druggists. Typically located in midwestern cities such as Cincinnati and St. Louis, where the botanico-medical movement was strongest, druggists such as William S. Merrell, T. C. Thorpe, George M. Dixon, William J. M. Gordon, and F. D. Hill began branching out to become wholesale suppliers of crude drugs and botanical preparations. By the 1840s, botanic retailers in Boston, including William Johnson and B. O. and G. C. Wilson & Co., entered the wholesale business, and New York's Hosea Winchester, a former Shaker, began dispensing Thomsonian and Eclectic remedies from his store on John Street.[59] In addition to selling preparations to physicians, many botanic druggists entered the patent medicine business and sold directly to patients. B. O. and G. C. Wilson specialized in manufacturing patent medicines such as Wilson's Sarsaparilla, Wilson's Cherry Bitters, and Wilson's Dysentery Syrup. Lowell, Massachusetts's druggist, James C. Ayer, one of the most prolific patent medicine entrepreneurs, advertised his long list of medicines, including Ayer's Cherry Pectorals and Ayer's Vermifuge, in entire columns in the nation's major daily newspapers. Pittsburgh's B. A. Fahnestock began producing his own line of patent medicines, including Fahnestock's Vermifuge.[60]

The late 1840s saw some important developments in botanical pharmaceutical manufacturing, and indeed in the history of the pharmaceutical industry in general. Prior to this time, dispensing botanical medicines was not simple or easy. Despite the advancements in wholesale botanical drug preparation and distribution, most botanic practitioners, if they did not harvest the plants themselves, still ordered them in crude form—that is, in the form of herbs, leaves, roots, and other plant parts. Then they had to compound them for each patient from supplies in their saddlebags. Patients typically took large doses of syrups, teas, and other preparations that had a very disagreeable taste. Indeed, distributing and administering botanical medicine was more difficult than, say, pouring a teaspoonful of calomel. This began to change in the 1830s and 1840s when American druggists learned how to isolate the alkaloids—the so-called active ingredient—from some of the popular indigenous species favored by the Eclectics, following a process pioneered in the late eighteenth century by European pharmacists who discovered how to make quinine from the cinchona tree. This process enabled smaller doses of more concentrated medicines to be distributed and administered.[61] William S. Merrell, a chemist from New York who opened a drugstore in Cincinnati in 1828, made a breakthrough in the production of concentrated remedies in 1847. Merrell claimed to discover, based on instructions from Eclectic physician John King, how to isolate the alkaloid of mayapple, transforming it into a resinous material he called podophyllin. As a substitute for calomel, podophyllin quickly became an "indispensable and highly important Eclectic remedy." Dr. John Uri Lloyd, an influential Eclectic author and practitioner in Cincinnati, later called it "perhaps the most prominent of Eclectic drugs." Merrell's accomplishment brought hope to these physicians that they might be able to match the convenience and efficacy of regular physicians' pharmacopoeia.[62]

Merrell's successful marketing campaign prompted many drug firms to enter the business of manufacturing what they called "concentrated remedies," which included alkaloids, resins, resinoids, and oleoresins, for the Eclectic market. The Cincinnati firms T. C. Thorpe, H. H. Hill, and George Dixon entered the business in the early 1850s, and the industry quickly spread to the East Coast. The New York firms of B. Keith & Co., William Elmer's American College of Pharmacy, Hosea Winchester, and Tilden & Co. soon followed. In addition to podophyllin, drugmakers soon claimed that they had learned how to create alkaloids of culver root (Leptandrin), blue flag iris (Iridin), bloodroot (Sanguinarin), goldenseal (Hydrastin), black cohosh (Cimicifugin), and some two dozen other plants. Allopathic physicians and some Eclectics criticized many of these preparations by calling into question the manufacturing methods used to produce them, but there was no doubt that they were important advancements, not only in Eclectic pharmacy but for pharmacy in general. Initially specializing in Eclectic preparations, Merrell eventually began selling them to allopathic doctors as well. After the Civil War, William S. Merrell & Co. grew and expanded, and Merrell became a founding member of the National Wholesale Druggists' Association.[63]

The technological advancements made by the Shakers and Tilden & Co. and the manufacturing of podophyllin and other alkaloids served to substantially increase the demand for crude drugs. Although statistics that could illuminate the size of this industry are not available, Edward Fowler, the Shaker agent in charge of the New Lebanon herb business, estimated in 1852 that the quantity of manufactured plant medicines used in the United States had doubled over the previous decade.[64] The American Pharmaceutical Association noted in 1860 the "general increase on the Atlantic seaboard, as well as in the West, of the use of so-called Eclectic remedies; this practice among regular practitioners is an indication of greater liberality, and a disposition to avail themselves of all the resources at their command, while it has induced a greater number of pharmaceutists to prepare them as the demand rises."[65] The growing demand for crude drugs increasingly came from a handful of manufacturers, a development that had important implications for the merchants of Southern Appalachia. Prior to the 1840s, anyone who wanted to engage in the crude-drug business, as Cowles found out, was limited by distribution problems owing to geography. What manufacturing existed was performed on a relatively small scale by druggists around the country. It was simply not profitable to make dozens of different shipments, each consisting of a box or two of plants, to small-scale druggists and practitioners in various locations. The emergence of large-scale botanical drug firms with national and international ambitions created opportunities for businessmen like Cowles to specialize in extracting wagonloads of plants from America's fields and forests.

The first years in the trade were anything but smooth for Cowles. As his father warned, success meant that he had to navigate the notoriously difficult botanical drug markets. He had to know, often without a purchaser or a purchase price, how much to pay his storekeepers for a wide variety of plants so that he could realize a profit by reselling them. Anticipating the market prices for each plant required a working knowledge not only of the demand for the plant but also how much of the plant was currently on the market nationwide. He had to ensure that the roots were correctly gathered and dried and that they would reach their destination without getting wet or lost. In order to attract orders, he assumed the liability of shipment, and this frequently meant trouble. In the winter of 1849, for example, he shipped eighteen bales and five boxes of roots and herbs to a Boston drugmaker. When he finally heard from the company, representatives said that at least two bales had been damaged so badly en route that they were now worthless. Furthermore, they said, the quality of the roots in five other bales was so poor that they could not sell it and would therefore not buy it.[66] "The root business so far has made us so much trouble and no Money that our friends persuade us to quit it but we will stick another year at least," he wrote to one of his buyers in 1851.[67]

Poised to ride the wave of botanical reform, however, Calvin J. Cowles soon found ready buyers for his crude drugs across the Northeast and Midwest. Analysis of his account books reveal that from 1850 to 1860, he sold some 150,000 pounds of crude drugs favored by Eclectics to roughly thirty parties in the emerging botanical drug network. Indeed, he sold roots and herbs to them all. The most common plants, not surprisingly, were bloodroot (17,000 pounds), lobelia (13,000 pounds), lady's slipper (11,000 pounds), mayapple (8,000 pounds), and wild ginger (7,000 pounds). Over half of the roots and herbs Cowles sold in the

1850s went to two firms: the Shakers and Tilden & Co. Five different communities of Shakers purchased a total of 40,000 pounds of crude drugs from Cowles; New Lebanon (17,000 pounds) ordered the most. Henry Tilden also purchased 40,000 pounds. At least four of Cowles's buyers were patent medicine makers. Between 1851 and 1855, James C. Ayer and B. A. Fahnestock purchased more than 5,000 pounds of blood-root from Cowles to make their blood purifiers. Philadelphia's John R. Rowand, an MD who became the proprietor of a variety of patent medicines in the 1830s, purchased over 12,000 pounds of blackberry roots from Cowles over a two-year period to make his Syrup of Blackberry Root, which he advertised as an "inestimable remedy for bowel complaints." Cowles also sold crude drugs to wholesale botanic drug houses and emerging leaders in botanical drug manufacturing in the West and the East. William S. Merrell purchased some 11,000 pounds of twenty-two different species of plants over a two-year period. Jacob S. Merrill, who founded a wholesale botanical drug house in St. Louis in 1845, ordered 2,300 pounds of roots, barks, and herbs. The Boston firm of B. O. and G. C. Wilson and the New York firm of Coolidge, Adams, and Bond were two of Cowles's most consistent buyers.[68]

The Appalachian Pharmaceutical Landscape

While finding buyers for his crude drugs became easier for Cowles, obtaining the roots and herbs from the fields and forests of northwestern North Carolina was another challenge altogether. By the mid-1850s, Cowles had settled into a trading pattern that brought him a measure of success in this burgeoning new industry. He bartered with harvesters for some roots and herbs at his own store in Elkville, but the bulk of his supply came from country storekeepers to the west, on the Blue Ridge. Because he was located just out of the mountains, closer to turnpikes and railroads, he promised them cheap goods, procured from northern commission merchants, at low prices. By the late 1850s, he was purchasing roots and herbs from more than three dozen middlemen, mostly storekeepers. Responding to price lists posted at their local stores, mountain families on the Blue Ridge brought their harvests in sacks and bartered for a variety of goods, primarily fabric, coffee, powder, lead, and luxury items such as candy.

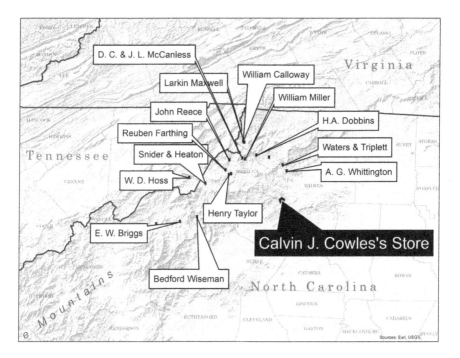

Location of Calvin Cowles's suppliers of roots and herbs, 1850–1857. (Map by author.)

Ginseng destined for the China market was consistently the most lucrative herb in the forest, earning anywhere from 25 to 60 cents per pound in the antebellum era. Other plants drew from 2 cents to 20 cents per pound, and their value varied from year to year.[69] Once or twice a year, each storekeeper took a wagonload of this produce down from the Blue Ridge to Cowles's store and exchanged it for boxes of goods. The storekeepers then took their goods back across the mountains to their stores to begin the bartering cycle again. Cowles, meanwhile, pressed his loads of roots and herbs from the Blue Ridge into three-hundred-pound bales and shipped them via wagon, railroad, and steamboat to his northern and midwestern buyers.[70]

Not only was Cowles tapping into growing demand by the pioneers in botanical drug manufacturing, but he was also helping to create a national market in crude drugs. It would not be too much of a stretch to say that Cowles—as one of the key suppliers of these medicinal plants—was instrumental in expanding the pharmaceutical industry in the

United States. An examination of the Shaker account books reveals that throughout the 1840s and 1850s, the Shaker herb businesses drew almost exclusively from their immediate environment to obtain their roots and herbs, either by growing them in their gardens or contracting with locals to harvest small amounts. Cowles was the outlier. Indeed, he was one of the first in the nation to supply these markets on a large, national scale, and he was able to do so because he was geographically positioned to take advantage of the wealth and variety of Appalachian flora. Due to the region's unique geology and ecological history, Southern Appalachia generally and northwestern North Carolina specifically contained some of the most botanically diverse temperate forests in the world. Appalachian biodiversity enabled Cowles to prosper.

By the time Cowles opened his store in Elkville, the diversity and abundance of plant life in the Southern Appalachians had already become legendary. The first wave of botanical explorers in the late eighteenth century, which included the likes of William Bartram, André and François Michaux, and John Fraser, had established the region as something of a botanical wonderland, containing a remarkably wide variety of flora.[71] Another wave, beginning in 1839, fixed the attention of American botanists on Western North Carolina, which would have significant implications for the development of the botanical drug industry there. In March, Asa Gray, recently appointed professor of botany at the new University of Michigan, was in Paris studying the herbarium of the late André Michaux. Gray, one of the emerging lights in American botany, was on a mission to examine the collections of American plants in foreign herbaria as part of his work on a comprehensive North American botany textbook when he noticed a peculiar specimen among a gathering of unidentified plants. The only clue to the flower's identity left by the Frenchman was a tag reading, "Hautes montagnes de Carolinie" (High mountains of Carolina). Intrigued, Gray christened the new genus Shortia after Dr. Charles Short of Transylvania University and wrote in his journal, "It is from that great unknown region, the high mountains of North Carolina."[72] Indeed, despite a few memorable journeys through the region in the late eighteenth century, much of this area remained unexplored by naturalists. But that began to change with another event in 1839 that renewed botanical interest in Appalachia.

While Gray was studying the Michaux herbarium, Moses Ashley Curtis, an amateur botanist from Hillsborough, North Carolina, set off on a four-month botanical expedition into the mountains. Curtis was an acquaintance of Elisha Mitchell, professor of geology at the University of North Carolina, and he had been to the mountains at least twice for short periods, so he was familiar with the region and aware that naturalists were only beginning to understand its rich flora and fauna. Disillusioned with his teaching job at a private school in Raleigh, Curtis hoped to make a name for himself in botanical circles. He explored the area around Grandfather Mountain and Black Mountain (now named Mount Mitchell after Elisha Mitchell) in July before moving on to the mountains farther west. Along the way, he identified several new species of plants and collected specimens previously catalogued by Michaux and others. Upon his return, he initiated a correspondence with Asa Gray and other botanists and helped generate renewed interest in Appalachian botany. Two years later, Gray, eager to find a living specimen of Shortia in the high mountains of Carolina, enlisted Curtis's help in planning his own botanical exploration.[73] "No living botanist . . . is so well acquainted with the vegetation of the southern Alleghany Mountains, or has explored those of North Carolina so extensively, as the Rev. Mr. M. A. Curtis," Gray later wrote.[74]

Following Curtis's advice and guidance, Gray, then professor of botany at Harvard College, explored the region around Grandfather Mountain in July 1841, just a few years before Cowles began purchasing medicinal plants there. Traveling south through the Great Valley amid flora he considered mostly "uninteresting," Gray finally made it to North Carolina; he "found a marked change in the vegetation on crossing the Blue Ridge." He was wholly impressed by the plant diversity around Grandfather Mountain. "The vegetation is essentially Canadian," he remarked, "with a considerable number of peculiar species intermixed."[75] In 1842, Gray's "Notes of a Botanical Excursion to North Carolina," published in the London Journal of Botany, enhanced the botanical reputation of the Southern Appalachians. Although he failed to find Shortia, he did succeed in identifying dozens of rare and undiscovered species that he included in his monumental Gray's Manual of Botany in 1851. Most important, Gray, who became the most significant figure in American botany in the nineteenth century, became a lifelong fan of the region's flora.[76] On the forested mountainsides of Appalachia, he later wrote, one can find "a greater variety of genera and species than any other temperate region, excepting Japan. And in their shade are the greatest variety and abundance of shrubs, and a good share of the most peculiar herbaceous genera."[77] Furthermore, he was the first to draw scientific attention to the East Asian–eastern North American floral disjunction discussed in chapter 1.[78]

Botanist Samuel B. Buckley, who had made a name for himself exploring the Peaks of Otter in Virginia in the late 1830s, traveled through the same region the year after Gray with Ferdinand Rugel, a German immigrant doctor.[79] Unable to procure guidance from Gray, Buckley turned to Curtis, who generously provided him with notes, maps, and contacts.[80] Buckley published his journal notes in the *Southern Agriculturist* and the *Cultivator* in 1845 and 1846. "The traveler cannot fail to be struck with the luxuriant appearance of the vegetation," he wrote.[81] Thus, the efforts of Curtis, Gray, and Buckley, among others, went far in publicizing the botanical richness of the Southern Appalachians. Anyone working in botany, including medical botanists, pharmacists, and physicians, would have been aware of the region's flora.[82]

The growing reputation of northwestern North Carolina as a botanical hotspot was certainly not lost on Calvin J. Cowles. Realizing that his location on the edge of the Blue Ridge Mountains gave him a leg up on the competition, he did not hesitate to sell potential customers on this fact. "We can get almost everything indigenous to the U. States," he told the medicine manufacturers B. O. and G. C. Wilson of Boston. "Our locality is in the Mountains midst a profusion of plants heretofore unexplored."[83] To the east around Elkville, he could find many of the plants native to the southern states, whereas only a few miles to the north and west in the high mountains, he could obtain species that grew in Canada. He once bragged to a potential London buyer, "We can get over one hundred sorts of Roots, Herbs, &c." from these woods.[84] He was not exaggerating—or not by much. Cowles's account books reveal that he dealt in some eighty-five different species of plants.[85]

Geography certainly made Cowles's entrance into the crude-drug industry possible, but he would not have been able to procure his supplies without the ethnobotanical knowledge of the region's inhabitants. Anthropologist Anthony Cavender has examined Appalachia as a "therapeutic landscape," a term he borrowed from cultural geographers to describe places that have "an enduring reputation for achieving physical, mental, and spiritual healing."[86] Indeed, Americans since the early nineteenth century have viewed Appalachia as a particularly salubrious region and have flocked to its cooler air, healing springs, and beautiful scenery to rejuvenate their health. However, the idea of a therapeutic landscape can also be used to examine how mountain residents themselves came to know the natural communities around them through a lens of health and wellness. Cowles was able to start selling "one hundred sorts" of roots and herbs because the people in the region already had a working relationship with those plants.

Like many rural Americans, the people of Southern Appalachia were firm believers in botanical remedies. In the antebellum era, as Cavender has found, the medical profession in the region was somewhat diverse ideologically, but most relied heavily on plant medicine. A survey conducted in 1850 revealed that of 201 practitioners in eastern Tennessee, 35 had graduated from a medical school and 42 had attended at least one course of medical lectures. Nearly half, 95, were self-taught doctors who learned medicine by reading medical books, most likely *Gunn's Domestic Medicine*. Furthermore, 25 were "botanics or steamers" (Thomsonians), and 2 were homeopaths.[87] According to Cavender, these physicians adhered to a "mishmash of humoral, miasmatic, and atmospheric theories of illness causation," and many of them practiced bloodletting, cupping, blistering, and other remnant therapies of the era of heroic medicine.[88] However, tinctures, ointments, teas and other preparations made from local flora formed the basis of most of their treatments.[89]

The health-care infrastructure was poorly developed in Southern Appalachia, and most rural residents rarely, if ever, saw a professional doctor, most of whom were clustered in the towns and cities in the region. "Nobody went to the doctor for anything except appendicitis or amputations," remembered Florence Cope Bush, who grew up in Western North Carolina around the turn of the twentieth century.[90] These people relied heavily on folk botanical knowledge, as well as domestic medical guides, to maintain their own health. "It is not a stretch to say that the two most widely read books in Southern Appalachia at one time were the Bible and *Gunn's Domestic Medicine*," Cavender writes.[91] Bush recalled in her memoir the great variety of plants her mother taught her how to use to treat

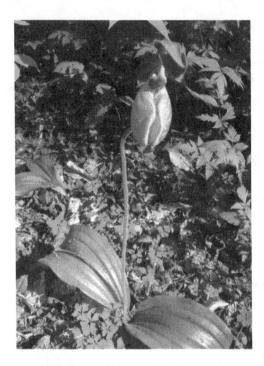

Pink lady's slipper (*Cypripe-dium acaule*). (Photo by Daniel Manget.)

common ailments: cockleburs for colds and coughs, sassafras for strengthening the blood, spignet for kidney ailments, and catnip and boneset for fretful babies and nervous disorders. "Everything we needed was all around us."[92] Cavender has identified a core of around fifty-eight commonly used plants in Appalachian folk medicine, while Judith Bolyard, who examined practices in eastern Kentucky, has identified around ninety.[93] It must be said that mountain residents did not rely exclusively on botanical remedies. Their therapeutics were a combination of herbal medicine, commercial medicines, including patent medicines, and other mineral- and animal-based medicines, but they maintained a special relationship with plants as a primary means of maintaining their health.

Like many Appalachian people, the Cowleses were firm believers in botanical medicine and often suspicious of regular doctors. When his son suffered from a fever in 1849, Calvin wrote to his father Josiah asking for advice. "Don't go to a Doct. with it," Josiah replied. "Get some Red Oak, make a strong paste or plaster from the inner bark and apply it."[94] A few months later, when Calvin's wife suffered from headaches, the elder Cowles approved of treating her with a homemade tincture of lady's slipper (*Cypripedium acaule*), a favorite prescription employed by Thomsonian physicians.[95]

When Cowles first branched out from ginseng and sought to find more stable markets for medicinal plants, the first plant he marketed was lobelia, the most revered herb in the Thomsonian arsenal. Throughout his copious correspondence with his buyers, Cowles demonstrated a perceptive knowledge of both botany and medicine. He read the American Journal of Pharmacy, and he did not hesitate to sell drug manufacturers on the medical virtues of certain plants. "Turkey pea has become a great medicine among the 'Eclectics,'" he told one potential buyer.[96] "Devils shoe string . . . is of great repute here in venereal diseases," he told another.[97] His experience with botanical medicine undoubtedly helped him navigate drug markets and, in some cases, expand them.

Euro-American settlers of the Southern Appalachians initially obtained some of this knowledge, either directly or indirectly, from the Cherokee. Cavender has found that rural residents drew heavily on Native American plant medicine, even while they rejected Indians' explanation of the causes of disease. When a group of Moravians arrived in the North Carolina backcountry from Pennsylvania in the 1750s, for example, they adopted ethnobotanical knowledge from local residents, who had learned it from the Indians. They referred to no fewer than fourteen different medicinal plants as a "snakeroot." According to one of the settlers, this was because "practically all plants which the Indians are known to use as medicine are called 'Snakeroot.'"[98] Early botanists traveling through the region often discovered plants they sought when locals recognized the description of a common medicinal, or even a plant they "disregarded."[99] Asa Gray discovered *Silene stellata,* for example, after locals showed him a specimen they called Thurman's snakeroot used by an "old Indian doctor" to treat snakebites.[100] When Cowles posted his advertisements offering to purchase these plants, he typically did not elaborate about where they could be found and what they looked like. He simply assumed that locals knew how to find them. And so they did.

Learning how to heal themselves with plants required mountain residents to develop a detailed knowledge of the various plant communities around them. Most knew how to recognize and find common plants like boneset, pennyroyal, sassafras, pokeweed, heal-all, and others that grew at the edges of nearby fields and along roadsides. Other plants,

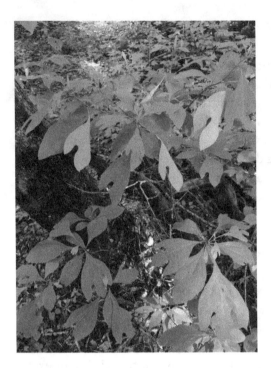

Sassafras (*Sassafras albidum*).
(Photo by author.)

however, grew deeper in the forest and could be gathered on demand only by those who knew the forest landscape well. While some plants, such as ginseng, blue cohosh, and Seneca snakeroot, grew in higher-elevation forests dominated by northern hardwoods, others, such as goldenseal, preferred lower-elevation forests. Blue flag preferred open, wetland areas, and pinkroot grew in the soil of low-elevation forests with a neutral pH, whereas wild ginger was found mostly in acidic soils in higher-elevation forests.[101] There were at least a few people in each Appalachian community with this kind of ecological knowledge, and they were more than likely women, as women were the primary conduits through which knowledge of medicinal plants passed down through generations, an appendage to their role as caregivers and healers.[102]

Cowles built his business not only on locals' knowledge of medicinal plants but also on the custom allowing such plants to be harvested from the wild on anyone's property. Like fish, game, and ginseng, they were considered the property of the harvester rather than the landowner.[103] The persistence of large swaths of unimproved land in the mountains helped preserve this custom from its frontier phase. In 1850—over half a century after initial settlement—unimproved acreage outnumbered improved acreage by a ratio of more than five to one in the area in which Cowles procured his roots and herbs, whereas in North Carolina as a whole, the ratio was nearly half that.[104] Cowles did not refer to the forests as a "commons,"—he preferred the term backwoods—but he realized that the concept was key to his extraction efforts. "We procure most of our Drugs from the woods," he told a London herb dealer, whereas "you raise yours in extensive gardens." He asserted that his methods enabled him to purchase a much wider variety of plants.[105] Without this custom, his business would not have met with the success it did.

This commons culture, combined with the floral diversity and abundance of the mountains, enabled Cowles's root business to provide drug manufacturers with a level of flexibility in their supply chain that they could not get from either northern forests or physic gardens. There were so many different types of wild plants readily available in large quantities that manufacturers could afford to take a risk on new trends in medical science without Cowles or any other suppliers having to invest land, labor, and capital in cultivation. Furthermore, manufacturers could place an order for certain plants that might never have been cultivated before without having to wait for cultivation methods to be perfected. Demand for many of these plants was so inconsistent that cultivation was largely impractical. Consumer demand for certain plants waxed and waned according to the popularity of the theories that supported their use. For example, American hellebore (*Veratrum viride*) was not used until the early 1850s when a South Carolina doctor demonstrated its effectiveness in treating pneumonia and typhus.[106] Shortly thereafter, Cowles sold seven thousand pounds of hellebore to manufacturers. In one year, 1856, Cowles purchased some sixteen thousand pounds of "staggerweed" (probably *Delphinium staphisagria*) because it held promise in treating venereal diseases, but in no other year did he buy any.[107] Thus, rather than serve as a hindrance, the commons was a key factor in enabling the commodification of many medicinal plants.

The emergence of Southern Appalachia as a significant supplier of medicinal plants to the growing transatlantic trade network was made possible by a combination of cultural, technological, and ecological forces. Changes in therapeutic practices stimulated mass demand for crude vegetable drugs. Better transportation and improved manufacturing technology provided the means of delivering them, and the Southern Appalachian commons supplied them. However, not all Appalachian residents had access to these markets in the 1850s. The botanical drug trade was yet in its infancy, not extensive throughout the region, and people living outside of Cowles's network might not have had the same opportunities to market the mountain commons as those inside it. While virtually all mountain residents could still find some ginseng and perhaps a little snakeroot and pinkroot to trade, their options were limited. The Civil War, however, would initiate widespread changes to the industry and bring these larger markets to more of the mountain region. By 1861, the Southern Appalachian region was only beginning to emerge as a significant supplier of crude drugs, but the events of the war and its aftermath would put the region on the pharmaceutical map.

4

Mountain Entrepreneurs

The Civil War and the Botanical
Drug Boom, 1861–1919

PERHAPS NO INDIVIDUAL OTHER THAN CALVIN COWLES HAD A GREATER
role in making Western North Carolina the center of the postwar herb
trade than Mordecai Hyams. Born into the Jewish community in Charleston, South Carolina, in 1819, Hyams developed an interest in botany,
perhaps influenced by the Charleston circle of botanists that included
Francis Peyre Porcher and Henry Ravenel, and began collecting plants in
his early twenties. He claimed to have studied at the University of South
Carolina, although no record exists of him there.[1] The outbreak of war
found him teaching school in Florida, and the forty-one-year-old enlisted
in the Confederate army as a private. Due to his botanical knowledge, he
was detailed to Charlotte, where he was employed by the Confederate
government to oversee the collection of roots and herbs under medical
purveyor Marion Howard. In this role, he assisted in the procurement of
crude botanical drugs from Cowles and others during the war. After the
Confederate defeat, Hyams moved to Wilkesboro, where he attempted to
continue in the root and herb business for two years, occasionally buying
and selling roots to Cowles to help him balance his books.[2] Wilkesboro
proved too remote, however, its transportation facilities too primitive,
so for the next five years, Hyams traveled through the region, collecting
herbs for several different companies in Piedmont towns, including M.
M. Teague of Marion (1867–1868) and Phifer and Turrentine of Statesville (1869–1870).[3]

Located near the western end of the Western North Carolina Railroad line, Statesville proved a better commercial location, and Hyams soon found an employer in the town with ambitions as grand and creative as his: brothers David and Isaac Wallace, Jewish dry goods merchants. In 1871, the Wallace Brothers firm constructed a two-story warehouse and hired Hyams to manage the root and herb branch of their business. Under Hyams's management, Wallace Brothers quickly became North Carolina's largest botanical drug wholesaler. By 1876, the company could boast of being the largest such concern in the world.[4] Hyams was so successful that when Detroit-based drug giant Parke, Davis & Co. opened an herb depot in Charlotte in 1888, it hired him away from Wallace Brothers to manage it. Within a year, he conducted $35,000 worth of business before the Wallaces purchased the entire stock of the depot, closed it, and brought Hyams back to Statesville.[5]

Hyams's story illustrates one way the Civil War spurred the development of crude-drug production in the South. Wartime necessity stimulated a surge in the popularity of botanical medicine—and specifically indigenous botanical medicine. Lacking a pharmaceutical industrial infrastructure and languishing under pressure from the Union naval blockade, southern physicians found ways to replace foreign imports like quinine with native southern plants. The Confederate government, led by Surgeon General Samuel P. Moore, implemented a program to develop the region's indigenous medicines. The effort met with mixed results and ultimately died with military defeat, but it did have important long-term impacts on the trade in crude botanicals. First, it introduced more southerners into the business of harvesting and processing medicinal plants, some of whom became leaders in the business following the war. Second, the United States' wartime policies facilitated the expansion of existing drug firms in the North and introduced new ones to the business. When the war ended, the pharmaceutical industry entered a period of rapid and sustained expansion that drove up demand for crude indigenous medicines nationwide, along with all kinds of other mass-produced medicines. As normal commercial relations resumed, southerners like Hyams drew on their wartime experiences to supply the burgeoning demand for crude drugs. Influenced by the model established by Calvin J. Cowles and attracted by the region's floral abundance, these entrepreneurs turned the Southern Appalachian region into the nation's most important supplier of crude botanical drugs.

Wartime Pharmacy in the North

As discussed in chapter 3, a network of wholesale and retail druggists and botanical manufacturers had emerged prior to the Civil War to supply physicians disposed to prescribe botanical remedies. Business grew as demand rose, and some antebellum firms became sizeable. Tilden & Co. employed around forty individuals, while the Shakers utilized the labor of dozens, if not hundreds, across their six herb-producing communities to produce their medicines.[6] However, despite the advances made by botanical drug manufacturing in the 1850s, the industry was still in its infancy. Most drugs consumed by patients were still compounded by either physicians or retail pharmacists, and most physicians were allopathic practitioners who relied heavily on mineral-based medicines. Indeed, in the years following the war, the botanical drug industry and the pharmaceutical industry in general would look much different.

The outbreak of war disrupted the supply of crude vegetable drugs from the South. The abrupt halt of medicinal plants flowing north made many pharmacists realize their growing dependence on the South generally and Appalachia specifically for medicinal plants. New York druggist John Maisch, a vice president of the American Pharmaceutical Association who became the chief chemist for the US Army drug laboratory in Philadelphia, reported to the American Pharmaceutical Association (APA) in 1864 that he could barely find many native medicinal plants, including American hellebore, bloodroot, and black cohosh, around Philadelphia. "In years gone by, senega [Seneca snakeroot], spigelia [pinkroot], serpentaria [Virginia snakeroot], ginseng and probably other drugs used to be collected in the East, but have become almost completely extinct there, so that we had been compelled to look to the South for a sufficient supply, and since this source has been shut off, [we must look] to the young and growing states of our great West," he told the Cincinnati convention.[7]

Yet, despite these concerns, most northern pharmacists did not suffer appreciably from the war's disruption. While Tilden & Co. and the Shakers were abruptly deprived of the roots and herbs they had obtained from Cowles, they adjusted their practices accordingly and continued to rely on the produce of their gardens for the manufacturing of extracts. Shaker account books at New Lebanon indicate that their wartime business not only did not suffer much from the war; by 1863, their business was producing more extracts than they had before the war and even received new orders from California and Chicago.[8] In general, although it deprived some of their southern supplies, the war had little effect on the ability of the North to produce botanical medicines. They simply utilized other sources located in friendlier territory.

The biggest change wrought by the war on northern drug manufacturing was in the area of mineral-based chemical drugs. As medical historian Michael Flannery has found, the needs of the army drove the expansion of chemical drug manufacturers. To subdue and conquer roughly 750,000 square miles of Confederate territory, the US government had to reckon with the logistics of supplying medicines and health care to a growing number of soldiers located increasingly farther from their home territory. Following the appointment of Jonathan Letterman as medical director of the Army of the Potomac in June 1862, a reliable three-tiered system of hospitals, consisting of field hospitals, post hospitals, and general hospitals, served the Union army for the duration of the war. In order to supply medicines to these hospitals, the surgeon general created a system of medical purveyors and medical storekeepers responsible for the distribution of drugs to the hospitals according to the official standard supply table of the US Army. (The system was initiated by Clement Finley and later reformed by his successor William A. Hammond.) This supply table mandated that field hospitals keep on hand some 80 medicines. Most were mineral-based chemicals; six were made from foreign plants; and only one (extract of Seneca snakeroot) was made from indigenous plants. General hospitals carried a few more indigenous remedies, 5 in total out of around 130 medicines.[9] The most commonly prescribed medicines among Union physicians included quinine, ipecac, ether, chloroform, calomel, and various opiates.[10]

Botanical medicine was almost entirely left out of the Union army's medical apparatus. The term *botanic* was met with derision among the Union medical community. Indeed, the army's allopathic physicians guarded the army from perceived threats of "quackery" posed by unorthodox physicians. Anyone attempting to substitute indigenous plant medicines for their cherished minerals was viewed as an irregular and fired. Surgeon General William Hammond himself fell victim to this tension when in May 1863 he issued the infamous Circular No. 6, which removed calomel and antimony from the supply table. Believing the move was a capitulation to botanical quackery, orthodox physicians viewed it as professional treason, and a chorus of criticism arose that ultimately led to his court-martial and dismissal in March 1864.[11] In such a professional atmosphere, indigenous plant medicines had little place in the Union army.

The desire for lucrative army contracts fueled the growth of private and public drug laboratories. According to Flannery, while many chemical drug firms derived material benefits from wartime demands, Rosengarten and Sons, Powers and Weightman, and Squibb were the firms that benefited the most from army contracts, especially the growing demand for quinine, an antimalarial drug derived from the South American cinchona tree.[12] Under Surgeon General Hammond, the army also got into the business of manufacturing drugs, establishing at least two large drug laboratories in Philadelphia and New York. In March 1863, the US Army took over a drug lab owned by Philadelphia drugmakers Powers and Weightman and appointed John M. Maisch to head it.[13] Such labs served as training grounds for several pharmacists who would grow to influence after the war.

In short, the Civil War gave pharmaceutical manufacturing in the North a shot in the arm, but botanical medicine did not benefit immediately.

Wartime Pharmacy in the South

In the South, however, the war had a more significant impact on botanical medicine, at least in the short term. Physicians, patients, and apothecaries found themselves cut off from northern pharmaceutical suppliers by official US policy and from foreign suppliers by the Union naval blockade. A few foreign drugs, patent medicines, and northern-made goods continued to trickle in throughout the war due to the efforts of blockade-runners and overland smugglers, and a thriving illicit trade developed for valuable drugs like quinine and morphine.[14] However, the majority of southerners were forced to turn to southern fields and forests for their remedies. One surgeon posted in a small-town hospital during the war recalled having virtually no access to commercial medicines. "I perused my dispensary and called into requisition an old botanic practice that had been handed down as a relic of the past," he told Atlanta druggist Joseph Jacobs in the 1890s. "I confess to have received valuable aid and very many useful hints in regard to the medical virtues of our native plants."[15] Jacobs interviewed several pharmacists and physicians who operated in the South during the war and reported to the American Pharmaceutical Association in 1898 that they had found ready substitutes for commercial medicines growing around them. Instead of digitalis, an imported plant-based drug that had (and still has) powerful cardiopulmonary effects, they prescribed bloodroot, wild cherry, and pipsissewa. In place of calomel, they used mayapple, dandelion, and butterfly weed. And instead of using quinine for intermittent fevers, they used tulip tree, dogwood, and willow bark, among others.[16]

Necessity also forced the Confederate government to find substitutes in botanical medicine which, as a result, occupied a more lofty position in the Confederate medical apparatus than it did in the Union. To supply the army's need for drugs, the Confederate government established a system of medical purveying depots. By November 1864, there were thirty-two such depots stretching from Richmond to San Antonio, including one in Charlotte under the direction of a Virginia surgeon, Marion Howard. Purveyors like Howard were charged with procuring and distributing crude drugs to army hospitals, where hospital stewards compounded the medicines for use on soldiers in the field.[17] They also obtained manufactured medicines from ten drug laboratories constructed around the South by the Confederate government beginning in January 1862.[18] Under the direction of A. Snowden Piggot, the drug laboratory in Lincolnton, North Carolina, manufactured tinctures, extracts, and other products made from indigenous plants, in addition to carbonate of soda, chloroform, rum, sulfuric acid, and various opiates.[19]

Early in the war, purveyors procured a variety of medicines from nearby druggists and blockade-runners, but as the blockade tightened and existing stocks were exhausted, Confederate surgeon general Samuel P. Moore took measures to promote indigenous remedies. In April 1862, Moore issued a circular to all medical officers, imploring them to investigate "indigenous medicinal substances of the vegetable kingdom." "It is the policy of all nations at all times, especially such as at present exists in our Confederacy," he wrote, "to make every effort to develop its internal resources and to diminish its tribute to foreigners by supplying its necessities from the production of its own soil."[20] In early 1863, facing the reality of life behind the blockade, Moore revised the army's standard supply table and printed a supplement listing ninety-two native and nat-uralized plants to be used "when the articles of the original Supply Tables cannot be procured from the Purveyors, or when they are deficient in quantity."[21]

Moore viewed the development of indigenous botanical medicines as a wartime necessity, but it also fit within his broader goals of national self-sufficiency, as was true of many other southern nationalists. He was no botanic sectarian. Although Moore did not see botanical medicine as inherently better than regular medicine, he nevertheless helped stimu-late a movement that brought the cause of the former into alliance with southern nationalism. At the same time he revised the standard supply table, Moore authorized Francis Peyre Porcher to write a guide to the medicinal uses of indigenous plants in the South. A Charleston medical botanist and graduate of the Medical College of South Carolina who had built a scholarly reputation in the 1850s for his microscopic study of dis-ease, Porcher was among those who believed the South should develop its own indigenous medicines. In 1847, he completed a detailed study of the medicinal plants and ferns in Berkeley County, South Carolina.[22] In August 1861, he penned an article for *De Bow's Review* in which he laid out 119 plants with medical value, urging southerners to learn them. "Much may be supplied by the Southern States if proper attention is directed to the subject," he wrote.[23]

Porcher was working as a field and hospital surgeon in the opening year of the war when Moore tapped him to write the book on southern resources. Working with amazing speed, he published *Resources of the Southern Fields and Forests* in late 1863. It was Porcher's magnum opus, a massive repository of botanical information that included four hundred known medicinal plants.[24] In addition to the knowledge he had gleaned from years of research and the work of other scholars, he relied heavily on the knowledge of Native Americans and of enslaved African Ameri-cans on his family's plantation in Berkeley County, South Carolina. In fact, according to historian Martia Goodson, as many as one-third of the plants he mentioned came from the slaves' materia medica.[25] No plant held more promise than bloodroot. "I employ no vegetable substance more constantly," he wrote. Yet Porcher was no sectarian either. He admitted that he employed very few vegetable medicines. "My endeavor is not so much to avoid a great multiplicity of agents, as to do no injury with any," he wrote. "The more full and accurate our knowledge, the more skillful is our application, whether the substance used be vegetable or mineral."[26]

Porcher's book met with critical acclaim and generated much discussion. In a letter to Porcher, Charlestonian Henry Ravenel, one of the South's most distinguished botanists, wrote: "The connection between practical Medicine and Botany opens a vast, very vast, and almost unexplored field, and your book lays the foundation for its study and application."[27] South Carolina's William Gilmore Simms, one of the South's most famous literary sons at the time, lauded Porcher's effort and envisioned the development of the South's botanical resources as a long-term goal. He encouraged southerners to turn to the "resources of the Southern fields and forests . . . not merely as expedients during the pressure of war and blockade, but continuously, through all time, as affording profit, use, interest and employment to our people."[28] Reflecting the religious nationalism of the early nineteenth century, Simms told the *Charleston Courier* that Porcher's book "takes rank with absolutely necessary histories of the country; and where they exhibit little else than the strifes, the struggles, the wars, and the miserable politics of society, this volume throws us back upon God; shows us what have been the blessings and bounties we owe to his hands; shows us where to turn for resource at the hour of need."[29] The book's popularity was initially hindered by limited distribution, so it was not widely read by the public during the war. Growing interest prompted Porcher to revise and republish the book in 1869, offering valuable information to many southern crude-drug suppliers that emerged after the war.[30]

By late 1863, the infrastructure was in place to provide a steady flow of crude botanical drugs through the Confederate medical apparatus, but obtaining those supplies was another challenge altogether. Orders were given to medical purveyors to appoint "from one to three trustworthy agents to go through the country in their districts, to collect and encourage the Country people to cultivate, collect, and prepare the indigenous plants needed."[31] Some enterprising men and women began cultivating valuable plants like poppies, but the vast majority of plants were only to be found growing wild. Beginning in the summer of 1862, purveyors published price lists for some sixty plants in newspapers, calling on loyal southerners to aid "The Cause" by harvesting them. The prices offered were much higher than they had been before the war, presumably due to wartime inflation. In some cases, the CSA offered three to four times what Cowles had paid prior to the war: whereas Cowles paid 6 cents per pound of bloodroot in the 1850s, for example, the Confederate government offered 40 cents. Similarly, it offered 75 cents per pound of mayapple and 25 cents per pound of wild ginger, whereas Cowles paid 6 and 12 cents, respectively.[32]

Because many of the records of the Confederate Medical Purveyor's Offices were burned along with the city of Richmond in 1865, it is virtually impossible to know where the bulk of the roots and herbs sold to purveyors were harvested. However, it appears that the Appalachian region emerged as an important supplier of the Confederate drug trade. Virtually all the plants requested by medical purveyors in North Carolina could be found in and around the mountains, and Porcher frequently identified "the mountains" as the heart of the range of many medicinal plants.[33] One Confederate botanist working in Western North Carolina during the war recalled that "the collections became rather larger than anticipated."[34] Indeed, the region clearly had a lot to offer the medical purveyors and the Confederate experiment.

As he had done with the Shakers and other buyers before the war, Calvin J. Cowles used his location near the Blue Ridge to solicit orders from Confederate medical purveyors. As early as December 1861, Cowles sent a list of his roots and herbs to Dr. James J. Waring, the medical purveyor attached to a depot in Goldsboro, North Carolina. "On the list, you may find some things that you can not get elsewhere, many equivalents of scarce and expensive medicines," he told Waring.[35] He included a catalogue of Shaker preparations and tried to sell him on the medical merits of other plants, notably Balm of Gilead buds, star root, beth root, and turkey pea.[36] Waring responded in February with an order for bloodroot, American hellebore root, lobelia, Virginia snakeroot, pipsissewa—and hopeful promises of further orders. "A large quantity of the above articles is desired not only to furnish my department but the army generally," he wrote.[37]

In July 1862, Cowles responded to a newspaper advertisement from Marion Howard, the medical purveyor in Charlotte, offering to sell him some fourteen thousand pounds of plants, including five thousand pounds of mayapple, two thousand pounds of bloodroot, and one thousand pounds each of wild ginger, wintergreen, and black snakeroot.[38] Without waiting for a reply, Cowles began shipping Howard packages of bloodroot, sassafras pith, turkey pea, Balm of Gilead buds, eight hundred pounds of bloodroot, and one thousand pounds of American hellebore, which, according to Porcher, "grows in mountain streams."[39] In the fall of 1862, Cowles sent two wagonloads of roots, including twelve hundred pounds of wild ginger, to Howard, informing him, "It was dug in the mountains and can not be got elsewhere."[40] Cowles's location at the foot of the Blue Ridge helped him cash in on the Confederate effort to develop the resources of the southern fields and forests.

For thirteen months, Cowles sold the Confederate government a steady supply of roots and herbs, but in March 1863, Moore himself informed Cowles that "more indigenous plants are not needed at present."[41] In the same letter, Moore conveyed news that Waring had resigned his post. Cowles lost touch with the Confederates and never sold them roots again. As postmaster general in Charlotte, Cowles remained busy in that city for most of the year but relaxed his involvement with the trade, becoming more interested in minerals.

Doing business with the Confederate government was not as lucrative for Cowles as the antebellum network he established. The orders coming from Waring and Howard were nowhere near as large as those he regularly filled for the Shakers and other northern manufacturers. Furthermore, Cowles's relationship with the Confederate government was one of continual frustration. Howard refused to pay for at least one shipment of bloodroot because it was wet and moldy, a claim Cowles denied.[42] Their correspondence details one misunderstanding after another over missing and mislabeled packages, discrepancies in weights, and tardy payments.[43] In January 1863, Cowles traveled to the purveying depot himself where, finding Howard away, convinced his assistant to let him examine the books, whereupon he discovered that Howard had simply crossed off a shipment of two hundred pounds of bloodroot received from Cowles. Howard agreed to pay what was owed, but that did not improve Cowles's opinion of him.[44] "Dr. Howard . . . seemed to be affected with a moral distemper worse than ignorance," he told one acquaintance in the business. "He cheated me out of two whole pkgs and about 20% of everything else sold him, and Dr. Waring of Goldsboro neglected to pay for about $50 worth of goods he got of me."[45]

Cowles was not the only person knowledgeable of the botanical drug trade who was highly critical of the Confederate purveyors. Moses A. Curtis, the Hillsborough, North Carolina, botanist who helped revive botanical interest in the Southern Appalachians, accused the department of "ignorance and charlatanry."[46] In letters to Cowles, he indicted purveyors for, among other things, advertising for plants that did not grow in the South and using common names unknown in the region. In an unsuccessful attempt to expose the purveyors' lack of knowledge in the trade, Curtis placed an anonymous advertisement in newspapers, offering to pay 50 cents per pound for all the bittersweet, or *Solanum dulcamara,* sent to him. He hoped to prove that bittersweet, a plant requested by the purveyors, did not grow in the South, but the joke was on him when Cowles shipped him a few hundred pounds of the herb. "I was taken not a little by surprise," he told Cowles. "I knew very well that the plant had never been found in the U. States by any botanist."[47] Cowles replied that he himself had introduced it to his father's garden in Hamptonville in the mid-1840s, and now it is "found trailing about the doors of Cabins on Beaver Creek."[48] He was so pleased with Curtis's attempt to "expose their ignorance," he charged Curtis only $10 for the plants.[49] Curtis also accused the Confederate government of setting prices for roots and herbs that reflected the medical value of the plants rather than the effort it took to find it, which did little to ensure that the variety of roots and herbs they needed would be collected. "It is evidence on their prices that these gentlemen did not understand the business they had undertaken, and that they would not be able to authenticate half the species on their list," he wrote.[50] While paying 75 cents for the relatively common mayapple, they paid 20 cents for skunk cabbage, a rare plant in North Carolina, and 50 cents for ginseng.[51]

In assessing the historical significance of the Confederate effort to develop the resources of southern fields and forests, it is important to be mindful of the yardstick we use to measure it. Historians have almost unanimously examined the Confederate effort from the perspective of medical progress and thus have little to say about its long-term impacts. Norman Franke, whose 1956 dissertation was the first scholarly examination of the subject, was critical of the Confederate pharmacy for failing to introduce any new indigenous plants into the materia medica.[52] Michael Flannery has been more conciliatory, referencing a "reasonable and concerted effort to deal with the harsh realities of providing a well-stocked supply table of reliable remedies."[53] It was a reasonable effort, albeit one plagued by inefficiencies and, in some cases, incompetence. Yet as Flannery briefly touches upon, perhaps the greatest long-term impact of the Confederate pharmaceutical program was that it raised the stature of botanical medicine in the South, which helped to sustain the growth of the crude vegetable drug trade following the war. Furthermore, the wartime effort introduced many southerners to the practice of gathering roots and herbs for the market and the business of selling them, and it provided a handbook, Porcher's *Resources of the Southern Fields and Forests,* to guide the new industry. When normal North-South trade relations resumed, many would draw on their experiences to make Appalachia the nation's most important supplier of indigenous medicinal plants.

The Post–Civil War Botanical Drug Boom

After the Civil War, changing demands and the stimulating effects of the Union army's medical apparatus brought dramatic expansion to the pharmaceutical industry. Rural physicians increasingly chose to purchase commercially made medicines rather than rely on locally gathered plants. In Appalachian communities, doctors jumped on the commercial bandwagon.[54] One merchant in Ashe County, North Carolina, reported in 1877 that he was developing a lively business with local physicians in commercial medicines. He was supplying six physicians in the county with "all the medicines and drugs they are making use of."[55] Specialized retail drugstores became more common fixtures in American towns, and they increasingly received their stock from wholesale drug houses for cash, rather than commission.

Many pharmacists who gained experience working with the Union army, such as Eli Lilly, E. R. Squibb, Frederick Stearns, John Wyeth, John Maisch, and others, went on to create successful drug manufacturing firms after the war, almost exclusively in northern and midwestern states. Many other chemists and drugmakers, most notably the Detroit-based firm Parke, Davis & Co., rushed into the business during the postwar years to capitalize on the growing markets for pharmaceutical products. Technological innovations during and after the war further enhanced the profitability of pharmaceutical manufacturing by, for example, improving the extraction process and the making of compressed and coated tablets. Following the war, pharmacists became more organized and made significant strides toward recognition as scientific-based professionals. Under pressure from trade groups, states began to regulate the industry, and wholesale druggists organized trade associations to better coordinate the activities of their members: first the Western Wholesale Druggists Association in 1876 and, less than a decade later, the National Wholesale Druggists' Association.[56] All of this occurred within two decades of the war's end; thus was the modern pharmaceutical industry born.[57]

The general thrust of this rapid postwar expansion was in the direction of chemically prepared, mineral-based drugs, but botanical preparations from indigenous plants played a role. In fact, the spirit of eclecticism and medical sectarianism continued to promote the use and manufacture of botanical medicines. As Edward Kremers and George Urdang noticed some sixty years ago, every successful drug firm that emerged out of the postwar period began by producing lines of vegetable tinctures, extracts, and other botanical preparations. Wholesale drug firms that specialized in botanical preparations emerged primarily in the Northeast and Midwest, including Wilson and Burns and Cheney, Myrick, and Hobbs of Boston. These joined other botanical specialists like Tilden & Co. and Coolidge, Adams, and Bond to supply physicians and drug stores.[58] The Shakers continued to sell their lines until at least the 1880s, when their herb businesses began to diminish due partly to increased competition and partly to the waning influence of Shakerism in general.[59]

Marketed directly to the consumer, patent medicines, many of which touted their indigenous vegetable origins, became a "veritable craze" following the war.[60] In 1859, the proprietary medicine industry manufactured roughly $3.5 million worth of medicines per year. By 1904, the annual manufactured value of proprietary medicines jumped to $74.5 million annually.[61] The number of different nostrums marketed nationwide rose from twenty-seven hundred in 1880 to some thirty-eight thousand by World War I.[62] Historian James Harvey Young attributes this surge partly to the restoration of the Union (or, more specifically, the reunification of northern patent drugmakers with their southern consumers), partly to the emergence of patent drugmakers in the South, and partly to the revolution in journalism and advertising that followed the war.[63] The ongoing transportation revolution, especially the expanded railroad network, also played a role, lowering transportation costs. Consumers demanded products like Pinkham's Vegetable Compound, Samaritan's Root and Herb Juices, and Dr. Bristol's Sarsaparilla.

Many of the companies that placed advertisements in newspapers appealed to consumers' therapeutic sentimentalisms. St. Louis–based Z. H. Zeilin & Co., the proprietors of Simmons Liver Regulator, assured customers that this "unrivalled Southern Remedy is warranted not to contain a single particle of MERCURY, or any injurious mineral substance, but is purely vegetable, containing those Southern Roots and Herbs, which an all-wise Providence has placed in countries where Liver Diseases most prevail."[64] The Swift Specific Company, an Atlanta drugmaker, attempted to sell its blood purifier by telling consumers that the ingredients came from "the mountains, from the forests, from the swamps," assuring them that "S.S.S. is made entirely of nature's gentle-acting, healing, purifying roots, herbs, and barks."[65] The sheer frequency with which patent medicine makers used these selling points suggests that the public's desire for natural indigenous remedies was greater than ever.

The southern mountains specifically were fast becoming a reliable source of crude vegetable drugs to pharmaceutical companies and patent medicine makers. Quantitative evidence that could shed light on the precise size and scope of the trade is surprisingly scarce, but anecdotal evidence is plentiful. Wendover Bedford, a New York pharmacist who drafted the committee report on the drug market for the American Pharmaceutical Association in 1874, found that "the trade in botanic articles appears to be increasing each year" and that "the East and North are fast giving way to the South as a source of supply to the wholesale trade."[66] He also noted that shipping practices had changed since the war. Whereas southern dealers had previously shipped their herbs in bags, they were now packing them into bales with the use of cotton presses. Louisville druggist Lewis Diehl told the APA at its annual meeting in 1870, "In many of the Southern States this branch of trade appears to attract considerable attention since the war, mainly in mountainous and swampy sections."[67] He noted that the mountainous region in eastern Kentucky supplied a large amount of medicinal plants to western druggists and cited brisk trades in East Tennessee and around the foothills town of

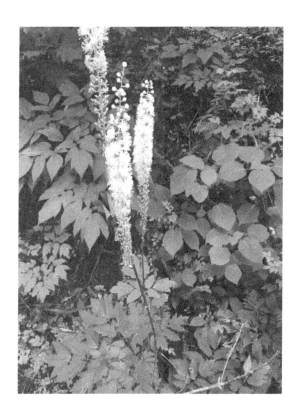

Black cohosh (*Actaea racemosa*). (Photo by Daniel Manget.)

Jack-in-the-pulpit (*Arisaema triphyllum*), also known as Indian turnip. (Photo by author.)

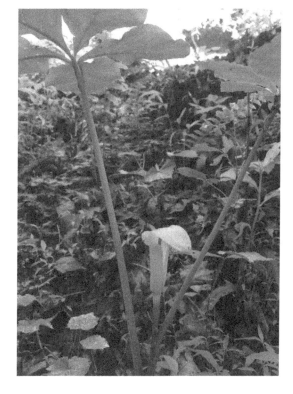

Walhalla, South Carolina. Diehl also took notice of a growing trend in the drug supply chain. Whereas the neighborhoods around Louisville once supplied druggists and wholesale dealers in the city with their crude vegetable drugs, the city now depended heavily on wholesale jobbers in the northeastern United States, many of which, as we will see, purchased supplies from Western North Carolina.[68] One North Carolina physician estimated in 1871 that four-fifths of the medicinal plants utilized by the large manufacturers came from the Piedmont and mountains of North Carolina.[69] That same year, one Boston newspaper claimed that the city's root and herb dealers had tripled their business over the previous three years. Three of these dealers purchased a combined $200,000 worth of crude drugs annually, most of which came from North Carolina and Tennessee.[70] Thus, it is clear that as the demand for crude vegetable drugs increased after the war and the national market expanded, eyes turned to the southern mountains.

And the mountains provided. In 1869, state geologist W. C. Kerr estimated that the gross income derived annually by harvesters from the root and herb trade in the mountains of North Carolina was $250,000.[71] And over the subsequent two decades, the medicinal herb trade grew and expanded to heights unparalleled before or since. *Branson's North Carolina Business Directory* from the years 1869 to 1890 lists medicinal herbs in the top five commercial staples of nearly every mountainous county.[72] The trade in roots and herbs became so important to economic life in some Western North Carolina communities that one member of the North Carolina Board of Agriculture reported in 1896 that "bales of these herbs may be seen collected about the country stores as bales of cotton are seen in the middle and eastern regions."[73] A look at the prominent merchants in the trade can give form and color to this otherwise opaque business and illuminate the influences of both Appalachian biodiversity and the Civil War in stimulating it.

Drug Dealing in Western North Carolina

Like many businesses in the South, Calvin Cowles's root and herb business suffered from the war. His stocks were exhausted, as he had made no attempt to replenish them with the cessation of orders from the Con-

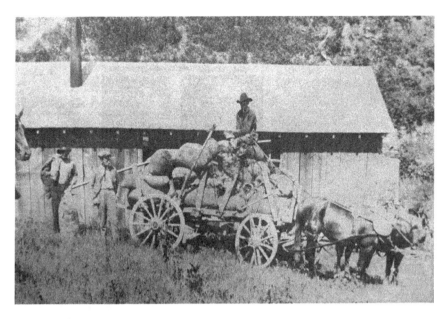

Men preparing a load of roots and herbs in a horse-drawn wagon in Western North Carolina, date unknown. (North Carolina Collection, Pack Square Library Special Collections, Asheville, NC. Reprinted in Ina Van Noppen and John Van Noppen, *Western North Carolina since the Civil War* [Boone, NC: Appalachian Consortium, 1973], 349.)

federate government, and he had little money to restart it. "Our business is torn up badly," he told B. Keith & Co. in 1865, "but still have vitality enough left to do a small business."[74] In the months following the Confederacy's collapse, Cowles reestablished contact with his northern buyers and offered them a diminished variety of roots and herbs, requesting that they advance him the money to pay for shipping. He instructed his son, Arthur, to travel to stores around Elkville and buy up all the roots and herbs he could find.[75] He also wrote to several acquaintances in the botanical drug trade, including Surgeon General Moore, asking to buy up what roots and herbs were left in the medical purveyor depots in Charlotte, Montgomery, and Columbia.[76] Whether Moore responded is unclear from the existing record. But by the fall of 1865, Cowles had cobbled together enough stock to send small shipments to familiar buyers— Tilden & Co., the New Lebanon Shakers, William S. Merrell, and B. O. and

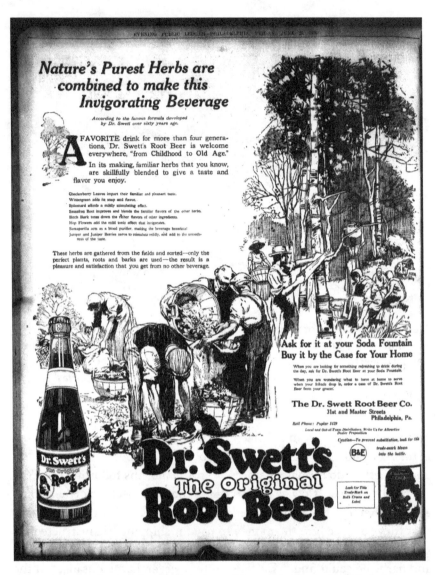

Advertisement for Dr. Swett's Root Beer. (*Evening Public Ledger* [Philadelphia], 23 June 1920.)

G. C. Wilson—as well as a few new customers, most notably George W. Swett, a Boston wholesale dealer in botanic medicines who began marketing Dr. Swett's Root Beer in the 1870s.[77]

Despite his partially successful reentry into the botanical drug trade, Cowles was gradually pulled in other directions. He endured a series of personal and political misfortunes after the war. His wife, Martha, died in April 1866 from a prolonged illness, and later that year, he was defeated by a single vote in an election for state senate that reeked of corruption. Although a slaveholder, Cowles was never in favor of secession, and during the war, he had become involved with the peace movement led by newspaper editor William W. Holden. During the 1866 election, he was painted by conservative governor Jonathan Worth as a staunch Unionist and was "very badly treated" in portions of the Forty-Fifth district.[78] Yet he became active in the state's Republican Party, led by Holden, and was elected a delegate to the state's 1868 constitutional convention, riding the wave that elected Holden governor that year. Holden appointed him president of the convention, and Cowles married his daughter, Ida Holden, later in July. Following the convention, Holden appointed him to head the US Branch Mint in Charlotte, and Cowles became increasingly involved in developing the mineral resources of Western North Carolina, which took him further away from the root business that had helped him become one of the state's political leaders.[79]

The Cowles root and herb dynasty did not die out immediately, however. For several more years, it continued to grow under the management of his son, Arthur D. As Calvin had done in 1846, Arthur moved west to Gap Creek to open his own store in partnership with his father. The store and herb warehouse he constructed in 1868 became the largest building in Ashe County.[80] Cowles sold a variety of about two hundred roots and herbs to many of the same buyers who had patronized his father, and he added a few more, including the large wholesale botanic druggists Garrison and Murray of Chicago, before the establishment was burned in the Chicago fire of 1871.[81] Yet by the time he opened his store, competition for the root and herb trade in northwestern North Carolina had already begun to accelerate.

Several firms jumped into the business following the war, all of which, according to one observer, "received their tuition and induction in

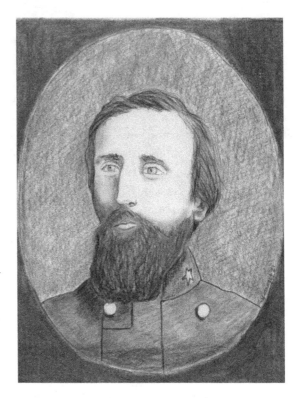

George Washington Finley Harper, ca. 1864. (Sketch by Natalie Manget, based on a photo in Walter Clark, *Histories of the Several Regiments and Battalions from North Carolina in the Great War, 1861–65* (Raleigh: E. M. Uzzell, 1901).

this trade directly or indirectly from Mr. Cowles."[82] Within a year of returning from fighting for the Confederacy, George Washington Finley Harper jumped with both feet into the trade. Born in 1835 to a prominent merchant in Lower Creek, Caldwell County, North Carolina, near the foothills town of Lenoir, Harper grew up tending his father's store. Although store ledgers do not indicate that he dealt in many roots or herbs prior to the war, he undoubtedly knew about the business carried on by Cowles, just thirty miles to the northeast.[83] In the spring of 1862, Harper joined the Fifty-Eighth North Carolina regiment and fought for the remainder of the war, receiving a wound in the battle of Resaca near Atlanta in the spring of 1864.[84] After his parole in May 1865, he returned to Lenoir, took charge of his father's store, and immediately expanded his dealings in roots and herbs. It is unclear why he decided to enter the root and herb business. In an area that struggled for economic traction, with little money stirring, he may have found it unavoidable. After all, the rural residents of northwest North Carolina had grown used to being able to trade them, and in order to compete with neighboring merchants for the barter trade, he had little choice. He and his father may have also been influenced by their wartime experiences with the Confederate medical purveyors.

Harper established a brisk root business over the ensuing years, following the same pattern as Cowles. Bartering for some roots and herbs at his store in Lenoir, he purchased most of his commodities from storekeepers across the Blue Ridge in the same territory as Arthur Cowles, including S. M. Silver in Yancey County; Henry Taylor in Valle Crucis, Watauga County; and Hugh Dobbins and Joel Norris in Ashe County. He maintained regular correspondence with these associates and even hunted and fished with them on occasion.[85] These storekeepers made regular trips to Harper's Lenoir store, where they exchanged their roots and herbs and other country produce for goods. Harper maintained itemized lists of daily barter transactions from the mid-1860s through the 1880s in his "produce books," which are scattered among two different collections at the University of North Carolina's Southern Historical Collection. They reveal that from 1868 to 1871, Harper sold some $28,000 worth of roots and herbs to many of the same wholesale drug firms in New York, Boston, Baltimore, and Cincinnati that purchased from Cowles.[86] Like Cowles, Harper regularly touted the botanical features of his native Appalachia. We can get "almost anything that grows from this climate to that of Canada," he told one buyer, "which is identical to Watauga, an adjoining county to us."[87] Harper's diary reveals that a few of these buyers made personal visits to his store. In 1869, he even went on a botanizing tour of Watauga County with Gardner S. Cheney, the Boston wholesaler who founded the firm Cheney, Myrick, and Hobbs.[88]

By the mid-1870s, Wallace Brothers of Statesville had emerged as one of the nation's largest wholesale botanical drug suppliers. Under the expert guidance of Mordecai Hyams, mentioned at the beginning of this chapter, the Wallaces began a widespread and systematic extraction of roots and herbs from the mountains of Western North Carolina. With a price list of roughly two hundred plants, the Wallaces sold 160,000 pounds of roots, herbs, barks, seeds, and flowers annually in the early 1870s, but Hyams and the Wallaces were poised for rapid expansion. In 1873, Hyams prepared an exhibit of indigenous medicines for the annual meeting of the APA, and attendees were duly impressed. The committee on specimens reported to the main body that they had "found more

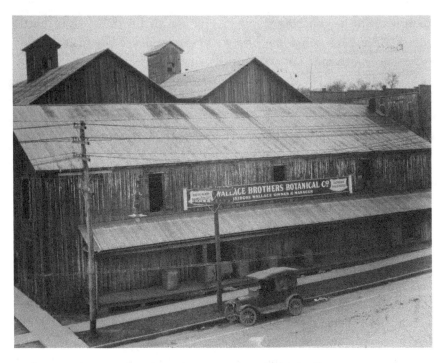

Wallace Brothers Botanical Company, ca. 1900-1910. (William Jasper Stimson and Benjamin Alston Photographic Collection [P0049], North Carolina Collection Photographic Archives, Louis Round Wilson Library, University of North Carolina at Chapel Hill.)

material for study in this extensive collection of herbs, roots, &c. than in any other portion of the room."[89] Three years later, Hyams prepared another exhibit for the Centennial Exhibition in Philadelphia, which won a bronze medal for its "extent, variety, and general perfection of the exhibit," and two years after that, another exhibit at the Paris Exposition won another medal. These exhibits brought international attention to the Statesville firm as well as to Western North Carolina in general.[90]

From the mid-1870s through the end of the 1880s, Wallace Brothers' herb business, selling primarily to patent medicine makers as well as wholesale druggists, grew by leaps and bounds. Business quickly doubled following the Philadelphia exhibition, and the Wallaces expanded sales to England, Germany, Austria, Prussia, and other European nations.[91] They abandoned their retail dry goods business to specialize in collecting and selling herbs and, in 1881, constructed a three-story, forty-four-thousand-square-foot warehouse. A glance at their books suggests why this was necessary. In 1879, for example, they received an order from Germany for ten tons of mayapple roots. Another buyer ordered an unlimited amount of liverwort and another ordered two tons of dried maidenhair ferns.[92] One observer in the early 1890s noted that in one month, the Wallaces sold fifty thousand pounds of mayapple, five thousand pounds of black cohosh, twelve thousand pounds of wild cherry bark, twelve thousand pounds of pennyroyal, eight thousand pounds of witch hazel, eight thousand pounds of yellow dock, and eight thousand pounds of unicorn root, among others.[93] These were voluminous shipments that dwarfed Cowles's and Harper's business combined. By the late 1880s, the Wallaces were dealing in roughly two thousand varieties of plants, selling 2 million pounds and collecting $100,000 (some $2.2 million today) annually.[94] They had become the most well-known wholesale root and herb dealers in the country. Raleigh physician Dr. William Simpson told the APA in 1894 that they were "the firm doing the largest business as herbalists in the world."[95]

Observers noted the Wallaces' location at the edge of the mountains as the reason for their voluminous business. In 1877, Hyams himself said that "the botanic resources of N. Carolina are more than all the other States combined in the extent and variety, and the medical products are inexhaustible."[96] Simpson noted that there were eighty-eight indigenous plants in the primary and secondary list of the official US *Pharmacopoeia,* and "all but one are found in North Carolina."[97] Some believed that the medicinal plants growing in the state were more efficacious than plants from other localities. In 1871, Lenoir physician Andrew Scroggs told the North Carolina Agricultural Society that drugmakers preferred the roots and herbs found in the state because "they possess an inherent intrinsic medicinal value beyond those coming from other sources."[98]

Like Cowles and Harper, the Wallaces contracted with country stores throughout the Blue Ridge, but whereas Cowles dealt with just two dozen or so country stores in four counties, the Wallaces purchased herbs from some four hundred stores in thirty counties.[99] Hyams estimated that the people gathering herbs for him numbered in the "many thousands."[100] One source claimed the number was around forty thousand.[101] Hyams frequently traveled the roads and turnpikes through the mountains and foothills, tromping through the woods looking for new and rare herbs. In the process, he played a key role in expanding botanical knowledge of the region. "Many of these medicinal plants were unknown as being indigenous," he explained to the North Carolina Agricultural Society, "and discovered by perseverance and industry, not enumerated in any botanic books of the present day."[102] Whereas Cowles was content to rely on rural residents' existing ethnobotanical knowledge, Hyams initiated an educational outreach campaign to instruct collectors how to find certain plants and the proper ways of harvesting and preparing them for the market. He also grew a test garden near his Statesville herbarium that served as a laboratory where collectors could come to learn more about herbal care and preservation.[103] Thus, one of the reasons Wallace Brothers was able to take the business to heights Cowles or Harper had never seen was Hyams's botanical training and educational outreach.

Hyams's familiarity with the mountain flora earned him national fame as a botanist. In 1887, he became the first botanist to discover *Darbya umbellata* (now *Nestronia umbellula*) since Moses A. Curtis found it growing in the 1840s, and he was the first to find *Iris florentina,* a species of white iris, growing in the United States.[104] In 1878, Hyams sent waves of excitement through the botanical world when news reached Professor Asa Gray of Harvard that Hyams, or rather his son, had discovered the holy grail of American botany, *Shortia galacifolia* (discussed in chapter 3), growing on a forested hillside near Marion in McDowell County. This was the plant that Gray had discovered in Michaux's Parisian herbarium but failed to find in the wild on two botanizing expeditions in North Carolina. In May 1878 Hyams, traveling with his son, Charles M. Hyams, a budding botanist in his own right, asked the younger man to climb a hillside and gather whatever was in flower. He returned with a peculiar plant that the elder Hyams had never seen. Indeed, no botanist had seen it since Andre Michaux in 1788. Hyams sent the specimen to a botanist friend in Rhode Island, Joseph Crogdon, who forwarded it to Gray, and the Harvard botanist was elated. This "has given me a hundred times the satisfaction that the election to the [French Academy of Sciences] did," he wrote to Crogdon.[105] Gray quickly contacted Hyams and arranged to meet him and his son in Statesville the following May, whence they would journey to the place of discovery to the west. When Gray saw the *Shortia* blooming amid a sea of galax plants, he felt like he had recovered "a long

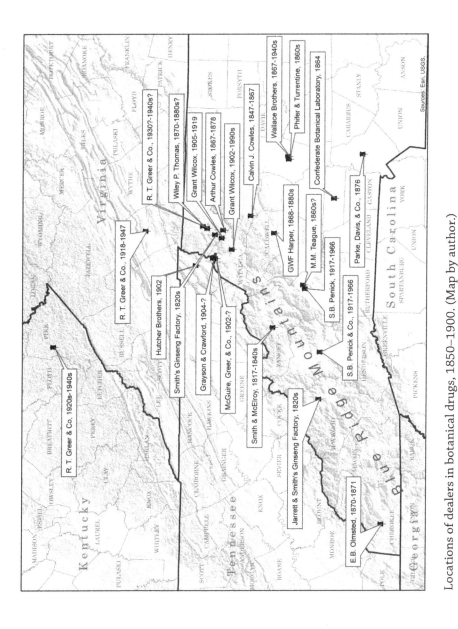

Locations of dealers in botanical drugs, 1850–1900. (Map by author.)

lost child."[106] Gray was also duly impressed by the botanical business carried out by the Wallaces. "A visit to the root and herb warehouse belonging to Wallace Brothers and under the charge of Mr. Hyams," he wrote, "furnished evidence that this branch of industry has reached an extent and importance of which few are aware."[107]

The Panic of 1893 proved devastating to Wallace Brothers, ushering in a significant shift in the business of Appalachian medicinal plants. The panic hurt many merchants in the business, forcing fellow Statesville herb dealer Louis Pinkus, for example, to sell his herbarium to the Wallaces in 1894. For a time, the Wallaces believed they could withstand the downturn, but margins had always been thin for them, and as they expanded, their debt load had increased to unsustainable levels. By 1895, they could no longer meet their short-term obligations to nervous New York creditors, and they filed for bankruptcy, generating widespread concern throughout the mountains. According to one newspaper, citizens "of all classes" in Statesville were "thrown into an unusual state of excitement" by the news.[108] The *Hickory Press* called the failure the "worst calamity that has befallen Western North Carolina. The effect of it permeates every nook and corner" of the region. "There is not a store in the country or at a crossroads in this section but what buys roots and herbs."[109] Pressure to revive the company mounted, and within a few months, David and Isaac Wallace had succeeded in garnering enough financial support from northern capitalists to form another company, the Wallace Brothers Company. After selling off land and buildings to satisfy creditors, the new firm purchased the remaining stock of roots and herbs and continued in a somewhat diminished capacity.[110]

The Wallace Brothers Company continued to purchase roots and herbs into the 1940s, but it would never again enjoy the near monopoly of the Western North Carolina trade it had in the 1880s. From the 1890s through World War I, a handful of other merchants who lived on the Blue Ridge and who had participated in the trade with the Wallaces emerged to fill the vacuum left by the bankruptcy and reorganization. Ashe and Watauga Counties became a hive of activity, as merchants jostled to take control of the botanical drug trade. George W. Greer, who grew up in Watauga County gathering roots and herbs for his family in the 1870s and selling them to Arthur Cowles and the Wallaces, formed a partnership with J. Q. McGuire, an Ashe County merchant. After the Wallaces' bankruptcy, Greer began traveling throughout the region buying up roots and herbs, helping to make West Jefferson a collection center for the new industry. In 1904, he branched out into Marion, Virginia, and the following year, to Pikeville, Kentucky, partnering with McGuire and Riley Thomas Greer to form the R. T. Greer Herb Company, which conducted a thriving business in these three locations until the 1950s.[111] Grant Wilcox also started a small root and herb business in Ashe County where, in 1905, he dealt in some 115,000 pounds of roots and herbs.[112]

Thus, the 1890s represented a changing of the guard in the botanical drug business. Not only did a new wave of Blue Ridge entrepreneurs take over the business from those in the Piedmont, the nature of the trade changed as well. As the automobile became a more common fixture in the mountains and as cash replaced barter in trade, country stores were no longer the only collection points for roots and herbs. Greer and Wilcox purchased their products directly from the harvesters for cash, often sending trucks through the countryside to procure them. Interestingly, the records of the Valle Crucis Company, which operated a store near the Mast General Store in Valle Crucis, Watauga County, from around 1909 through the 1940s, do not contain the slightest hint that they were engaged in the trade, despite the fact that the valley was a major supplier of roots and herbs beginning with Calvin Cowles in the 1850s.[113] This is likely because the valley's herb gatherers could now sell them directly to dealers for cash. Roots and herbs disappeared from the records of country stores. Although the size and volume of the trade had shrunk considerably since the 1880s, the crude-drug business continued to provide an economic boost to northwestern North Carolina.

World War I and the Revival of Botanical Medicine

Despite the efforts of Blue Ridge entrepreneurs, the botanical drug trade entered the twentieth century somewhat diminished from its heyday in the 1880s. The outbreak of World War I, however, helped stimulate a reawakening of sorts in the flora of Western North Carolina. As had happened during the American Revolution and the Civil War, the outbreak of war in 1914 disrupted drug markets and sent druggists and merchants searching for new sources of plants. Over the previous half century, London, Hamburg, and Trieste had emerged as centers of the trade, as drug

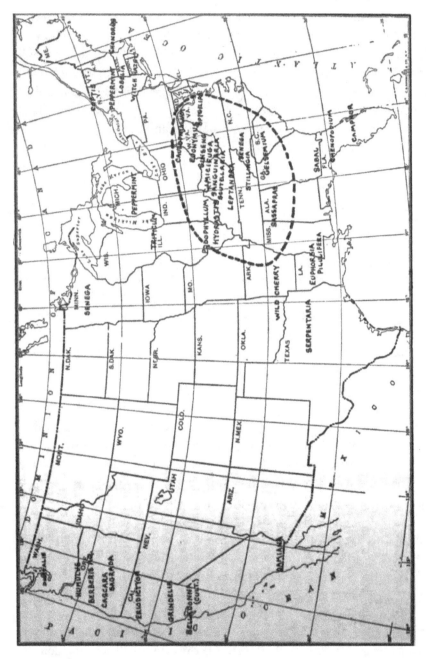

Map of drug-producing areas in the United States, 1919. ("Geography of U.S. Botanical Drugs," *Pharmaceutical Era,* March 1919, 63–66.)

houses there purchased many crude drugs from around eastern and western Europe and western Asia and sold them around the world, including in the United States. With these supply lines in question, demand for indigenous American plants that could be used as substitutes skyrocketed—and prices rose accordingly. "The European war and the scarcity of botanicals heretofore imported from abroad exerted a powerful effect upon the market for such drugs, and as a result all eyes were turned toward our native production," declared the *Pharmaceutical Era* in 1919.[114] As had happened in the Confederacy during the Civil War, nationalists called on country people to supply the nation's drug needs, and it was clear to all involved that Southern Appalachia would be an important supplier. Rising interest in what some called "pharmaceutical geography," or the study of the natural origins of medicines, brought greater appreciation for the southern mountains as the "chief source of American botanical drug supplies."[115] A 1919 map showing the "habitat of plants producing American crude drug supplies" distributed by the *Pharmaceutical Era* included a large circle around the Southern Appalachian region. Inside the circle, the author had handwritten the names of numerous medicinal plants, while the rest of the map was relatively blank.[116] A US Department of Agriculture survey estimated later that year that some three-quarters of the crude botanical drugs harvested in the United States came from inside this circle.[117] Instead of a giant blank spot, which typically characterized Appalachia's geographic position on maps, the region was the center of attention.

Watching these events unfold with avid interest, Sydnor Barksdale Penick was determined to profit from wartime demands. Penick's life story could have come straight from a Horatio Alger book. He was a twelve-year-old orphan in 1895 when he moved from his hometown of Culpepper, Virginia, and began working for Strother Drug Company, which sold patent medicines from its factory in Lynchburg, Virginia, as an errand boy. He proved a quick study and an ambitious businessman, and eight years later, the company chose him to open a wholesale branch in Bristol, Tennessee, where he sold patent medicines to nearby retail druggists. After two years in Bristol, however, stiff competition caused the branch to close, delivering a severe blow to Penick, who had recently married and had a child. But the young Virginian was resilient and resourceful, and around 1906, he decided to make a career change that would have significant implications for the botanical drug trade. While in Bristol, he had witnessed throngs of country people bringing in loads of roots and herbs to local stores and learned that these stores were, in turn, selling them to crude-drug firms across the mountains in North Carolina, probably Wilcox and Greer. Believing he would have more success in the crude-drug business, Penick left for New York to seek a job with the emerging wholesale drug firm of J. L. Hopkins & Co., and by 1912, he had risen through the ranks to become a trusted financial officer. But Penick wanted his own business.[118] In May 1914, just three months before Gavrilo Princip assassinated Austrian archduke Francis Ferdinand and precipitated World War I, he borrowed $8,000 from family to add to his own $5,000 in order to establish a crude-drug business in the small mountain town of Marion, North Carolina.

Rushing to take advantage of the rising prices of botanicals during the war, Penick distributed price lists widely across the region, from West Virginia to North Georgia, offering anywhere from 10 cents to 40 cents per pound for crude drugs such as dandelion root, pleurisy root, peppermint leaves, wild cherry bark, mayapple, Balm of Gilead buds, and burdock root. He implored "farmers and their helpers" to "put forth their utmost efforts as a patriotic duty and as a means of helping to win the war."[119] His supplies came from wherever he could procure them: from Watauga County, North Carolina, to India and South America. Some of the more sought-after plants he purchased, including digitalis, belladonna, and poppies, came from extensive gardens located around the United States, but those he purchased from the mountain South continued to come from their native habitat. His fleet of trucks and agents regularly toured the mountain roads purchasing roots, herbs, barks, flowers, and other crude drugs directly from harvesters who procured them from the forest commons. By the time the United States entered the war in 1917, Penick had constructed a large warehouse in Asheville and moved the headquarters of his business to New York.

World War I would ultimately launch Penick to worldwide success. By the 1930s, his company had grown to tremendous proportions, having branched out to deal in various chemical drugs, but the heart of his indigenous plant collection remained Southern Appalachia. By the 1940s, according to the *Saturday Evening Post*, Penick was purchasing roots and herbs from around thirty-five hundred families scattered around Southern Appalachia.[120] Claiming to be the "world's largest dealer in botanical drugs," his company owned an estimated $10 million in assets by 1947 and did roughly $20 million worth of business annually, selling crude drugs to some twenty-five thousand wholesale drug manufacturers around the world.[121] In 1929, Penick was elected president of the American Drug Manufacturers' Association.[122]

Penick's was not the only business to receive a boost from World War I. In 1919, Grant Wilcox moved his business from Ashe County to the growing and more well-connected town of Boone in Watauga County, where he would continue to operate until the 1980s.[123] R. T. Greer Herb Company also expanded during the war. Wartime prices brought great profits to Greer's two main branches in Pikeville, Kentucky, and Marion, Virginia. In 1918, the company constructed another herb warehouse in southern Ashe County, North Carolina, a propitious location following the arrival of the Virginia-Carolina Railroad and a timber boom around the town of Todd. The new warehouse was part of a thriving new village called Brownwood, built by a local landowner in the 1910s to take advantage of the timber boom.[124] The warehouse became the largest commercial concern in the community outside of the timber business. Buck Cooper, a longtime resident, later remembered that the lines of wagons that would line up in the summer to unload their roots and herbs stretched a half mile down the road.[125]

R. T. Greer Herb Company met with great success throughout the 1920s. Unlike Penick, Greer never branched out into other regions or other drugs, remaining exclusively focused on botanicals in Southern Appalachia. Between 1918 and 1922, one historian has estimated, R. T. Greer purchased some $600,000 worth of roots and herbs annually through all three of its branches.[126] Greer's business records indicate that the company grew throughout the 1920s, and by 1928, at the height of its influence, it was purchasing close to $1 million annually from harvesters across the Southern and Central Appalachians.[127] Greer frequently received roots and herbs via the US Postal Service from people across the South, but the bulk of his roots and herbs were procured at the warehouses, where individual harvesters as well as country storekeepers would bring their produce. The company's check register suggests that it purchased roots and herbs from at least six hundred different people in one month alone in 1928 (March).[128] The company baled these roots and herbs and sold them to some of the largest pharmaceutical companies in the United States, including Ely Lilly;

Parke, Davis & Co.; and McKesson, Robbins, and Rexall. It also sold to companies in Canada, China, Australia, and across Europe.[129] The strength of these companies ensured that root digging and herb gathering continued to be an important component of the economic and social life of mountain communities through the 1920s and '30s.

As was the case with so many other facets of American life, the Civil War was a watershed moment for the crude-drug industry in the Southern Appalachians. By stimulating the growth of large-scale pharmaceutical manufacturers in the North and introducing many southerners to the business, the war helped expand the market for a wide variety of medicinal plants. The trade reached the height of its influence in Western North Carolina from around 1870 through the 1890s under the dominance of Wallace Brothers. Available sources do not indicate that other subregions of Appalachia engaged in the trade in anywhere near the volume of Western North Carolina at this time. In 1894, for example, observing the great success of North Carolina merchants, the Tennessee commissioner of agriculture, T. F .P. Allison, lamented that the collection of crude botanicals in his state had been "entirely overlooked." He commissioned botanist August Gattinger, a resident of East Tennessee, to write a book on the medicinal plants of Tennessee, hoping that it would "prove of great commercial value to the State."[130] After the 1890s, due to the influence of Western North Carolina merchants, the trade accelerated throughout the rest of Southern Appalachia as collection centers opened in places like Bristol, Tennessee; Pikeville, Kentucky; and Marion, Virginia. Indeed, the business of collecting crude botanical drugs, with its modest origins in 1850s Elkville, reached unprecedented heights in the decades after the Civil War, leading to the rise of some of the largest botanical drug firms in the nation. With the collapse of Wallace Brothers in the 1890s, a wave of new entrepreneurs—veterans of the trade on the Blue Ridge—started several herb companies, some of which grew to rival the influence of the Wallaces due to the boost they received from World War I.

The effects this had on mountain communities were tremendous, as the trade turned a vast array of Appalachian medicinal plants into commodities. However, to understand these impacts and how local conditions continued to shape the commodification process, we must zoom in a little closer to the communities that helped extract them.

5 | Nature's Emporium
Root Diggers and Herb Gatherers in Post–Civil War Appalachia

AT FORTY-SEVEN, JOSIAH CLINE WAS TOO OLD TO FIGHT WHEN THE Civil War broke out. With a one-year-old son and a pregnant wife, Cline decided to try and ride the war out in the high mountains of Pocahontas County, West Virginia. He had two more children during the war. The 1870 census listed him as a farmer, but he owned no land and had just $20 in personal property. He traded ginseng for virtually everything he and his family needed to survive. From 1869 to 1874, Cline brought in a load of ginseng to Isaac McNeel's store in Mill Point almost every two weeks beginning in June, totaling nearly $300. With his ginseng, he purchased thirty-nine bushels of corn, 264 pounds of wheat flour, 612 pounds of bacon, and various amounts of butter, powder, shot, nails, and many other goods. Indeed, he was no farmer. He was a root digger.

Cline's experience was not uncommon among those who harvested roots and herbs during the unprecedented boom in the late nineteenth century. For every enterprising individual who decided to buy and sell roots to northern manufacturers, there were hundreds, if not thousands, of men, women, and children who harvested them from the fields and forests. Unfortunately, due to a lack of comprehensive sources that can help us re-create the entire scope and extent of the trade across the region, any historical investigation into the late nineteenth-century boom is necessarily limited. Therefore, we must adjust our analytical lens to the community level. This allows us to make better use of a limited set of sources and draw bigger conclusions related to the social and environmental contexts of the root and herb trade. It also enables us to observe

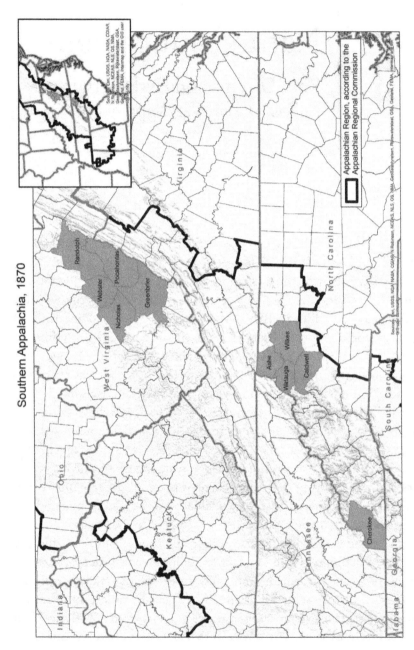

Southern Appalachia, 1870

Appalachian Region, according to the Appalachian Regional Commission

Clusters of communities under study in Southern Appalachia. (Map by author.)

the numerous interactions between and among humans and nonhuman communities that defined and regulated the commons. This chapter zooms into three clusters of communities within Southern and Central Appalachia: southwestern North Carolina around Cherokee County; northwestern North Carolina, including the counties of Watauga, Ashe, Yancey, and Caldwell; and southeastern West Virginia, including the counties of Pocahontas, Webster, Randolph, and Greenbrier. It does not claim that these communities are typical of the rest of Southern Appalachia. And it is not necessarily a comparative study. Each community produced different sets of sources, and so the same questions cannot be satisfactorily answered of all three. Rather, this is an attempt to create a collective portrait of roots, herbs, and people in late nineteenth-century Appalachia and shed valuable light on a rather understudied aspect of this pivotal era in Appalachian history.[1]

The Ginseng Trade in Southwestern North Carolina

In September 1870, E. B. Olmsted said good-bye to his wife and four sons in Washington, DC, and set off by rail, heading west into the Appalachian Mountains.[2] Like many of his fellow countrymen, the former disbursing agent for the US Post Office was chasing rumors of the vast riches that could be made dealing in ginseng, but he had more pressing reasons for venturing into the fastnesses of the southern mountains. He was in serious legal trouble. Three years earlier, Olmsted apparently spent some time in Cherokee County, where he obtained the deed to twenty-two thousand acres of land in a shady deal with the state of North Carolina.[3] After witnessing throngs of diggers selling roots to country merchants for relatively little money, he returned to Washington, DC, to attend to some unfinished business—which, it turns out, was also illegitimate. The following year, he absconded with $75,000 in postal employee earnings and disappeared into the West Virginia woods, leaving his family in Washington while federal officials searched for him. For over a month he wandered along the Chesapeake and Ohio Railroad, then under construction in West Virginia, where he undoubtedly came into further contact with people involved in the ginseng trade. After his arrest in Richmond in October 1868 for embezzlement, he turned over some of his lands to the federal government in exchange for his release from prison. His abysmal financial outlook and memories of ginseng being mined from the earth like gold prompted him to approach the New York wholesale drug firm Lanman and Kemp with a business proposal: front him $1,000, and he would be the firm's ginseng agent in Murphy, the Cherokee County seat.[4]

Despite objections from his wife and a thorough lack of experience in the southern ginseng trade, Olmsted was hopeful that he could purchase enough roots from diggers and country merchants to turn his ill fortunes around. And so he made his way on the Orange and Alexandria Railroad, past Manassas Junction and Appomattox Courthouse and across a landscape still scarred by four years of war. From Lynchburg, he traveled west across the Blue Ridge to Bristol, Tennessee, and down the western slope of the Great Smoky Mountains. In Cleveland, Tennessee, just north of the Georgia line, he bought a horse and continued his trek east over the Unaka Mountains, arriving in Murphy, the county seat of Cherokee County, North Carolina, eleven days after leaving Washington. There, despite the remoteness of the location, Olmsted would have found even more evidence of the destructive aftermath of the Civil War. Abandoned farms littered the countryside. Currency was almost nonexistent. Small communities survived by bartering what little they could produce. Indeed, the one market that offered hope for economic security was ginseng, and Olmsted knew it. "My neighbors would hail me a public benefactor," he wrote to his business partners, "for they hardly see any money at all since the war."[5] Olmsted's ginseng journey, preserved in correspondence to his partners, opens a rare window into the post–Civil War economy of southwestern North Carolina.

At first glance, it appears odd that Lanman and Kemp were interested in ginseng. With its history stretching back to 1808, the partnership emerged in 1858 when David T. Lanman, the inheritor of a large firm, joined with Irish immigrant George Kemp. By the 1860s, the company had become one of New York's leading wholesale drug suppliers, taking advantage of the mid-nineteenth-century shift in drug production and distribution. Lanman and Kemp supplied drugstores, primarily in the Northeast and Midwest, with stocks of medicines purchased from all over the world. It also distributed a few patent medicines, including a fragrant toilet water called Florida Water, around the Western Hemisphere. However, the firm did not specialize in botanic preparations and dealt in few indigenous plants. It was interested in the ginseng trade, it turns out, solely for the purpose of obtaining highly valued opium from China.[6]

The community into which Olmsted landed in the fall of 1870 was still reeling from the effects of the Civil War. Prior to the war, the economy of Cherokee County showed signs of tremendous development. Throughout the 1850s, its population increased 34 percent, the number of farms doubled, and its average farm value jumped 61 percent, from $844 to $1,400.[7] Moreover, the number of livestock, the region's other marketable commodity, skyrocketed. By 1859, the county produced 21,075 hogs, 5,702 cattle, and 9,270 sheep, making it the second-leading livestock producer in Western North Carolina.[8] However, depredations by irregular partisans from both sides of the conflict, depressed markets, and the general lack of law and order that existed during and after the war delivered a major setback to the economy. One of the hardest hit in Western North Carolina, the county lost some 40 percent of its improved farmland, over half of its livestock, and more than 10 percent of its population in the war-torn 1860s. Furthermore, the county lost an astonishing 65 percent of its total farm values.[9] The surrounding countryside experienced similar declines. In Western North Carolina and North Georgia between 1860 and 1870, the average farm lost 25 percent of the value of its livestock, including 45 percent of its hogs. Production of the other staple crop, corn, was cut by 40 percent.[10] Observing the effects of the war in Murphy during his famous thousand-mile walk to the Gulf of Mexico in 1867, the venerable wanderer John Muir remarked that it was "the most primitive country I have seen. . . . The remotest hidden parts of Wisconsin are far in advance of the mountain regions of Tennessee and North Carolina."[11] Their agricultural economy devastated, many Cherokee Countians turned to ginseng.

Indeed, Olmsted had stepped into a community whose economic life was very much defined by ginseng. Muir noticed its attraction to one of his hosts in the area, whose pantry contained only corn bread and bacon. "Coffee is the greatest luxury which these people knew," he wrote in his journal. "The only way of obtaining it was by selling skins, or, in particular, 'sang,' that is ginseng, which found a market in far-off China."[12] In an 1872 report, US commissioner of agriculture Frederick Watts reported that Cherokee County produced seventy-five thousand to eighty-five thousand pounds of ginseng that year, purchased from diggers for 25 to 27 cents per pound of green, unwashed roots.[13] Export data suggest that such a harvest would have comprised some 8 percent of the nation's total ginseng exports that year.[14] Such a harvest would likely have involved the participation of a substantial proportion of the farming households in the county.[15] In addition, locals made more money from ginseng that year—from $18,750 to $22,950—than they earned from farming and manufacturing wages, orchard products, garden products, and other forest products combined.[16] Indeed, ginseng was one of the few commodities that offered hope to the people of Cherokee County.

Observers in the region noted this growing dependence on roots in the years following the war. On a visit to Western North Carolina in 1867, a correspondent for the *New York Herald* reported on the "wretched class known as the 'poor whites' that abound in the mountains, and are met at the wayside at every turn."[17] He noted that many of them survived by digging ginseng. That same year, a correspondent for the *Raleigh Sentinel* reported that the trade in ginseng and other medicinal roots "carries comfort to many a mountain home of the poor and destitute, and is nearly their only means of raising money, these roots being nearly the only marketable thing they have."[18]

Olmsted was just one of thousands who sought to get rich off of ginseng in the South following the Civil War. From the 1860s through the 1880s, the same time frame that saw the expansion of the botanical drug industry, the Southern Appalachian region experienced arguably the largest ginseng boom in its history. In the three years that followed the war, the United States exported 1.4 million pounds of ginseng, a sum that nearly equaled the total exports of the 1850s. Exports continued to climb after the war, reaching their peak in the 1880s. From the beginnings of the trade through 1861, ginseng exports averaged 250,000 pounds per year, but from 1862 to 1890, the annual average jumped to nearly 400,000.[19] Although state-by-state ginseng production was not consistently documented until well into the twentieth century, it appears safe to say that the southern mountains, from West Virginia down to northern Georgia, formed the heart of the postwar ginseng boom.[20]

Although Olmsted understood the potential ginseng offered, profits proved more difficult to realize than he had thought. Indeed, he found his plans thwarted at virtually every step. On his way south, stopping in

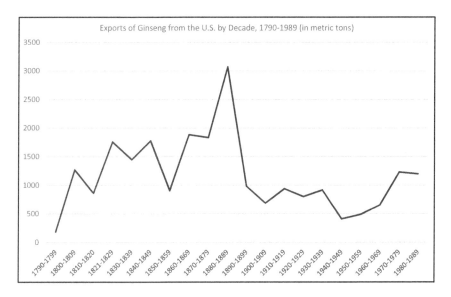

Ginseng exports from the United States, 1790–1989 (in metric tons). (Statistics compiled by author from annual communications on exports from the treasury secretary to the US Congress. Prior to 1817, these can be found in the American State Papers, Commerce and Navigation. After 1817, they can be found in the US Congressional Serial Set. These statistics are corroborated by Alvar Carlson, who also used statistics from the US Treasury Department's reports on foreign commerce and navigation. See Carlson, "Ginseng: America's Drug Connection to the Orient," *Economic Botany* 40, no. 2 [April-June 1986]; and Franklin A Hough, *Report upon Forestry, Prepared under the Direction of the Commissioner of Agriculture, in Pursuance of an Act of Congress Approved August 15, 1876,* vol. 2 [Washington, DC: Government Printing Office, 1880].)

Lynchburg, Virginia, and Bristol, Knoxville, and Cleveland, Tennessee, he consistently received the same daunting message: "There was no 'Sang' in the place."[21] When he finally arrived in the heart of ginseng country, he found Cherokee County crawling with agents representing firms from Atlanta, Philadelphia, Baltimore, and New York, and he was "greatly disappointed at finding so much competition."[22] He had hoped to purchase the dried root for 20 cents per pound at country stores, but he quickly found that this was impossible. Some of the larger dealers, specifically three brothers named Smith, offered 60 cents per pound of green root, and Olmsted soon realized that it would be "useless to think of getting it cheaper for cash."[23] While some stores continued to deal in ginseng, an increasing amount bypassed the stores altogether. He learned that agents who purchased the root for the large firms lived among the diggers the entire year, cultivating relationships that translated into unwritten contractual obligations on the part of the digger to sell to that agent for an agreed-upon price. "The whole country has changed within three years," Olmsted lamented. "The diggers have ascertained the value of roots and do not dig at old prices."[24]

While Olmsted did not appreciate the new competition, diggers certainly benefited from it. Not only did their root fetch higher prices, they no longer had to dry it themselves—"they refuse to go through the trouble"—because they could easily unload it green.[25] Olmsted found that other dealers had constructed clarifying establishments, or "factories," as an earlier generation called them, to process the roots (see chapter 2 for more on clarifying). The Smiths had some twenty of them scattered from Qualla Town to Franklin, Ft. Hembree, and Valley Town. These establishments, located on watercourses where the ginseng could more easily be washed and steamed, were primitively constructed of waddle and daub and featured stone furnaces. One of the Smith brothers told Olmsted that he had shipped some fifty thousand pounds of clarified roots the previous year. Realizing he would need to emulate this procedure if he hoped to succeed, Olmsted asked Lanman and Kemp for $100 to construct one of these establishments, but it never materialized.[26]

It is clear that because they were "the only people who come in contact with the living plant," astute diggers were able to use their skill at finding ginseng to manipulate the trade for their own benefit.[27] Most important, they could obtain high prices for the roots at the expense of merchants and overeager dealers like Olmsted, who were reliant upon the diggers not only for the actual supply of ginseng but also for any knowledge about the supply. Because he had no idea of the precise state of ginseng availability, Olmsted was forced to accept whatever the diggers told him. "My diggers are well at work but say the root is so hard to find they can't make wages at 20¢ for green 'sang.'"[28] A successful ginseng dealer told Olmsted that he had given up focusing attention on market prices, instead just paying "enough to induce the diggers to work."[29] Thus ginseng diggers, in some cases, could dictate the terms of their own labor.

Olmsted's foray into Cherokee County reveals the changing racial dynamics of the area's ginseng commons. Cherokee people had been digging and selling ginseng from the forests of Cherokee County since at least the construction of William Holland Thomas's Murphy store in the early 1830s (discussed in chapter 2), and evidence suggests that those who resisted removal efforts continued to do so after the Civil War. According to the 1870 census, there were nearly five hundred Cherokee still living in Cherokee County, while more than twice that number resided on lands purchased by Thomas in nearby Jackson County.[30] Many of these Cherokee, according to James Mooney, the ethnographer who lived among them in the 1890s, depended heavily on "ginseng and other medicinal plants gathered in the mountains" to procure what supplies they needed from nearby traders.[31] The difference between the 1830s ginseng commons and that of 1870 is that more whites were engaged in the trade. Store records from thirty years earlier suggest that the Cherokee were the primary harvesters of ginseng and other roots (see chapter 2). However, when Olmsted arrived to inspect the twenty-two thousand acres to which he still claimed title in 1870, he was surprised to find "Indians and white men" digging all over it.[32] In 1890, a resident of Graham County, which had been carved out of Cherokee County in 1872 and included a Cherokee community, reported to the North Carolina Department of Labor that "this part of the country is very badly behind in farming. Not one-fifth of our county is settled, and not many men in this county understand farming. Their delight is fishing, hunting bear, deer, and other game for meat and furs, etc., and digging ginseng root."[33] Ginseng now dominated the economic life of many, both Cherokee and white.

Finding himself an outsider looking in, Olmsted formed a partnership with a local man, John Williams, who knew "almost every old digger and the country people whom he can get to dig" ginseng.[34] A successful merchant and trader in Murphy before the war, Williams had been "robbed by rebel scouts" and lost everything during the war. After fleeing to Cincinnati, he returned after the surrender and used ginseng to recoup some of his losses. Within five years, he had "3 houses, stables, slaughter houses, and a vacant lot; stock and goods to the value of $2,500 and is free from debt."[35] Williams and Olmsted took turns riding a circuit from Hiawassee to Blairsville, Georgia, up through Murphy, and over into western Chero-

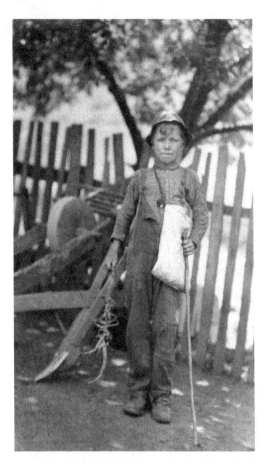

Boy with a large ginseng root. (Image No. 418, Claude Matlack Collection, 1982.01, Photographic Archives, University of Louisville, Louisville, KY.)

kee County, to purchase roots directly from the diggers. This proved difficult, however. "The diggers live so far apart and in such rough mountains, and besides get so little each that it is slow work," Olmsted told his partners.[36] An average day's work yielded only two pounds per day.[37]

By the end of the season in November, Olmsted had cobbled together enough dried and clarified ginseng, purchased from diggers and from other dealers, to send a wagonload over the mountains back to New York. But the season's business did not meet expectations. "You will be sadly disappointed in the quantity I get this year," a dejected Olmsted wrote to Lanman and Kemp. He confided that "in many respects my entire ignorance [concerning the traffic in ginseng] was such that no sane man, were he aware of that ignorance, would understand to engage in it on his own account, nor employ one so little informed to engage in it."[38]

In the fall of 1870, Olmsted had stepped into a market dominated by diggers and a community increasingly oriented around harvesting ginseng.
He was wholly unprepared for such an immersion. He had traveled south
to take advantage of the depressed southern economy, only to discover
that it was he who was on the raw end of the deal.

The fate of E. B. Olmsted, who does not appear in any censuses of
Cherokee County, is unknown, but his expedition into the mountains
reveals some important insights into the post–Civil War ginseng commons. In some communities devastated by the war, the ginseng trade
took on a whole new level of importance—both to the diggers themselves and to the merchants who sought to trade in it. For merchants, it
offered a readily available avenue to stability, as Chinese demand for the
root did not wane in the years after the war. Even with the increased supply from the southern mountains, the price paid by exporters continued
to climb, from $0.56 per pound in 1860 to $1.20 in 1865 and reaching
$2.03 in 1883. For diggers, ginseng offered a degree of economic empow-
erment in an otherwise powerless time. One astonished writer for the
New York Herald noted in 1867 that successful North Carolina diggers
could make as much as $3 a day: "They only make two [dollars] at the gold
mines near Morganton; so it is better than gold digging, in North Carolina at least."[39] It was the commons custom that enabled this trade to
reach such large proportions. In areas like Cherokee County, with a sizeable amount of undeveloped land and a pattern of absentee ownership,
those who lived far from settlements were able to access large tracts of
forests—including those owned by Olmsted—to find their roots without
worrying about crossing property lines. In 1860, although all of it was
privately owned, less than 10 percent of the land in Cherokee County was
improved, leaving roughly nine hundred square miles of unimproved forests with the potential for ginseng exploration.[40] And as Olmsted's story
illustrates, diggers had considerable control over the terms of their own
labor. Olmsted could not even compel diggers who harvested ginseng
from his own lands to sell to him.

Gender and Herb Gathering in Northwestern North Carolina

In much of Appalachia in the 1860s and 1870s, ginseng was one of the
very few marketable plants available from the forest commons. The com-

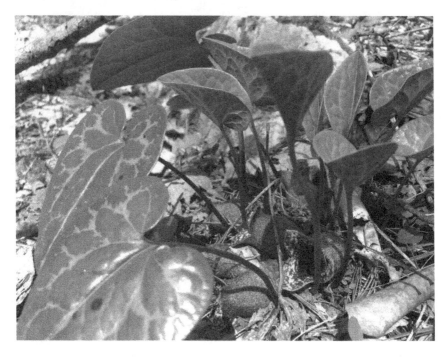

Wild ginger, or heartleaf ginger (*Hexastylis virginica*). (Photo by author.)

mercial reach of the botanical drug houses in the Piedmont did not extend to the far southwestern portion of North Carolina, and few other merchants purchased roots other than ginseng. Olmsted, noting that "Pink Root, Lady Slippers, May Apple, Spikenard, and Sarsparilla are abundant here, also bloodroot and snakeroots," inquired into the possibility of purchasing them but, receiving no instructions from Lanman and Kemp, did not buy them.[41] In northwestern North Carolina, however, due to the concentration there of botanical drug entrepreneurs and unparalleled biodiversity, commons users benefited from an expanded gathering commons. Ironweed, jewelweed, carrion flower, Carolina allspice, morning glory, skullcap, and even privet leaves could now be made to pay.[42] The marketability of so many new plants, combined with depressed markets, a lack of currency, and the lingering effects of the Civil War on the livestock industry, brought increased reliance on the Blue Ridge commons for market exchange.

Indeed, the forests of northwestern North Carolina became a great

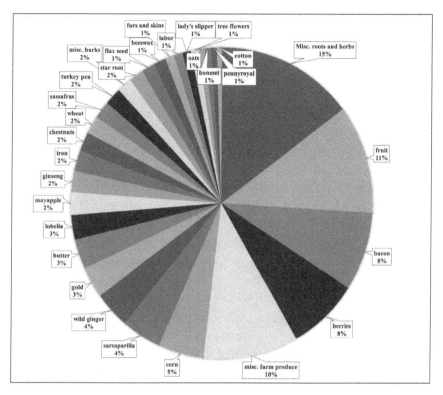

Items bartered at G. W. F. Harper's store, Lenoir, North Carolina, 1872–1875 (by value in dollars). (Chart by author.)

emporium where hundreds of different varieties of plants could be found and readily exchanged for store-bought goods made in the large factories of industrializing America. A statistical analysis of Lenoir merchant George W. F. Harper's store records from 1866 to 1875 confirms that roots and herbs were indeed "the life of Western North Carolina," as the *Raleigh Sentinel* proclaimed.[43] They comprised 45 percent of the total value of the barter business conducted by Harper. Customers made more money selling medicinal roots, leaves, seeds, barks, and flowers than by trading fruit, butter, wheat, corn, bacon, or berries *combined*. Harper purchased some three dozen different species of medicinal plants, and ginseng barely cracked the top five in terms of overall value. The most important were, in order of total revenue generated: American sarsaparilla, wild ginger, lobelia, mayapple, ginseng, sassafras, turkey pea, and star root.[44] Indeed, Harper's records confirm that the commons users in northwestern North Carolina had significantly more opportunities to find valuable plants than in many other parts of Appalachia.

The commodification of so many different plants disrupted accepted gender roles, creating new opportunities for women to participate in the marketplace and ultimately turning more men into gatherers. But this shift did not come quickly. Cultural expectations of gender roles had long influenced the way men and women used the forest commons. Women gathered edible and medicinal plants; men hunted and fished. These expectations had deep roots in both Western and non-Western cultures: indigenous peoples from New England to the Southeast and Euro-American communities alike had long adhered to a gendered division of the commons. Root digging and herb gathering was a natural extension of the woman's role as the family's primary caregiver and healer.[45]

Due to the gendered stigma associated with it, rural men did not take pride in root digging and herb gathering because it did not conform to their masculine ideals. Men prided themselves on their hunting abilities, on the number of bears or panthers they had killed, on the quality of their hunting dogs. They saw themselves as hunters and woodsmen, and herb gathering had little to do with their notions of masculinity.[46] During the Civil War, commentators championed it as a task for women and children to contribute to the war effort. The *Carolina Watchman,* for example, called specifically on women and children to "make money for themselves and render a great public benefit by collecting these plants."[47] Surgeon General Moore even issued a circular instructing the medical purveyors to assist the "ladies throughout the South" in the cultivation of garden poppies and the collection of other herbs.[48] This stigma continued after the war. The *Southern Cultivator* insisted in 1888 that gathering herbs was "work for women and children."[49] Indeed, herb gathering was never promoted as a task for men.

Ginseng, however, was an exception, and the fact that many men readily dug ginseng suggests that more subtle forces were at work shaping the gendered commons. Because ginseng was seen as a commodity that brought cash and was therefore not the same activity as gathering medicinal herbs for use at home, digging it became more acceptable as a masculine use of the commons. Indeed, gendered expectations often dictated the verbiage used to describe the activity. Men did not "gather" or even "dig" ginseng; they almost always "hunted" it. Puncturing these conventions enough to convince men to harvest lobelia leaves or mayap-ple root proved to be more difficult. These gendered expectations of com-mons use persisted into the twentieth century, even as the botanical drug trade accelerated. Referring to root digging and herb gathering in the early twentieth century, one dealer commented, "The men, in gen-eral, consider such occupations beneath them, and, ostensibly, trade only heavy and bulky products, such as barks of the larger trees, and bring in the other products with an apologetic 'Here's some yarbs the women got.'"[50] However, as medicinal plants gained a market value, some men overcame their initial reservations and began to gather other roots and herbs on a regular basis. The sociologist James Lane Allen relayed the story of one eastern Kentucky community during a season in the 1880s when the corn crop failed. The local storekeeper advised the people to gather mayapple. "At first only the women and children went to work, the men holding back with ridicule. By-and-by they also took part, and that year some fifteen tons were gathered."[51] The necessities of survival often hastened this cultural shift, but the underlying forces of commodifica-tion were ultimately responsible.

Women, in the meantime, found root digging and herb gathering empowering, even if it was circumscribed by custom. As an acceptable way to generate revenue independent of their husbands, the task helped some women support their families and others live independently of them. Michael Flannery has found that gathering herbs for use in the army was one of the ways Confederate women, whose public role was limited by southern custom, could actively participate in the war effort.[52] In her 1892 memoir, *How It Was: Four Years among the Rebels,* Nashville resident Julia Morgan recalled a journey she made in the late spring of 1862 into the mountains of East Tennessee. Persuading some local women to accompany her on jaunts collecting wildflowers in the moun-tains, she learned that many of them made up for the loss of men to the war by digging calamus, ginseng, angelica, and other roots and herbs, in addition to gathering huckleberries, blackberries, and dewberries.[53] Joseph Jacobs, a successful Atlanta pharmacist who is best known for his early role in promoting Coca-Cola, recalled in a speech to the American Pharmaceutical Association, "The grandmothers of those days revived the traditions of Colonial times."[54] These remarkable women "learned from experience that barks were best gathered while the sap was running, and when gathered the outer and rougher portion should be shaved off and the bark cut thinly and put in a good position in the shade to dry; that the roots ought to be gathered after the leaves are dead in the fall, or better, before the sap rises; that seeds and flowers must be gathered only when fully ripe, and put in a nice dry place, and that medicinal plants to be secured in the greatest perfection should be obtained when in bloom and carefully dried in the shade."[55] While such practices served to reinforce the boundaries of the feminine and masculine commons, they also reveal the opportunity that many women found in the emerging botanical drug trade.

After the guns fell silent, women in northwestern North Carolina drew on their wartime experiences to engage the depressed postwar economy. Lenoir, North Carolina, merchant George W. F. Harper's store records provide perhaps the best glimpse—albeit a somewhat hazy glimpse—of the gendered division of the commons. Because convention dictated that men were in charge of commercial transactions, most store ledgers typically listed only men's names, regardless of who dug or traded the plants. If a woman was married, her account was typically considered part of her husband's. Harper's barter daybooks, however, included women's names. Despite conventional gendered accounting methods, fully one-third of the transactions recorded in Harper's barter books were conducted by women, as indicated either by a female identifier ("Mrs." or "Miss") or an obviously female name. Yet female customers comprised well over half of those transactions conducted solely with roots and herbs. Women were statistically more likely to trade these commons commodities, men more likely to trade private commodities.[56] The store ledger from the Taylor and Moore Store in Valle Crucis, Watauga County, tells a similar story. In the early 1870s, just over half of the customers who traded in roots and herbs were women. Those women sold roughly 45 percent of the roots and herbs purchased by Henry Taylor, the store's co-owner.[57] The actual volume of roots and herbs harvested by women was likely much higher than Taylor's and Harper's books suggest, as male customers still often traded roots dug by their wives or daughters.

Many widows, including war widows, depended on the gathering commons to maintain a level of subsistence in the absence of their husbands. From 1872 to 1874, Wiley P. Thomas, who owned a store in Jefferson in Ashe County, sold at least eight thousand pounds of roots and herbs, worth somewhere between $1,500 and $3,000, to Arthur Cowles or, occasionally, directly to northern buyers. His ledger reveals that less than 15 percent of his customers traded in commons commodities. Most of those customers used roots and herbs to supplement their farm production, trading a few dollars' worth alongside their bacon and buckwheat. However, there were nearly two dozen customers who used roots and herbs to cover their entire purchase, and several of them were women.[58] Three of Wiley Thomas's customers were identified as widows, and they all relied exclusively on roots and herbs for their purchases. Mary Gardinett, for example, sold a bag full of roots every two or three weeks for a period of eight months, with which she purchased coffee, domestic cotton fabric, spectacles, and shoes, among other goods.[59] Farther south in Haywood County, Mary C. Cathey, who lost her husband during the Peninsula Campaign in 1862, sold a load of ginseng, averaging around $2, every month in 1870 and 1871.[60] As a source of income, roots and herbs were much more easily obtained than raising a farm surplus, and it helped widows—a larger segment of the population in the post–Civil War years—acquire purchasing power.

Two stories that circulated in northwestern North Carolina in the late nineteenth century provide further insight into how women used roots and herbs to secure financial independence from men. Sometime in the 1830s, Watauga County native Betsy Calloway married a recent arrival from Kentucky, James Aldridge, who quickly developed a reputation for being a great "marksman, trapper, and backwoodsman," identities associated with the traditional masculine commons. For close to fifteen years, he lived with his family (the couple had seven children) in a small cabin under the Grandfather on Hanging Rock Ridge. Then a woman arrived from Kentucky, claiming to be Aldridge's real wife, and that revelation destroyed his relationship with Calloway. She took to digging ginseng and other roots to gain financial independence from Aldridge. She became known as a "master sanger," often digging ginseng with her youngest child strapped to her back; she also worked several sugar orchards across the mountains and sold maple sugar for 10 cents a pound and maple syrup for 10 cents a gallon. Aldridge eventually left her, but with the proceeds of ginseng and maple products, Calloway purchased clothes and other necessities, kept a comfortable house, and,

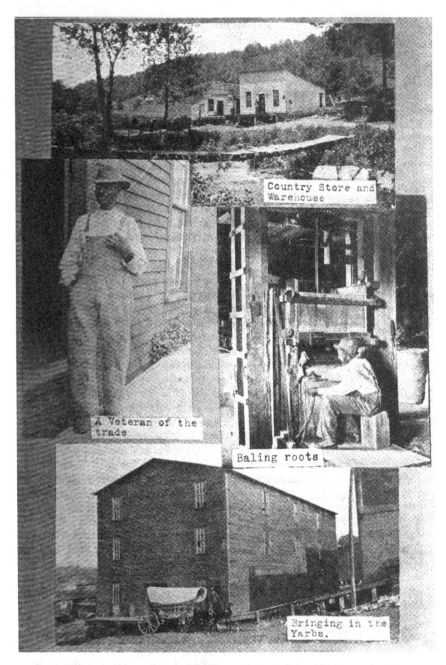

(*Above and opposite*) Snapshots from the Blue Ridge. (Claire Ewing and Elwood Stanford, "Botanicals of the Blue Ridge," *American Druggist and Pharmaceutical Record,* June 1919, 30–31.)

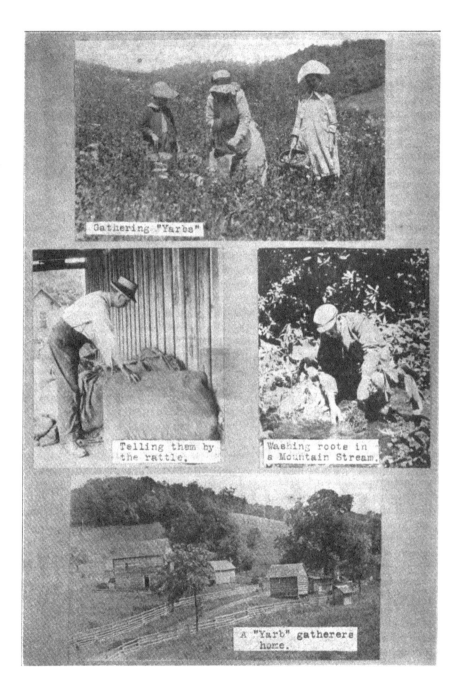

Gathering "Yarbs"

Telling them by the rattle.

Washing roots in a Mountain Stream.

A "Yarb" gatherers home.

according to the memory of the old-timers, "took care of all preachers who came to her home."[61]

In an unfortunate twist of fate, Betsy's sister Fanny also had seven children by her husband, John Holtsclaw, before he eloped with Delilah Baird. Baird, from Valle Crucis, was aware that Holtsclaw was a married man, but he promised her that they would move to Kentucky and away from his past. However, after deceiving her into thinking they had traveled across the mountains, he settled into a crudely built cabin at the base of Beech Mountain not far away from Baird's family. Holtsclaw kept his mistress secluded while he hunted and roamed, but she took to digging "great quantities" of ginseng, which brought her over the surrounding mountains. Eventually realizing her actual location, she reestablished contact with her family. Instead of leaving Holtsclaw, Baird continued to sell ginseng and maple sugar, eventually making enough money to purchase Holtsclaw's 480 acres along the Elk River for $250.[62] Indeed, many women like Calloway and Baird used roots and herbs as well as maple products to interact with the commercial economy to obtain a certain degree of economic freedom.

This story of northwestern North Carolina brings into focus a dynamic of the root and herb trade that had long been obscured from the historian's view: the forces of gender shaped the ongoing process of the commodification of roots and herbs. Notions of masculinity and femininity in the mountains created expectations that men would dominate animals and women would tend to plants. However, as plants gained a market value far above their use value, and as survival increasingly depended on finding other sources of income, those expectations began to break down. Ginseng was the first to follow this process; others would follow.

Class and Ginseng in Southeastern West Virginia

One sunny December day during the otherwise harsh winter of 1861–1862, a mysterious old man appeared out of the woods near Fayetteville, West Virginia, riding an ox into a camp of Union troops under General William Rosecrans. The man appeared to be a "veritable Rip Van Winkle," with long hair, a long beard, and homespun clothing that had been reduced to rags. He had somehow evaded the pickets and was now guiding his ox down the muddy road, hawking his forest products in an

English-African dialect that no one could quite understand. Captain H. R. Brinkerhoff immediately identified him as a ginseng digger but suspected he was a Confederate spy disguised by "elaborate makeup." Because no one stopped him or questioned him, he "leisurely" disappeared out of sight and into historical obscurity.[63] During the Civil War, there were numerous encounters like this between sang diggers and Union and Confederate soldiers in the forests of West Virginia.

As it did elsewhere in Appalachia, ginseng proved a critical source of income allowing West Virginians of various loyalties to obtain store-bought necessities as the effects of the war rolled across the Southern Highlands. Some were able to use ginseng to remain aloof from wartime hostilities, at least for a time. Penn Kirk remembered that as a boy in the Shenandoah Valley he escaped the cannon blasts to dig ginseng in the mountains with his brother. "We had this interest in woods life, and loved it enough to follow it so ardently there was no mortal could tell," he recalled. "But hither we would hie, spend long days out of sight of the rest of the world as it were, and listen only to the sounds that echoed in the tree tops from time to time."[64] In the fall of 1861, Confederate partisans arrested John O'Brien and his son Miles on suspicion of disloyalty. Upon questioning the two, Confederate interrogators found that O'Brien had been born in Harrison County, later moving with his family to Kanawha County and then up the Elk River to Webster, where he "lives remote from settlements in the woods, and makes his living by hunting and digging ginseng."[65] Concluding that he was "ignorant of all things going on in the settlements," but showed a "great respect for the old Commonwealth," his captors discharged O'Brien and his son after they swore loyalty oaths.[66] In the fall of 1862, partisans calling themselves the Caskie Rangers arrested and imprisoned fifty-one-year-old Isaac Scarborough for suspected disloyalty. Scarborough was on his way to Kanawha, a Union stronghold, to sell a load of ginseng when the Caskie Rangers stole his horse and his ginseng and apprehended him.[67] Statistics indicating how many people like O'Brien and Scarborough roamed the forests of southeastern West Virginia during this time are nonexistent, but it appears safe to say that there were dozens if not hundreds of people in each community who came to rely heavily on ginseng during the war.

Webster County—due to its abundant fish, game, and ginseng—became something of a haven for people seeking to escape wartime hostilities and economic devastation. Formed in 1859, Webster had the lowest population density in the state, a mere three persons per square mile, and ginseng fueled the county's economy for years. At the time of the county's formation, the county court set the price of a pound of ginseng as equivalent to one pound of coffee or one deer or wolf pelt and ordered that taxes and judgments could be paid in ginseng, cash, pelts, or coffee.[68] For the first five years of the county's existence, because of the outbreak of war, it lacked organized government, earning it the appellation "The Independent State." While the county voted overwhelmingly to remain in the Union during the secession votes of April 1861, its inhabitants were more interested in maintaining their autonomy. Thus, when the Union army invaded the area in late 1861, they engaged in partisan resistance against it. Although sources are extremely scarce, it appears that some people went to the area because it offered the freedom of life in the woods and a haven from war and economic ruin. Indeed, Webster County, according to one observer, was a "hunter's paradise, as deer, bear, and all kinds of game were abundant, and every family could, if they desired, have venison for breakfast by simply going out in their yard or 'patch' and shooting such game as they wished."[69]

It ultimately proved impossible to avoid the war in southeastern West Virginia, as Webster, Pocahontas, and surrounding counties were hit hard by the conflict. The area experienced fighting by both guerrillas and regular armies, including in the battles of Cheat Mountain, Greenbrier River, and Camp Allegheny in the late summer and fall of 1861. It remained under Confederate control until the fall of 1863, when the Union army, under the command of John Echols, defeated a Confederate force under William W. Averell at the battle of Droop Mountain in the Greenbrier Valley.[70] The agricultural economy was devastated. During the war-torn 1860s, the average farm value in Pocahontas County was cut in half.[71] One voyager through neighboring Webster County recalled traveling fourteen miles through the mountains "without coming to a house; although prior to the war many excellent farms were cultivated along the route."[72]

After the war, with its economic effects still lingering, the forests would be filled with many more people like the O'Briens who turned to the woods to preserve their rural worlds in the face of dislocation and economic catastrophe. Before the Civil War, Preston Grant was an overseer on a tobacco plantation in Rockbridge County, Virginia, and lived in

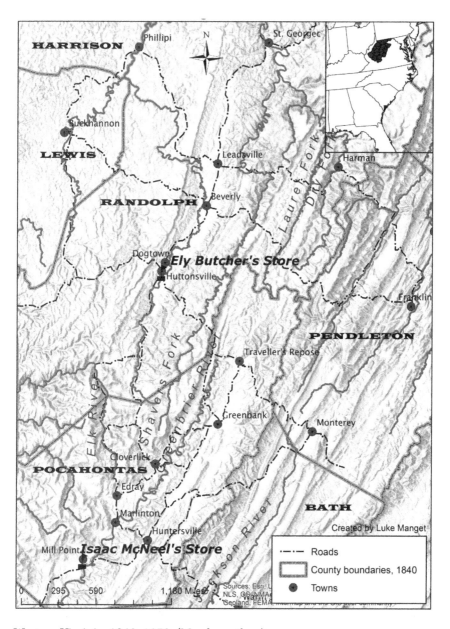

Western Virginia, 1840–1870. (Map by author.)

a modest house with his ten children in the Shenandoah Valley. His job came to an end with the abolition of slavery, so he moved his family into the mountains of Pocahontas County and rented a farm on the north side of Droop Mountain. There, according to family lore, the Grants raised a garden and kept sheep, hogs, and occasionally a cow, but they also depended heavily on hunting, fishing, and digging ginseng. His daughter Sally became an expert sang digger who, according to her granddaughter, "went sangin' many and many a day." Sally started her own family in 1875 in neighboring Greenbrier County and soon instilled in her children a love for "sangin'" that was carried through generations.[73]

While many families continued to rely on root digging and herb gathering as a way to supplement their farm production, in parts of Appalachia, the class of landless people who were entirely dependent on roots and herbs for survival expanded. Nowhere was this class as conspicuous as in southeastern West Virginia. An examination of the store records of Mill Point, Pocahontas County, merchant Isaac McNeel provides a fascinating glimpse into this shifting class dynamics of root digging. McNeel dealt in virtually no ginseng before the war, but between 1871 and 1874, he took in $900 worth of the root. It was the most commonly bartered item, and in the revenue it generated for local customers it was surpassed only by wool ($,1500) and beef products ($953). McNeel took in roughly $13,000 in various forms of payments at his store, of which some $11,500 can be identified from his store ledgers. Customers purchased $2,800 worth of goods in cash and $1,800 worth by trading their labor, mostly hauling and millwork. The rest, $6,800 (60 percent), was paid in barter. Some three-fourths of the barter business, or $4,600, came from sources raised on a private farm. These included, in order of importance, wool, beef products, butter, hog products, corn, wheat, tobacco, eggs, and chickens. Nearly one-quarter, or $1,500, of the barter business was conducted with commons commodities, of which ginseng comprised 60 percent. Other commons commodities included maple sugar, fish, venison, furs and skins, and chestnuts.[74]

While ginseng may have comprised less than 10 percent of the overall economy of Mill Point, it was vitally important for a handful of customers. Two dozen of McNeel's 430 customers provided two-thirds of all the ginseng traded at the store, and those two dozen customers used ginseng to pay for more than 90 percent of their store purchases. Instead of

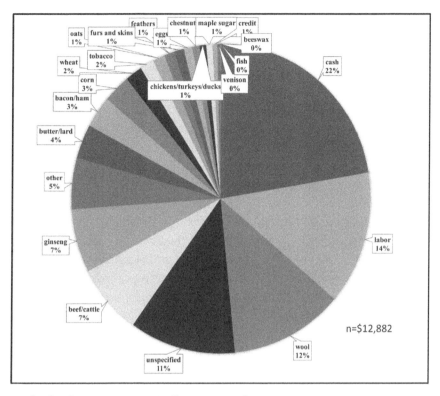

Methods of payment at McNeel's store, Pocahontas County, West Virginia, 1871–1874 (by value in dollars). (Chart by author.)

being merely one widely used component of a landscape of subsistence that incorporated both forest and farm, as was evident at Ely Butcher's Randolph County store before the war, ginseng was the sole source of revenue for a smaller subsection of the population. For the purposes of analysis, I will call these full-time gatherers what contemporaries often called them: "sang diggers." Of the thirteen sang diggers who can be identified by the 1870 census, six owned no land, five owned less than $500 in real estate, and two owned more than $1,000 in real estate. All were middle-aged (from thirty to fifty-six years old), had sizeable families (from four to eight children), and were listed as farmers. Additionally, they were virtually all affected by the war in some way. Allen Grimes had started a promising career as a shoemaker before the war, but by 1870, he was a small farmer who relied solely on ginseng for his store purchases, trading some $65 worth in two years. Some, like Robert D. Silva, were war veterans who returned to find few prospects in the war-torn economy. Silva was a twenty-two-year-old farmhand in neighboring Webster County when the war broke out. After a two-year stint in the Fortieth Virginia infantry, he returned to his native Pocahontas County, rented a farm, and, along with his wife and six-year-old son, began digging ginseng to cover virtually all the family's store purchases. Almost every month starting in July, he brought a load of ginseng, ranging in value from $2 to $15, to McNeel's store and traded it for coffee, powder, tools, eggs, calico, and a variety of other goods.

Like Silva, Samuel J. Brown found his future highly uncertain when he was mustered out of service in the Union army in August 1865. Before the war, he had worked on his father's farm in Greenbrier County, West Virginia. At age nineteen in 1862, he traveled over the mountain to Sutton to enlist in the Union army, an act of courage that would have earned him the scorn of many of his secessionist neighbors. After spending six months in a military prison in Alexandria in 1864 for being absent without leave, he returned to his regiment for the war's duration. Despite having no land or employment prospects, he married within months of discharge and tried to settle into a life as a farmhand on a Pocahontas County, West Virginia, farm. By 1870, the couple had an infant son but owned no land and had only $150 in personal property. The small farm he rented produced barely enough food for the family, so he turned to the forests. Brown and his wife, probably with their son strapped to her back, must have spent much of their time in the summers and falls tromping through the hardwood forests in search of ginseng. From 1872 to 1874, Brown traded some 180 pounds of fresh, green ginseng, or $54 worth, for corn, tobacco, coffee, sugar, fishhooks, and other necessities at a McNeel's store.[75]

Although all of McNeel's ginseng customers described themselves as farmers to the census takers, the title legitimately belonged to only some. It is clear from store purchases that some had working farms that provided enough food to live on but no marketable surplus. Grimes, for example, used ginseng to buy plow points, a cowbell, and a milk pail. However, some sellers used the root to buy large amounts of farm produce, indicating that they made little effort to maintain their own farm. Josiah Cline, mentioned in this chapter's opening vignette, was a prime example of this type of sang digger. McNeel's records indicate the existence of a group of people who did not maintain a farm but instead relied on ginseng and, to a lesser extent, other commons commodities to purchase food. In short, harvesting the commons became less a subsidiary practice conducted by farmers and their families and more an occupation in and of itself. Commodification had finally led to specialization.

Additionally, after the war southeastern West Virginia began to attract large numbers of outsiders who came looking for ginseng and other marketable roots. In the mid-1870s, Bernard Mollohan, a successful builder and surveyor in Webster County, reported with disdain to the *Weston Democrat* (Lewis County) about "a crowd of strange men from other counties with sang hoes and knapsacks on their backs, in search of ginseng on the mountains of Webster and Pocahontas counties."[76] Indeed, from the late 1860s through the 1880s, Pocahontas and surrounding counties became something of a haven for itinerant sang diggers, which may explain why large numbers of McNeel's ginseng customers do not appear in local census records. There were a few reasons for this. Unlike many areas of the state closer to the Ohio River and the Big Sandy, where the initial frontier ginseng boom had taken place, southeastern West Virginia forests generally had not faced the kind of pressure other areas had, and ginseng was still abundant when the war ended. The area had the lowest population density in the state and some of the highest and least accessible mountain ranges. Furthermore, through the 1880s, the area had largely escaped the large-scale deforestation that was sweeping across the state. Between the 1850s and 1870s, two trunk railroad lines penetrated West Virginia's mountains. The Baltimore and Ohio ran across the northern edge of the state, and the Chesapeake and Ohio bisected the state's south-central mountains. Once these were completed, independent railroad companies, allied with timber and coal companies, created an elaborate web of feeder lines that extended deep into the West Virginia interior, where large-scale timber extraction proceeded apace. In the 1880s, track mileage doubled. It doubled again in the 1890s. Much of the early industrial expansion, however, occurred in the more accessible and settled portions of the state in the north and west.[77]

As ginseng disappeared from the more accessible and settled portions of the state, diggers were increasingly compelled to travel for miles with their sang hoes and camping gear into the most remote stretches of forest. University of Kentucky botanist Harrison Garman observed in the 1890s that "only he can expect to find the largest and finest roots who has strength and inclination to tramp and climb in all sorts of out-of-the-way nooks, where commonplace men and the ubiquitous hog and cow rarely penetrate."[78] Thus the tactics used to hunt ginseng began to change. One West Virginia resident remarked in the late 1870s that many families "will unite and go into the unsettled regions where they can find ginseng, erect temporary dwellings of logs, and stay until they have dug all the ginseng in the vicinity, or until the season is over, and then go back to their homes."[79] Cecilia McKnight Brown was one of these people. Growing up in mountainous Letcher County, Kentucky, in the 1860s, Brown later recalled going "senging" in groups of fifteen or twenty into the remote Black Mountain area along Kentucky's border with Virginia. The groups would typically camp out under rocky cliffs and lean-tos for a week or two at a time, spending the days scouring the hills for the increasingly rare plant. They ate "jenny cakes," made by stirring together corn meal, salt, and water and cooking it on a buckeye board over an open fire. They also feasted on wild game and trout.[80] In the antebellum era, rural residents like James B. Hamilton were likely to find the plant growing on nearby hillsides, so they needed to spend only a few hours in their spare time searching for the root. In the decades following the war, those easy to reach plants were no longer available, and harvesters had to go to greater lengths to access them. By the 1890s, the high mountains of southeastern West Virginia remained the last bastion of old-growth forests in the state, and they became the favorite hunting ground of many a digger from the surrounding counties.

From the 1870s through the 1910s, railroads penetrated the most remote stretches of West Virginia, as well as Kentucky, East Tennessee, and Western North Carolina. They were followed by large-scale coal and timber companies intent on extracting the rich resources of the mountains, thus beginning a drama that has been documented by many able Appalachian scholars.[81] Some mountaineers were attracted to the money offered by wage work, but others, proud of their independence, found such work disagreeable.[82] During this transitional period, some mountain residents tried to maintain their independence from wage work by digging roots and herbs. John U. Greer, born and raised in the mountains of Pike County, Kentucky, grew up digging ginseng in the 1870s and 1880s and continued digging his entire life. Even after the Consolidation Coal Company and other companies opened up the Elkhorn coalfield around the turn of the twentieth century and after his five sons entered the mines in the 1920s, Greer refused to work for wages. He moved onto a son's property and spent much of his time digging ginseng. His grand-daughter remembered "sanging" as "one of his favorite things to do."[83]

In the 1880 census, as industrial extraction began to accelerate, a small handful of families in mountain districts listed their occupations as "sang diggers" to the census takers. In one area around Cabin Creek in the Kanawha coalfields of south-central West Virginia—an area that would gain infamy during the coal wars a few decades later—six individuals identified themselves as sang diggers, including members of the Conley family. James and Nancy Conley had lived somewhat of a vagrant life as tenant farmers, moving from Tazewell in southwest Virginia to near Roanoke sometime in the 1850s. James and an older brother joined the Confederate cause, and James died in Richmond in 1865, leaving Nancy a widow with six children still under her care. Following the war, Nancy moved her family west to her eldest son's house in Putnam County, West Virginia, where they apparently supported themselves by digging ginseng. The 1880 census found them in yet another location, Cabin Creek, identified as sang diggers. By this time, one son, William, had gotten married, had three young children, and moved into a nearby house. He and his wife also identified as sang diggers. Another self-professed sang digger was Johnson Gipson, who grew up the son of a tenant farmer in East Tennessee. In 1880, he was living with his twenty-six-year-old wife and two-year-old daughter, evidently relying on ginseng for a living.[84]

For someone to identify as a sang digger was to acknowledge that the general catchall label "farmer" no longer applied to them. Interestingly, these self-identified sang diggers all lived in neighborhoods dominated by wageworkers. Most of Gipson's neighbors were railroad workers, whereas the Conleys' neighbors were virtually all coal miners. This simple fact illustrates the erosion of the subsistence landscape that once supported rural life in these areas. Forests were turned into industrial operations, crop prices dropped, and ginseng disappeared from the easy-to-reach places. The farm and forest economy became untenable, and residents turned to more specialized work. Some turned to wage work, while others, perhaps those who desired more independence, came to rely on finding what little ginseng remained, as well as what other roots and herbs they could find. Telling the census takers they were "sang diggers" was perhaps an act of defiance against the dependence of wage work. But it was to be a short-lived identity. Ginseng could barely support such an existence any longer, and many sang diggers found they could not avoid wage work forever. By 1900, William Conley had become a coal miner. His brother James turned to doing odd jobs and working periodically as a laborer, and their younger brother Harvey became a junk dealer. Gipson became a railroad hand in Grundy County, Tennessee.[85]

End of an Era

By the turn of the twentieth century, the imminent extinction of ginseng was a common topic around the country stores. It was "as scarce as hen's teeth," one observer noted.[86] Arthur Harding, a ginseng dealer who had traveled extensively around West Virginia and Kentucky in the 1890s, estimated in 1908 that the collection of wild ginseng was only 10 percent of what it had been in the early 1890s.[87] Export totals reflected the growing scarcity. After averaging nearly 400,000 pounds per year from 1865 to 1889, annual exports fell to just 216,000 in the 1890s and would continue to fall. Simultaneously, prices paid by exporters skyrocketed, jumping from $1.17 per pound in 1880 to $2.13 in 1890 to $4.71 in 1897.[88] Writers began to refer to the ginseng trade in the past tense, and mountaineers reflected nostalgically on the days when ginseng was plentiful.

Other medicinal herbs were on the decline as well. Lady's slipper, plentiful during Cowles's first two seasons, nearly vanished from the books after the war, although demand for it was still high. Harper regularly responded to inquiries about the plant with statements like: "We have not seen as much as 100 lbs of it this season. It is unusually scarce."[89] Lady's slippers struggle to attract pollinators because they do not reward them with nectar. Consequently, only 5 percent of plants develop fruit, and those that do rely on wind to disperse thousands of tiny seeds that must find the right combination of microclimate, soil, and symbiotic fungus to germinate.[90] In 1903, Henry Kraemer, a botanist with the US Department of Agriculture, could not find a specimen of the longtime medicinal pinkroot (*Spigelia marylandica*), which led him to conclude that

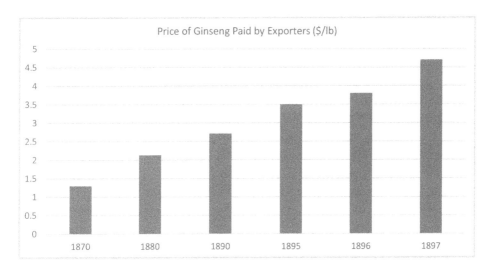

Prices of ginseng paid by exporters, 1870-1897 (dollars per pound). (Graph by author from data in G. W. Koiner, *Annual Report of the State Board of Agriculture of Virginia* [Richmond: J. H. O'Bannon, 1900].)

it was now "exceedingly rare" in its historic range.[91] Goldenseal (*Hydrastis canadensis*) and Virginia snakeroot (*Aristolochia serpentaria*) had also retreated further into the woods. Kraemer blamed the industry and the harvesters, but he also pointed a finger at the "destruction of forests, by cutting and fires."[92]

The disappearance of ginseng and other herbs was felt across the ecosystem, from humans to box turtles. For humans, it contributed to the erosion of subsistence landscapes, sending some further afield in search of the plant. "It was a sad day for the people when the 'sang' grew scarce," wrote James Lane Allen in 1892. "A few years ago one of the counties [in Kentucky] was nearly depopulated in consequence of a great exodus into Arkansas, whence had come news that 'sang' was plentiful."[93] Some turned back to farming, but many entered wage work in the railroads and extractive industries. In 1897, the *Clinch Valley News* lamented the "passing of the sang digger," writing, "The click of the 'sang' diggers hoe is almost a thing of the past, except in a few communities."[94] Even as early as 1888, West Virginia native Major J. C. Alderson, reporting for the *Wheeling Register* on the "wheels of progress turning in the forests and mountains," noted that the southeastern part of the state "used to be a great ginseng country, and a very large proportion of the population in years passed supported themselves off that root. Now, however, the ginseng is about exhausted, and the 'sang diggers' have gone to logging."[95]

The impacts of the root and herb boom on nonhuman communities are difficult to assess. The removal of certain herb species from the forest understory certainly diminished biodiversity, which threatened long-term ecosystem health and viability.[96] It also created ecological ripples that began as limited and localized effects. For example, in early summer, eastern box turtles favor the fruits of mayapples as a food source, and mayapples depend to a large extent on box turtles for their seed dispersal. Because the plant was one of the most popular commodities—harvesters regularly pulled out thousands of pounds of the root—box turtles may have suffered.[97] Likewise, the pipevine swallowtail caterpillar feeds on the leaves of two other highly prized botanical commodities, wild ginger and Virginia snakeroot, because these plants contain toxins that help protect the caterpillar from predation.[98] As the plants declined, this species suffered. Furthermore, heavy harvests may have influenced the nutrient cycling in the forests. According to the so-called vernal dam hypothesis, the roots of woodland herbs play an important role in absorbing nutrients that would otherwise be lost to rain runoff, cycling them back into the ecosystem.[99] Thus, harvests that removed thousands of pounds of roots from the forest floor had an impact, however subtle, on overall forest health.

In comparison to other extractive industries in the mountains like timber and coal, of course, these impacts were relatively ecologically benign. Moreover, harvesting plants from the wild was less disruptive to ecosystems than commercial monocrop agriculture, which required the reshuffling of entire assemblages of flora and fauna and more drastic reduction in biodiversity. However, the disappearance of individual species associated with the herb trade created ripples that spread through the ecosystem, and it is difficult to know where those ripples end.[100]

The post–Civil War herb boom certainly had noticeable impacts on both the nonhuman and human communities situated in the southern mountains. The war delivered a blow to the agricultural economy, leading many with limited resources to fall back on the forest for subsistence. In parts of Appalachia, ginseng became something of a savior for rural people. In areas of low population density like Pocahontas County, residents and transients became wholly dependent on the root, relying on it to furnish them food as well as other store-bought goods. Because it had grown so scarce, however, it took days and even weeks to obtain enough roots to make it financially worthwhile. Thus ginseng digging became the domain of a small group of specialists in certain areas, many of whom likely came from outside the immediate communities. In places like northwestern North Carolina, however, mountain people could find a much wider variety of marketable plants in the forest commons. As a result, harvesting roots and herbs was a much more widespread activity, comprising almost half of the barter business for some country stores. Some mountain residents used them to resist the pull into wage work. Women found unprecedented opportunity to engage with the market independent of men, and Cherokee people used roots and herbs to maintain their forest-based economy. Thus the forest commons served as both a safety net and a culturally preferred mode of production, ultimately helping to turn the Southern Appalachian Mountains into the nation's botanical-drug-producing region. Yet the postwar root and herb boom did not come without social and ecological costs. As we shall see in the next chapter, these changing dynamics of root digging generated tensions within mountain communities and led to a consequential development in the process of commodification: privatization.

6 | "Beasts in the Garden"
Class, Conservation, and Cultivation

IN THE SUMMER OF 1908, MILLARD COLLINS, THE TWENTY-ONE-YEAR-old son of a tenant farmer, set out to dig ginseng in the forests of Wise County, Virginia. Married just three months earlier, he had recently found himself in some legal trouble, and he needed a quick source of cash to pay a fine. He found a patch of the plant growing on a forested hillside. Undeterred by the makeshift fence surrounding the plants, Collins waded stealthily into the patch. Tragically for him, his foot kicked a tripwire that was attached to the trigger of a shotgun, which delivered a fatal discharge into his chest. The owner of the patch, Jones Wilson, discovered Collins's decomposing body eight days later and buried him in a nearby grave. A coroner's jury later exonerated Wilson, ruling that "Collins came to his death as a result of his own acts."[1]

Times had changed since the 1860s. The process of ginseng's commodification had entered a new phase, with consequences for people like Millard Collins. In 1865, ginseng was a commons resource, the property of the harvester, available to anyone who could find it growing wild within the mountainside forests. By the time of Collins's death in 1908, however, it had become a private commodity, protected as property of the landowner by a patchwork of state laws. The commodification of roots and herbs now demanded privatization. These laws were one part of a more widespread renegotiation of common rights, documented by several scholars, that took place across much of the East in the late nineteenth and early twentieth centuries. In the last quarter of the nineteenth century, southern states passed a wave of new laws aimed at regulating or enclosing the commons. Game and fish laws sought to both strengthen private property rights against trespassing and regulate the taking of fish and game from publicly accessible forests and streams. Stock laws adopted by localities around the South from the 1870s through the 1920s required livestock owners to fence in their livestock, effectively enclosing the open range.[2] In some ways, the privatization of ginseng and other herbs was part of these enclosure movements. Yet in other ways, it was stimulated by its own set of internal dynamics.

The motivations behind the renegotiation of the ginseng commons were a complex amalgamation: alarm over the disappearance of ginseng, concern for the value of timberlands, and the desire to derive larger, more consistent profits from ginseng. Some of the most influential opponents of common rights were speculators concerned that the growing class of vagrant sang diggers threatened the free use of their property. Another group, composed primarily of farmers and other smallholders, had watched ginseng disappear from the surrounding forests and wanted to conserve the plant on their property so they could continue to derive long-term profits from it. Still another group, consisting mostly of professionals and businessmen from mountain towns, hoped to cultivate ginseng more intensively, create private gardens, and stimulate a profitable industry. All proponents of privatization sought to use the power of the state to renegotiate common rights.

This renegotiation created winners and losers. Indeed, privatization led to the establishment of a ginseng-growing industry in Southern Appalachia that raised the incomes of those willing to engage it. Commons users, however, found it increasingly difficult to access the wild plants in the forests. Their landscapes of subsistence shrinking, many refused to acquiesce to the new property regime and to acknowledge the rights of private landowners to grow ginseng only for themselves, which aggravated tensions within communities. As ginseng gardens proliferated across Appalachia, they became focal points in the decades-long struggle over common rights. This process of privatization was messy and uneven. Chinese tastes, agroecological challenges, and local land-use practices all exerted influence over how this phase of commodification unfolded. By the second decade of the century, this shift was in full swing, and people like Millard Collins found themselves on the wrong side of the new system. They were now thieves and trespassers.

Regulating the Commons

The reasons for ginseng's disappearance in the late nineteenth century are complicated, but understanding them is crucial to understanding how and why privatization took place. Many contemporaries placed the blame squarely on rural people for overharvesting. Beginning in the 1890s, writers, conservationists, and agriculturists who lived outside of the region accused ginseng diggers of being "the principal agents in the extermination of the native supply" of the root.[3] One writer attacked them for "maiming the goose that laid the golden egg through igno-rance."[4] The issue, critics asserted, was that in their effort to take as much root as they could from the forest, greedy sang diggers placed short-term profits over the long-term viability of the plant. It was, in effect, a classic tragedy of the commons precipitated by selfish commons users. Maurice G. Kains, a Cornell University–educated conservationist, horticulturist, and agrarian, explained it this way: "They exercise no judgment whatever in collecting. They take even the tiniest roots whenever they see them . . . and the plants are thus given no chance to reproduce themselves."[5] These characterizations—stereotypes—were very much in line with how pro-gressive conservationists, businessmen, and other stakeholders described other rural commons users: too ignorant to effectively manage resources. Yet the rapid decline of ginseng is a much more complicated—and much more interesting—story, and it suggests that this blame has been some-what misplaced.

First, we must recognize that habitat destruction due to livestock expansion and timber and coal extraction had a more devastating impact on medicinal herbs in some areas than rural harvesters. The timber industry wrought the biggest changes. Historian Ronald Lewis estimates that as late as the 1880s, as much as two-thirds of West Virginia remained covered by old-growth hardwood forests, but over the subsequent four decades, virtually the entire state was deforested as railroads rendered timber extraction more efficient and cost-effective.[6] Large operations financed by northern capital and facilitated by railroads began clearing forests in eastern Kentucky and West Virginia in the late 1880s, reaching Western North Carolina by the turn of the century. Throughout Appala-chia, timber companies acquired vast tracts of forestland and employed mostly clear-cutting practices to extract timber. By 1909, Southern

Appalachian forests were supplying upward of 40 percent of the total hardwood cut in the United States—at an enormous ecological cost.[7] Clear-cutting led to more devastating fires, increased erosion, deteriorating topsoil quality, and flooding, as the removal of trees hampered the ability of the forest to absorb excessive rainwater.[8] In 1909, a US Geological Survey employee sent to investigate the effects of industrial logging in the Watauga River valley, the area that had supplied Cowles with most of his roots, observed that the watershed was "torn to pieces."[9] These changes had catastrophic effects on medicinal herb populations, especially those such as ginseng that thrived only in shade.[10] Thus, habitat destruction accounted for much of the rapid decline of ginseng in the late nineteenth and early twentieth centuries.

Of course, overharvesting certainly played a role in ginseng's decline, but understanding why it became such a problem requires a look at how the relationships among people and between people and ginseng unfolded in the wake of the Civil War. Only then can we see the broader socioeconomic factors at work. As we have seen in chapter 2, by the late antebellum period, some individuals had begun to tend the commons more conscientiously, and some mountain communities attempted to regulate their own ginseng harvests. By refraining from harvesting the plant until September, they gave the plant a chance to reproduce. The success of this form of regulation depended on both market dynamics and socioeconomic conditions. But it ultimately hinged on trust, trust that other people in the community would also pass up digging a plant if it had not yet borne seeds. One of the great casualties of the Civil War in many mountain communities was trust. As pioneering Appalachian scholar Cratis D. Williams put it, "A great collective family had been split asunder," leaving mountaineers "socially and economically disorganized."[11] Mistrust—of neighbors, of politicians, of outsiders—was widespread in mountain communities. So, too, was mistrust of other forest users. As human populations were dislocated by the war, crop prices declined, slavery was abolished, and ginseng digging became the domain of full-time specialists, many of whom came from outside the region and were likely unknown to locals. Any cultural tools that communities may have used to internally regulate the ginseng commons were overwhelmed by circumstances.

Following the outbreak of war, most full-time diggers like Josiah

Cline (discussed in chapter 5) could not wait until fall to harvest the root. Indeed, they needed money as soon as possible, and storekeepers obliged them. Store ledgers that have survived from the postwar period indicate that storekeepers purchased roots, both green and dried, regularly throughout the growing season, from May through November.[12] These harvests undoubtedly accelerated the plant's decline and even affected the quality of the roots. In 1886, Morris Horkheimer, a ginseng dealer in Wheeling, West Virginia, who purchased ginseng from across the state, told an interviewer that the poorest-quality root came from Braxton, Pocahontas, Webster, and Randolph Counties because "the diggers have not allowed it to mature." He continued: "Out in the far interior, you see, there are people who make a business of it every season, hunting for and digging 'seng, and they so work this soil that it becomes exhausted. That gotten here in this Panhandle is better because it is not sought after so eagerly, and therefore has an opportunity to grow to some size."[13] Thus, due to the proliferation of full-time sang diggers and the increased competition that followed, hunters no longer waited until fall to harvest. Diggers could no longer trust each other to adhere to any unofficial season. As one observer put it, "When a patch of the root is found the hunter loses no time in digging it. To leave it until fall would be to lose it, for undoubtedly some other hunter would find the patch and dig it."[14] Thus ginseng's disappearance should more appropriately be chalked up to wartime dislocation and the failures of the broader market economy rather than the ignorance of rural people.

Rural people understood exactly what was happening to ginseng and why. The best source by which to assess local attitudes toward ginseng is a set of nearly two hundred questionnaires collected in 1898 by Harrison Garman, a botanist and entomologist in charge of the Kentucky Agricultural Experiment Station in Lexington. Wanting more information about the status of the plant in the state, Garman asked people in communities throughout Kentucky about the relative abundance of ginseng and whether any efforts had been made to cultivate it. The responses to these questionnaires shed important light on how white male smallholders viewed their evolving relationship to ginseng and the status of commodification.[15]

Many of Garman's respondents evinced a thorough and detailed ecological knowledge of ginseng's growing habits that could only have come from years of observation and experimentation. One "old man" relayed his experience in words that read like a botanist's notes. "The home of sang," he told Garman, is among limestone rocks on the north side of a hill with good shade, few weeds, and no grass. Plant seeds near the rocks in September without plowing, he advised Garman, and in twelve months, the plants will come up.[16] Elisha Bird developed a scale of ginseng health based on the type of trees growing on the land. He noted that ginseng grew largest and thickest in "sugartree land," or among the sugar maples. The roots were a little smaller on beech lands, and smallest on oak land.[17] Others claimed ginseng grew best on sandstone rocks, among butternut trees, and in other niches.

While several respondents gave only one-word answers, many took the opportunity to elaborate on human-ginseng relationships; collectively, the narrative of tragedy they created could easily have come from a progressive conservationist. Of the more than two hundred responses, only three claimed ginseng was relatively common in their county. The rest of the answers ranged from absent to "extremely scarce" to "not very abundant." Within the respondents' lifetimes, ginseng had virtually disappeared from their counties. "Thirty years ago, our county was full of ginseng but it is all gone now," one Bracken County farmer wrote. "The little seng hoes that were used by the hunters are rusty and of no use now."[18] In Powell County, ginseng "was very plentiful during and after Civil War," but no longer.[19]

Respondents blamed both sang diggers and deforestation for overharvesting. "Dug out" was a common refrain. "It will be exterminated if people can't quit digging it before berries is ripe," one declared.[20] Another admitted that "it is dug hear from time it's as high as your finger in spring on till fall."[21] Echoing a charge familiar to West Virginians, one blamed the destruction on the "men in our county [who] does nothing else in the summer but dig roots."[22] Others pointed to deforestation. "Disappeared with the forests," one aging farmer recalled.[23] All seemed to agree that the plant now grew only "in the wildest forests," and many associated it with mountains.[24]

At least a half dozen took the opportunity to tell Garman that they believed laws should be passed to protect ginseng. One farmer from the mountainous Pike County on the border with West Virginia even went so far as to assert that the plant "should be protected to extent of owners' own premises and even there till the berries are ripe first of October."[25] Such testimonies demonstrate that these men understood what was happening to ginseng. It was a tragedy unfolding in real time in front of their eyes. They advocated for conservation, but the fact that so many now depended on it made enforcing any conservation measures difficult.

Some Appalachian people turned to the state for help in the turbulent years following the Civil War. The first state laws to regulate the harvesting of medicinal roots from the commons came when North Carolina (1867) and Georgia (1868) both prohibited the digging of ginseng before September 1. Enshrining into law what had been a local custom in some communities, these prohibitions were intended to prevent the digging of ginseng until the plant could bear seeds. Indeed, concerns about overharvesting seem to have driven these initial laws. Introduced by a state representative from the ginseng stronghold of Transylvania County, North Carolina's law was specifically entitled "An Act to Prevent the Destruction of Ginseng in the Mountains of North Carolina."[26] However, neither North Carolina nor Georgia was prepared to prohibit harvesting on private property. Adding a caveat that effectively strengthened private property rights, North Carolina's law provided that "no man shall be prevented from destroying Ginseng upon his own premises."[27] Although it is not clear whether anyone was ever prosecuted under these laws, their passage suggests that some communities feared that the changing dynamics of ginseng digging after the war threatened to destroy the species, and they turned to the state to protect it. It should be noted, however, that no other Appalachian state would adopt a ginseng season for another three decades.

At least one community attempted to enlist the state's help in establishing a more exclusive commons. In 1870, a group of 257 "citizens of Pocahontas County," West Virginia, headed by farmers James A. Price and Joseph Beard, submitted a petition to the legislature calling for a law to prohibit nonresidents from harvesting ginseng in their county. There seemed to be widespread support among the county's farmers for such legislation; the number of names on the petition was equivalent to nearly half of all farm households. These petitioners were not necessarily in favor of ending common rights altogether. Rather, they hoped to limit access to members of their own communities, protecting the commons from the waves of alleged outsiders who were flocking to the county's forests. In effect, they wanted the state to empower their community to better manage their own commons. The legislature, however, was not supportive. The petition was referred to the Judiciary Committee, which reported that it would be "inexpedient to legislate for that purpose," and the issue was dropped.[28]

Enclosing the Ginseng Commons in West Virginia

While conservation was a goal of these early state ginseng laws, it was not the only one. The story of an 1873 West Virginia law indicates that some landowners were more concerned with protecting their standing timber. Within weeks of taking office following the 1872 West Virginia election, William J. Woodell, a Democrat from Pocahontas County, introduced "a bill prohibiting digging ginseng or other medical roots, or prospecting for the same on the land of another, without the consent of the owner." It would require diggers to obtain permission from the landowner before digging any roots. Categorizing a violation as a misdemeanor, it imposed a fine of between $10 and $50 dollars for violators and held open the option of two months in the county jail. Under this law, no one could assume the right to harvest herbs wherever they found them growing. They would have to obtain permission of the landowner, which empowered landowners to more effectively regulate the use of their land.

Conservation-minded men would later claim that West Virginia's law "provided for the future" by protecting the species from destruction, but nothing in the bill or discussions surrounding it suggest that concern about resource scarcity was even a peripheral issue, much less the primary reason for the initiative.[29] Woodell, a merchant and one of the top ten landowning residents of Pocahontas County, laid out the reason why he introduced the bill in the preamble: "In some sections of the state, the citizens are greatly annoyed and their property damaged by evil disposed and idle persons congregating in certain localities, under the pretense of digging and prospecting for ginseng, and snake root, &c."[30] Indeed, Woodell and his allies were concerned, first and foremost, with their economic interests. He promoted his bill as a means of protecting communities and their property from the "lawless" sang diggers.[31]

By "property," Woodell meant primarily timber. The timber boom would not occur in the mountainous southern and eastern sections of the state, including Pocahontas, Webster, and Greenbrier Counties, until the 1890s, but already in the late 1870s and 1880s, local and outside elites were speculating in land in anticipation of the arrival of the railroad and timber companies.[32] The oaks, hickories, spruce, pines, and other trees deep in the inaccessible reaches of the mountains were transformed into commodities by the promise of rail linkages to the mass markets of eastern cities. Ginseng and the commons culture it perpetuated posed a threat to the value of these commodities. Many landowners and speculators perceived, perhaps accurately, that those who dug ginseng were also more likely to use their trees for firewood, building purposes, medicinal barks, tanbark, honey, syrup, sugar, or any other number of uses. They were also more likely to set the woods on fire to create a better habitat in which to range stock and hunt game, a practice that extended deep into the pre-Columbian past.[33] Empowering landowners to curtail ginseng digging on their property would undermine this forest-dependent way of life.

"Woodell's Sang Bill," as House Bill 93 became known, generated widespread opposition in Charleston. According to the *Wheeling Intelligencer*, it was one of the most debated bills of the session.[34] Inside the statehouse, the bill faced stiff opposition from both Democrats and Republicans. Apparently feeling that the preamble mischaracterized ginseng diggers, Republican Anthony Smith successfully moved to strike the words "evil disposed and idle" from the bill. Legislators disagreed over penalties, jurisdiction, and the law's application to enclosed versus unenclosed lands.[35] Outside the statehouse, the bill met with even more resistance, as critics mobilized the language of commons defense. The *Wheeling Intelligencer* took a philosophical stand against it. One anonymous letter writer believed that the bill removed a critical social safety net from the state's poorest inhabitants. "What [does it matter] if by digging up a few roots that would otherwise rot in the ground, he can make a few dollars for the support of himself and family!" he wrote. "Oh charity! Veil your face in very shame. . . . I suppose the Legislature will next waste its valuable time in getting up a bill to prohibit persons from picking blackberries, &c."[36] Because most of the ginseng dug in the mountainous eastern and southern sections of the state came from land owned by speculators and absentees, many West Virginians saw the bill as class-based oppression, believing it would be a "step towards enslaving the industrious poor people and placing them in the power of the wealthier class of landowners."[37] One observer stated incredulously, "John Smith lives in New York and owns 10,000 acres of land in Wyoming County. Under the ginseng bill Davy Jones cannot go upon his lands and dig the roots of 'sang,' without his permission. . . . God created all men free, and He intended the uncultivated hills and hollows for their heritage."[38] Much like the opponents of stock laws that were mobilizing around the South, opponents of Woodell's Sang Bill drew on the political discourse of the commons to defend their way of life.

Facing stiff opposition from around the state, the bill was ultimately amended to apply to only three counties clustered in the state's southeastern corner—Greenbrier, Webster, and Woodell's Pocahontas County —but it contained a provision that enabled any other county court to enact the law upon receipt of a petition with just one hundred names on it.[39] Perhaps tellingly, no other county ever took advantage of this provision. "You may be sure that it will never be ordered by any county court," one observer accurately predicted. "There are people in [Mercer, McDowell, Wyoming, Boone, Cabell, Wayne, and Kanawha Counties] who make their living by digging ginseng, and they are of such a class and character as have but few moral restrictions upon them, and hence would feel no compunction of conscience in suspending a man to a leaning tree until he was three times dead, if he in any way aided or abetted the abridgement of their rights and liberties."[40] The amendment limiting the bill's scope helped it obtain the necessary votes, and it was signed into law by Governor John Jacob in December 1873, becoming the nation's first law to end the common right to harvest medicinal plants. Among those who voted for the bill were the delegates representing the three counties to which the law applied: Pocahontas, Greenbrier, and Webster.[41]

One of the most outspoken proponents of Woodell's Sang Bill in the state senate was Gideon D. Camden. Never afraid to mix his business goals with his political interests, Camden was one of a group of influential antebellum public officials from northern West Virginia, including Judge John J. Jackson, Peter Van Winkle, Judge William J. Jackson, and Jonathan Bennett, who speculated in land and invested in railroads and natural resource extraction. Following the war, as part of a bipartisan state elite that also included his nephew, future US senator Johnson

Newland Camden, he courted northern capital to open the West Virginia interior to development. Early in the 1873 session, Camden introduced an unsuccessful fence bill that would have required owners of livestock to fence in their animals rather than letting them roam at large in the forests. In November 1873, Camden gave a spirited speech in favor of Woodell's Sang Bill, which convinced a divided senate to pass it.[42] Indeed, people like Camden had financial reason to target those who lived off of the commons. In 1870, Camden owned $100,000 in real estate, including timberlands across the state, and by the time of his death in 1891, one newspaper could claim that he was "the largest landholder in West Virginia."[43] Speculators like Camden hoped to chip away at the resource base of this subsistence culture. The debate surrounding Woodell's bill thus indicates that the bill's proponents were not concerned with protecting ginseng from overharvesting; they wanted to force a legal and cultural shift in the way property rights functioned. As predicted, rural people in southeastern West Virginia reacted to the new law with indignation, viewing it as an assault on their rights. The following August, a group of representatives from Pocahontas, Webster, and Braxton Counties met in Webster for a "convention" and passed a resolution, written by a schoolteacher, condemning what they saw as an enclosure movement. In one of the most remarkable defenses of common rights from the era, it said, in whole:

> Whereas, the cows can roam the forests and eat grass on the common; the sheep can feed on the mountain sides by a natural and indefensible right, and
>
> Whereas, We, human beings, created in the image of our Creator, have been placed below the level of the cow and the sheep, the only brute put on a level with us being the hog, by the Democratic Legislature of West Virginia, depriving us of our natural right to dig ginseng; therefore
>
> Resolved, That the said Legislature was made up mostly of asses; and further
>
> Resolved, That although we are Democrats, we will never vote another Democratic ticket until the Sang Law is repealed.[44]

The fate of these resolutions is unclear from the historical record, but they suggest that the communities of Pocahontas and surrounding coun-

171

ties were deeply divided over the fate of the commons. Clearly, some landowners wanted to enclose their lands, while others just as vehemently defended rights of access.

The sources consulted for this book, which include court records, correspondence, journals, and scores of digitized newspapers, suggest that violent protests against ginseng enclosure were rare, if not altogether unheard of. People protested these laws primarily by disregarding them. Sources are somewhat unclear about just how effective enforcement efforts were, but it is unlikely that the laws were enforced with any vigor. One reason is that local governments lacked the personnel for the task. Game wardens were not yet a fixture in the countryside, so it was up to individual landowners to catch lawbreakers. Court records from Greenbrier County do not indicate that anyone was brought up on charges associated with the law over the subsequent decade. At least one observer expressed skepticism that it could be effective in protecting medicinal plants, as "it is so easy for roamers in the woods to gather ginseng and other roots without detection."[45] Thus, conflicts over the renegotiation of the ginseng commons played out in a thousand different ways in a thousand different locales, as landowners and commons users attempted to protect what they saw as their individual prerogatives.

It should be noted that ginseng was just one of many commons resources targeted by state laws. From the late 1860s through the 1880s, West Virginia passed a slew of game and fish laws that further regulated or ended commons practices. The legislature, for example, created seasons for many fish and game species (1867, 1868, 1870, 1882, 1887, 1891, 1897), prohibited the use of dragnets and fish traps (1867), prohibited the use of ferrets to catch and kill rabbits (1875), and forbade hunters from running deer with dogs in Webster County (1868). In 1875, the legislature required all hunters to purchase state-issued hunting licenses and created the position of game warden to enforce game laws.[46] Perhaps the most consequential piece of legislation aimed at common rights was an 1882 law that empowered local governments to prohibit hunting on their unenclosed lands provided that they could obtain the signatures of merely ten freeholders.[47] Thus, within two decades of the end of the Civil War, West Virginia instituted a wave of laws that sought to change the way people had traditionally used resources. Not solely about timber, the motivations behind these laws were a complex mixture of concerns regarding class, game species, and commodity production. Nevertheless, they had similar effects on local people. They all served to chip away at customary use rights in the forest.[48]

With the passage of this patchwork of laws, some large landowners in interior West Virginia effectively became managers of commons areas, controlling who could hunt, fish, and dig ginseng on their property. L. D. Fowler, a resident of Durbin in Pocahontas County, was a purchasing agent for the Wheeling-based Pocahontas Tanning Company from around 1900 to 1920. Among his jobs was managing the rather large volume of written requests for permission to hunt, fish, and dig ginseng on company lands. Fowler was generally liberal with his permissions, but locals knew what he wanted to hear. "We are not fish hogs, nor woods burners," one wrote, "but just out for a little recreation and catch a few trout at the same time."[49] Another informed Fowler that neither he nor his companion were "habitual hunters."[50] Requestors frequently sought to reassure Fowler that they were not the kind of people who depended on the forest for survival. They often informed him that they were residents of Pocahontas County. Some were adjacent landowners who promised to grant him reciprocal rights on their property. Fowler created a form template that essentially became a license to use the property of Pocahontas Tanning Company. It said, in part, "This permission is granted with the distinct understanding that no timber or bark is to be destroyed nor any fires built except for necessary cooking or camping purposes."[51]

Other landowners were not so generous. Around 1910, Howard K. Sutherland, a state legislator and large landowner from neighboring Randolph County, employed Ira Shockey to keep an eye on his standing timber and keep ginseng diggers off his property. In their correspondence, the two men complained about sang diggers and "fish hogs" coming onto Sutherland's property. The two even discussed the feasibility of passing a ginseng law that would apply to the entire state, as Randolph County was not one of the counties to which the current ginseng law applied.[52] Thus, with new power to effectively monitor the types of people who used the forests and regulate their use, landowners further restricted landscapes of subsistence.

Cultivation as Conservation

Large landowners and speculators, motivated by class concerns, were unmistakably behind the push for West Virginia's 1873 ginseng law. However, as ginseng disappeared throughout the 1880s and 1890s, many mountain farmers and small landowners grew increasingly concerned about the viability of the resource. Some championed cultivation as conservation. Concerned about the disappearance of medicinal plants, the editors of the *American Journal of Pharmacy* issued a call for the widespread cultivation of medicinal plants and the preservation of American forests. "The time is not far distant," the editorial prophesied, "when we will be as dependent upon the agriculturist for timber and medicinal plants as we are today for many of the food products yielded by plants."[53] But what did the cultivation of ginseng actually look like?

Adjusting to the plant's disappearance in the late 1800s, farmers began to assume greater stewardship over the ginseng plants on their property. Harrison Garman's questionnaire responses reveal this changing relationship. Virtually none of the respondents admitted to knowing anyone who "cultivated" it, but occasionally someone would let on that something was going on. One person told Garman that "it is not cultivated at all," but in the next sentence admitted that "tha is a cupple of men here that has a bed of gin sang. They have woodland and it is in it."[54] Trimbling County farmer Elisha Bird said he came across a few plants while clearing a hillside, raked away some of the undergrowth around it, told his boys not to dig it, and left it alone for three years to mature.[55] Pulaski County farmer Essex Spurrier decided against clearing a forested hillside on his property, pressed a few ginseng seeds into the forest floor where he'd found other ginseng growing, and placed brush around it to keep the livestock off.[56]

Interestingly, these men did not view what they were doing as cultivating. One respondent specifically objected to the use of the term, explaining that "cultivation means he hoes, plows, or something of the kind. My experience is that to cultivate it is simply to make the conditions of the soil something like it is where it grows in wild state."[57] For many, this meant simply tending a particular patch of ginseng in the woods. It could mean transplanting roots from the commons to a hillside near their own farm, manipulating the forest just enough to make it conducive to growth. Above all, it meant taking ownership of it, stewarding it. John Nuttall, who grew up in late nineteenth-century Fayette County, West Virginia, downstream on the Greenbrier River from Pocahontas County, remembered that farmers "conserved the sang on their own patent as money in the bank and did their sanging on some investors' patent."[58] Nuttall recalled an old farmer named Anderson Amick who "had some land unsuitable for farming but he had found some sang on it and thereafter whenever he found any sang in the woods, he dug it up carefully and transplanted it opposite his house to make that bit of land his savings bank that paid interest by way of the sang growing a little larger every year."[59] In taking increasing ownership over the ginseng on their property, people hastened the shift toward privatization and ensured that the struggle for ginseng conservation would play out on a personal level across the landscape as common rights were renegotiated.

The central challenge to such a renegotiation was that too many people were unwilling to acknowledge that ginseng was the property of the landowner rather than the harvester. Elisha Bird's ginseng patch was dug up before he had a chance to harvest it. Another claimed to have had his patch raided twice, after which he abandoned his effort. John M. Brooks, a farmer from mountainous Bell County, reported, "Some years ago an effort was made to grow it by some enterprising citizens, but some equally enterprising persons gathered it for them 'atween the days,' and so the effort was abandoned." He continued: "I have been trying to get others to try it, but the difficulty of preventing the depredations of the professional or habitual 'sanger' has hindered."[60] Respondents were all aware that ginseng was disappearing, and many had started to adapt to its loss by asserting a level of private ownership over the plants growing on their property, but they were operating in a landscape that still privileged common rights, and they came to view full-time sang diggers as the primary threat. These sangers, they believed, were operating outside the customary bounds of ginseng harvesting.

Full-time sang diggers, many of whom ventured in from other areas, continued to frustrate the local efforts toward privatization. Nuttall told the story of a family of sang diggers named Roe who came to Fayette County, West Virginia, to dig ginseng in the 1870s. Working from bases in abandoned cabins or under cliffs, they ventured up and down the hollows and valleys along the Meadow and Gauley Rivers, digging every plant they encountered, occasionally stealing from corncribs and killing free-ranging livestock. According to Nuttall, the Roes were social outcasts who did not interact much with the valley farmers. When Nuttall saw one, "I would wave a greeting but he would turn on his heel, knowing that he had no friend in Fayette."[61] At some point, the Roe family discovered Anderson Amick's patch and made off with $1,000 worth of ginseng while Amick was away from home.[62] Similar stories seem to have played out thousands of times across Appalachia during these pivotal decades, generating tensions within communities and hindering the process of privatization.

The continuing influence of the commons culture forestalled any serious attempts at cultivation. W. W. Profitt, a ginseng dealer in Yancey County, told the *Asheville Citizen* in 1887 that "it will not thrive artificially cultivated; but if protected in its natural locality, it will become abundant. But sang gardens, like cattle ranges, are common property, and are greedily pounced upon by searchers without regard to rights of ownership."[63] The next challenge for ginseng stewards, then, was to physically wrest the plant from the commons. Growing ginseng in the forest under natural shade was (and is) the easiest and cheapest method, and it was virtually the only known method until the 1890s, but because those patches tended to be raided by commons users, growers increasingly realized that in order to subvert the commons culture and obtain more profit from commodification, they would need to either locate their gardens nearer their homes, where they could be better monitored and protected, or enhance security measures over existing patches. "The average 'sang' digger has very little conscience, and questions not whether the roots are cultivated and rightfully belong to another," Maurice Kains told potential growers. "Therefore, unless the grower can place his beds beyond the sight and reach of the professional hunter of this root, he had better not attempt ginseng cultivation."[64] Physically wresting the plant from the commons, however, was not easy. It required re-creating natural growing conditions, negotiating fickle Chinese markets, and changing the culture of mountain communities.

Artificial cultivation began to attract considerable attention in the 1890s due largely to the efforts of two men, John Wilson Sears of Somerset, Kentucky, and George Stanton of Summit Station, New York. According to his own account, Sears was a farmer and ginseng dealer in the foothills community of Pulaski County. He watched with concern as the "expert 'sang digger'" dug out the plants from around his community and the "hillsides and valleys were . . . cleared up."[65] Sensing that demand would soon far outpace supply, he spent about $200 in 1891 on rootstock and seeds and started a small garden in the woods near his home. According to one newspaper reporter who interviewed him, Sears was "ridiculed by his friends and denominated a 'crank' by his acquaintances," but he persisted in his experiments, and within a few years, he was making nearly $1,000 a year selling his cultivated root.[66] For the first several years, Sears was a firm believer in replicating "nature's way of growing."[67] The key variables, he insisted, were soil and shade. His three-acre garden, enclosed by a wooden fence, was situated on a gently sloping, north-facing cove with elm, maple, and sycamore growing on the banks of a small stream among outcroppings of limestone. He kept the bed free of weeds and trimmed the tree branches on all the trees up to about ten feet.

Stanton began experiments with growing ginseng in the forest in 1887, but he quickly learned that ginseng would grow under an artificial lath screen. Within six years, after a succession of fits and starts, he had established thirty-two beds, each one three by sixteen feet. Each bed could produce roughly 350 roots weighing some forty pounds.[68] By the late 1890s, Stanton's ginseng "plantation" was reported to be the largest in the nation. In 1902, he helped create the New York State Ginseng Growers Association, and within ten years, the group boasted a membership of over one hundred growers.[69] Stanton and Sears had done the seemingly impossible—start a ginseng plantation.

Stanton and Sears spread the news of their successes to agricultural journals, newspapers, and any other periodical that would publish their stories. In 1894, the magazine *American Gardening* ran a story about the two men, and the article was reprinted in the *American Journal of Pharmacy*.[70] In an 1894 article for the *Pharmaceutical Era*, Stanton explained to readers the keys to early success: "forest culture on an extensive scale, proper location, thorough preparation of ground, liberal fertilizing, cottage to command view of plantation, guard, then push for all it is worth; there is money in it."[71] Sears published his own how-to, a pamphlet to sell seeds and stock titled *The Ginseng Culturists' Guide,* in 1902. He told potential growers that "one acre in ginseng will bring in as much money as a large farm cultivated to other crops, such as corn, wheat, oats, etc.

The cultivation is simple and easy when you once know the nature of the plant."[72]

In 1901, a grower from Skaneateles, New York, Charles M. Goodspeed, founded the magazine *Special Crops* as a clearinghouse of information by and for ginseng growers; the periodical soon embraced other medicinal plants like goldenseal. Within a decade, literally dozens of pamphlets written by growers were circulating throughout the country, offering sure-fire ways of getting rich with only an acre or two of land.[73] Optimism ran high. "The ginseng craze has spread over the country from ocean to ocean until the situation . . . has become serious," one newspaper reported.[74] By the first decade of the twentieth century, the most important centers of production clustered in western New York; Pulaski County, Kentucky; Marathon County, Wisconsin; and southern Missouri.[75] Most of the major growers made money by selling both dried ginseng to China and seeds and nursery stock to would-be growers. Both the publicity and the seeds and stock generated by these nurseries fueled the rapid growth of gardens across the northern and midwestern United States as well as throughout Southern Appalachia.[76]

The popularity of ginseng growing around the turn of the twentieth century can be partly explained by the emergence and growth of a new wave of agrarian philosophy among certain circles of progressives. The economic cataclysms following the Panic of 1893, the rapid growth of urban areas, the escalation of monopolies, and the seeming deterioration of the countryside in the late nineteenth century sowed extreme unease among many middle-class Americans who feared that the changing character of the United States portended dire social, economic, and environmental consequences. This unease manifested itself in many forms, including the back-to-the-land movement and certain aspects of the broader conservation and country life movements.[77] Concerned citizens believed that agriculture needed fundamental change. Farmers should become better businessmen, diversify, and implement scientific principles. A plethora of ideas circulated around the country offering different schemes for making farming and other rural pursuits more attractive and lucrative. Within this context, ginseng growing took on a missionary's zeal.

Perhaps no one had more influence in spreading the ginseng-growing gospel than Maurice G. Kains. A native of Ontario, Kains graduated from Michigan Agricultural College, now Michigan State, in 1895 and promptly enrolled in the agricultural college at Cornell University, where he studied horticulture under the renowned Liberty Hyde Bailey. Bailey was well on his way to becoming one of the most distinguished horticulturists in US history, but he was much more than that. As a writer, philosopher, founder of the nature-study movement, and later chair of Theodore Roosevelt's 1908 Commission on Country Life, he espoused a philosophy that, according to historian Allan Carlson, "redefined the agrarian mind in progressive, forward-looking ways."[78] He voiced his concerns that the rapidly accelerating industrial revolution threatened to unravel the rural fabric of American life, and he sought to steer the conservation movement in a more agrarian direction.[79] His 1915 manifesto, *The Holy Earth,* made the case that farming kept people in touch with nature on a spiritual level and that the loss of the family farm severed that tie. Yet Bailey, like his pupil Kains, did not advocate a return to a traditional agricultural lifestyle. He believed that cooperation among farmers, better use of business strategies, and a commitment to intensive and diversified farming under scientific principles could help resuscitate small farmers in the United States.

Kains certainly took Bailey's teachings to heart. Upon graduating from Cornell, he worked for the US Department of Agriculture as an expert in special crop culture, developing a fascination with ginseng culture that he spread to countless other farmers. His 1899 book, *Ginseng: Its Cultivation, Harvesting, Marketing, and Market Value,* went through three editions in four years and was for many years the most comprehensive and scientifically oriented book on ginseng growing. For Kains, ginseng was not simply a potentially profitable crop. It was a badge of progressivity. The ginseng grower, he insisted, "should always strive to be bigger than his business. . . . The reason he is in [the business] seems to prove him to be progressive and keep himself abreast of the times. He should endeavor to maintain this state by reading and discussing all matters pertaining to farm life."[80] Kains soon left government work for academia, teaching horticulture at Pennsylvania State University and Columbia University. Among his twenty-seven books on horticulture and agriculture, his most lasting legacy was the best-selling 1935 book,

Five Acres and Independence: A Handbook for Small Farm Management,
which became a how-to bible for generations of back-to-the-landers.[81]

Ginseng growers placed their faith in improved agricultural methods and relied heavily on the emerging alliance between university scientists and the state to help them unlock the secrets of ginseng culture. Sears corresponded regularly with Harrison Garman, soliciting opinions and advice from the Kentucky Agricultural Experiment Station director. Indeed, they learned much from each other. Sears helped persuade Garman to undertake his study of ginseng cultivation (which was published in 1898 as Kentucky Agricultural Experiment Station bulletin no. 78, *Ginseng, Its Nature and Culture*), and Garman convinced Sears to switch from forest culture to the artificial cultivation practiced by Stanton. Garman visited Sears's garden regularly and relied on his experience for much of the information he included in his bulletin. Sears invited anyone who was interested to come tour his garden, and it thus served as an unofficial demonstration farm, proving so influential that the Pulaski County ginseng industry rapidly expanded. By 1902, there were some ninety ginseng farms in the county alone, the value of which had risen in just two years from $12,000 to $160,000.[82] The same year, George Nash wrote (and Kains later revised) a bulletin for the US Department of Agriculture entitled *American Ginseng: Its Commercial History, Protection, and Cultivation*. Requests for information on ginseng growing flowed into state and federal agricultural departments, prompting a wave of investigations into the potential new industry. The agricultural experiment stations in Maine, Pennsylvania, and New York followed with their own bulletins in the first decade of the twentieth century.[83] With the help of this agricultural infrastructure, many believed, ginseng growing could be done by "any progressive, wide-awake farmer."[84]

Caught up in ginseng fever, many rural Appalachians believed ginseng gardens would bring quick riches. The *French Broad Hustler* struck an optimistic chord when it informed mountain farmers, "The possibilities from ginseng culture in the mountains of Western North Carolina is worthy of the most serious consideration on the part of all our farmers."[85] Ginseng gardens began popping up around the region, as small farmers like Jones Wilson—mentioned in this chapter's opening vignette—and Cherokee County's Elbert Bates enclosed parts of their land and, in some cases, built artificial shading.[86] Horace Kephart, a St. Louis librarian who

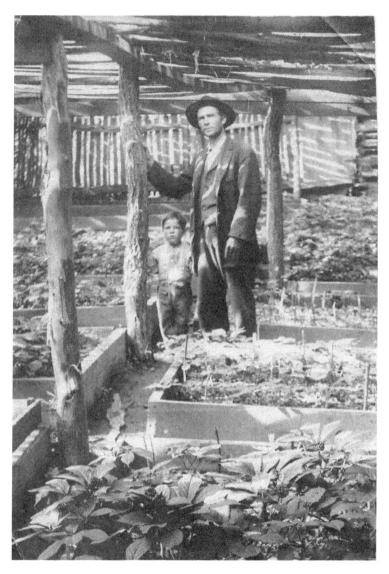

Will Morrow with ginseng patch, Haywood County, North Carolina, date unknown. (Haywood County Public Library.)

moved to the Smoky Mountains in 1904, noted that there were "several patches in cultivation" in his "neighborhood" of Hazel Creek. One grower informed him that two acres of the plant could generate $2,500 to $5,000 a year.[87] It is perhaps ironic that so many Appalachian people believed that their continued stability and independence on the land depended on ginseng culture when success in this endeavor depended heavily on instruments of the state and precarious global supply chains.

Despite ginseng's promise for small farmers, the largest growers in Southern Appalachia were not self-identified farmers. They were generally business-oriented men and women who lived in towns and perhaps owned a few acres of land in the country. W. L. Sandridge, for example, moved from Missouri to Bryson City, North Carolina, in the 1890s, where he worked for a time as editor of the *Bryson City Times*.[88] Caught up in ginseng fever, he quit his job in 1905 and started a ginseng garden, and within a decade, the *Asheville Citizen-Times* declared it the "largest ginseng farm in the United States," an unlikely but provocative description.[89] Marion C. Toms, a dry goods merchant in the mountain town of Hendersonville, North Carolina, started a ginseng farm in 1903 with his son Charles, a Hendersonville attorney, on land just outside of town. The *Bulletin of Pharmacy* hailed it as "one of the best in the country." In 1918, upon the elder Toms's death, a man from the town of Fairview purchased the entire garden and transplanted all the roots some fifty miles to his farm.[90] Other notable ginseng farms in the region were started by J. O. Harrison, a traveling salesman from Franklin, and Harlan P. Kelsey, a Boston landscape architect and horticulturist.[91] Archibald C. Sudderth, a photographer from Monterrey, Virginia, planted his patch on a town lot that measured no more than an eighth of an acre before he branched out into the suburbs. By 1910, he had ten thousand plants growing.[92] Indeed, the larger growers were not typically farmers. They were townspeople.

Despite the chorus of reformers calling on farmers to try the new crop, many agriculturists remained highly skeptical of ginseng culture. Some were concerned that demand was inelastic, believing an increase in supply would drive prices down for everyone. Others believed that the plant had no inherent value as a medicine, a skepticism that hinged on their views of the Chinese. "None but the singular and rice-eating Celestials can feel any of the effects from the use of it," one observer commented. "The belief among the Chinese is mostly superstitious. It is sort of fetish, its powers are supposed to be occult, of the nature of magic."[93] Ginseng's popularity depended on the "backward" Chinese, they claimed, and the progress of civilization would render such beliefs antiquated. In advising farmers against growing the new crop, the *Southern Planter*

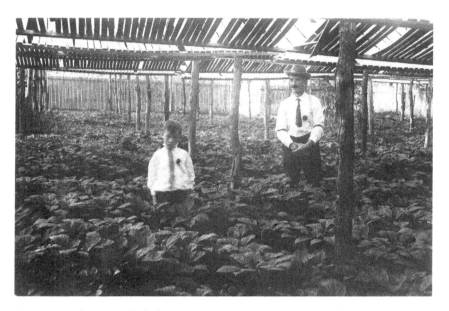

Ginseng garden near Gatlinburg, Tennessee, ca. 1900–1910. (Calvin M. McClung Collection, Knoxville Public Libraries.)

remarked, "As 'John' [Chinaman] becomes more civilized he will doubtless cease to buy the worthless stuff, and then there will be no market for it."[94]

After enjoying at least a modicum of respect in the mid-nineteenth century, ginseng largely fell out of favor with Western pharmacists. When the US *Pharmacopoeia* was revised in 1880, physicians and pharmacists removed ginseng, along with many other vegetable drugs, from its place on the secondary list.[95] Amid a cloud of anti-Chinese nativism, highlighted by the Chinese Exclusion Act of 1882 and the rise of the anti-Chinese Workingman's Party in California, ginseng was dismissed as "humbuggery" by the medical establishment. "We would warn our readers not to be seduced into wasting their time with any such crops," the *Southern Planter* asserted.[96] After initially promoting cultivation in the 1890s, the US Department of Agriculture under the new secretary James Wilson changed its tone. "Let ginseng alone," Wilson instructed farmers in 1904. "It is a delusion and a snare."[97]

To counter such criticism, growers found themselves defending both the medical virtues of ginseng and the intelligence of the Chinese.

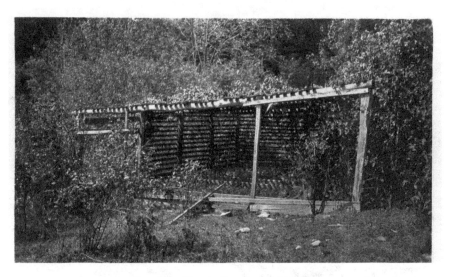

Ginseng garden in Cataloochee, North Carolina, 1935. (Courtesy of the Great Smoky Mountains National Park.)

The pages of *Special Crops* contained regular testimonies from growers, doctors, herbalists, and others who assured readers that ginseng was a worthy commodity. They even undertook an effort, if a fairly minor one, to promote the use of ginseng in the United States. Editor Charles M. Goodspeed assured growers, "After so conservative a people for a thousand years and more, have used anything in their religious rites, in their daily food, and made of it their most highly prized drink, and their one universal cure-all, they will not lightly throw it aside for western ideas; but, rather, the western world [will] take up the tried and proved remedy of the older east."[98] Harrison Garman was even more laudatory of Chinese medicine, displaying an openness that was rare for his time. In his 1898 bulletin, he defended the Chinese as at least "our equals in capacity for any sort of brain work" and admonished critics for dismissing their intellectual contributions. "The Chinaman has his philosophy of right living, and who shall say that it is not a better one than our own?" he asked.[99] The fledgling ginseng growing industry helped counter anti-Chinese nativism and pave the way for ginseng's greater acceptance as a medicine in the United States later in the twentieth century.

In 1904, swayed by the growing importance of the ginseng industry, the Medical College of the University of Michigan and the Hahnemann College of the Pacific, San Francisco, both homeopathic institutions, collaborated on the first scientifically based trials of ginseng. Seventeen "drug provers," or what some called the "Poison-Drinking Society," agreed to systematically ingest ginseng for a period of a few days and record the effects it had on their bodies. The provers reported a variety of powerful and curious effects, from eye pain, itchiness, and nausea to a lack of appetite, nocturnal emissions, and a "craving for drugs." Seven participants failed to finish the trials out of anxiety and fear. Despite these apparent negative effects, researchers were impressed by the plant's power over the body. Dr. W. A. Dewey concluded that the "employment of ginseng in the past, *where it has been most successfully applied and where it has obtained a reputation of value,* rests upon a purely scientific basis." He suggested that the plant should be used homeopathically to treat sexual disorders and other physical ailments in which "the mental sphere is involved."[100] These findings encouraged growers and other advocates, who called it the "most fascinating and greatest drug-proving experiment ever attempted in this country."[101] In a letter to the *Rural New Yorker,* one grower predicted that "a boom in the ginseng industry may be expected soon."[102] Yet despite the optimism surrounding the trials, the medical establishment and the general public remained skeptical. "No one has discovered any powerful drug in ginseng because there is none in it," the editor of the *Rural New Yorker* exclaimed.[103] Thus, despite the valiant promotion of Chinese medicine, the medical establishment remained hostile to ginseng for at least another half century. China would remain the sole buyer of American ginseng.

Back to the Forest: The Limits of Artificial Cultivation

When Stanton and Sears both demonstrated that ginseng could be grown in prepared beds under artificial shade, potential growers who had been wary of theft by diggers were encouraged. If it could be grown under artificial shade, it could be physically wrested from the commons. However, it soon became clear to growers that removing ginseng from the forest was more difficult than expected, due primarily to agroecological challenges and Chinese tastes.

The so-called open-field method posed numerous agroecological problems that growers constantly sought to overcome. Those who chose this method faced higher risk of disease and fungal infection. In 1906, J. R. Pirtle, a dentist from Hartford, Kentucky, who established one of the largest ginseng gardens in Kentucky, lost five hundred thousand plant tops to blight; 20 percent of these were killed entirely. The next year, although Pirtle sprayed the young plants with the fungicide Bourdeaux Mixture, blight again killed the tops of all his plants, ruining his entire year's crop.[104] When Sears started planting more in open gardens under artificial shade, his plants started coming up earlier in the spring, leaving them vulnerable to late frosts. In 1906, he lost many young plants to late frosts, but he noticed that those in firmer soil did not come up early and survived the frost, convincing him that growing in loose, rich soil was a mistake. This forced him to reassess his commitment to the artificial method.[105] Moles and mice also proved a consistent threat. Intensive cultivation in open gardens forced growers to examine and reexamine the biological relationships existing in their gardens. They received help from agricultural experiment stations and publications like *Special Crops,* the pages of which were filled with questions of how to deal with blight, disease, and other issues. Some felt that the effort was not worth it and continued to raise their ginseng in the forest.

Agroecology was not the only challenge to the artificial method of ginseng cultivation. As growers were constantly reminded in the first decade of the twentieth century, success in the industry depended on a precarious transpacific commodity network that was subject to all sorts of vagaries. After decades of relative peace and stability in Chinese ginseng markets, a series of events affecting trade relations between the United States and China stirred unease among those who had recently invested much of their time and savings into ginseng gardens. Following the Boxer Rebellion in 1900, prices dropped some 40 percent in just a few weeks as trade with China temporarily slowed.[106] Prices rebounded to unprecedented heights in 1904 when the outbreak of the Russo-Japanese War cut off the main supply of ginseng from Manchuria, thereby boosting demand for the American root, but this also proved temporary.[107] The biggest shock to growers came in 1905, when ginseng prices plummeted, threatening to derail the entire industry. New York exporters sent out circular letters to growers and dealers telling them that "there is absolutely no sale for cultivated ginseng. Do not send us any more." They explained, "This is the end of the great boom in ginseng."[108]

Prices slid by 40 percent. Demand for nursery stock and seeds dropped off. Nurseries suffered, and many got out of the business altogether.[109] Growers rushed to point fingers at a variety of culprits. Some speculated that an irresponsible grower had put diseased root on the market, thus spoiling the well. Charles Goodspeed, editor of *Special Crops,* believed that some growers were drying their roots too fast, partially cooking them in the process, while J. R. Pirtle believed the downswing was part of a new seasonal market cycle controlled by Chinese monopolies.[110]

The precarity of this transpacific commodity chain often distracted from the more existential threat that was ultimately behind the market instability. Chinese consumers did not like the cultivated root; they much preferred the wild. One New York exporter told Garman that "the whole trouble lies in the fact that cultivated root is a comparatively new product, and the Chinese as a people are notably backward in taking hold of anything new." Growers, he continued, needed to grow roots "that meet the ideas of the Chinese consumers and NOT the ideas of the growers. The kind that the Chinamen want is the root that most resembles wild root in appearance, quality, shape, handling, etc."[111]

Thus the conventional wisdom of generations of cultivators was turned on its head. Farmers and market gardeners had always believed that crop breeding in private gardens would lead to genetic improvement. That is, crops always improved with cultivation, as farmers learned how to select the best varieties and specimens for reproduction, thus enhancing the characteristics that consumers wanted. But these consumers were different. Many Americans could not understand why the Chinese preferred the wild root. "There is no good common sense in the idea that cultivation will injure or destroy the flavor of ginseng, while it improves the quality of every other plant of which we have any knowledge," one incredulous grower remarked.[112] But there was a difference. As discussed in chapter 1, there were physiological and psychological reasons the Chinese preferred the wild root, and by the late nineteenth century, they had developed two distinct grades of the root: wild and cultivated. They paid a premium, around 25 percent more, for the wild article. Following the 1905 scare, growers became more conscious about their methods, and many abandoned artificial shading altogether. Others sought better ways of cultivating ginseng intensively to look more like the wild root.

The combination of agroecological challenges and Chinese preferences increased the attractiveness of the natural method of growing, complicating the process of privatization. The fact that many growers preferred to grow in the forest did little to ease existing social tensions between commons users and growers. The pages of *Special Crops* and similar publications were filled with announcements of theft and requests for assistance in locating stolen ginseng. The *Progressive Farmer* cautioned growers, "The floating county scum, both black and white, is apt to watch a good ginseng nursery almost as carefully as its owner."[113] Growers used a variety of methods to deter ginseng thieves, all of which depended on the threat of violence. Many, including Sears, employed watchmen to live on the premises and protect the patch with "the aid of certain shot guns and dogs of discourteous disposition."[114] Some, like Jones Wilson, attached shotguns and alarm bells to tripwires surrounding their gardens. In 1905, C. A. Rowley started marketing a closed-circuit alarm system that became popular among some growers.[115] Thus, the Chinese preference for wild ginseng, in conjunction with the agroecological challenges to open-field cultivation, served to exacerbate the tensions over the Appalachian commons.

Amid ongoing conflicts between growers and commons users, growers succeeded in convincing several states to pass punitive laws aimed specifically at protecting the fledgling industry, thus initiating a wave of new legislation in the first decade of the twentieth century. Kentucky and South Carolina were the first. In 1902, Kentucky made it a felony, punishable by up to three years in the state penitentiary, to dig ginseng growing behind any kind of lawful fence, which could include barbed wire. The same year, South Carolina took the law a step further. While it did not go so far as West Virginia in privatizing all ginseng, it did protect any "intentionally planted" ginseng on private property, whether it was inside or outside an enclosure. How diggers could tell if it was "intentionally planted," however, remained unclear. The penalty was less harsh: a fine of less than $100 and no more than thirty days in jail.[116] Three states followed Kentucky's lead in making it a felony to dig ginseng behind an enclosure: New York in 1903 and Michigan and North Carolina in 1905.[117] Charles F. Toms, the Hendersonville attorney and ginseng grower who was elected to the state senate, was the driving force behind North Carolina's law. If he had had his way, North Carolina's law would have been much tougher. When he introduced the bill, Toms set the penalty for digging ginseng from an enclosure at from five to fifteen years' imprisonment, which was ten years longer than the maximum punishment for other forms of larceny.[118] Many legislators objected to the severity of the punishment, and an amendment eventually reduced the sentence to two to five years.

These were the first laws aimed at protecting ginseng since West Virginia's 1873 law, but their proponents were animated by different concerns. Rather than seeking to undermine traditional landscapes of subsistence and control the forest class, these laws were passed largely to protect the fledgling ginseng industry. Nevertheless, they both contributed to the same process of privatization. Combined with ecological changes to the commons (overharvesting and deforestation), privatization ultimately led to the physical and cultural reorientation of ginseng from a commons commodity to a private one. As ginseng gardens and patches proliferated and ginseng rapidly disappeared from much of the forest commons, the only plants that anyone could find were increasingly "owned" by someone.

North Carolina's law and the cultural shift it reflected was put to the test in 1909 when some four thousand ginseng plants were stolen from a garden owned by Dr. Chase P. Ambler of Asheville. A native of Ohio, Ambler had moved to Asheville in the 1890s as a recent medical school graduate to practice medicine on the many pulmonary patients who were flocking to the region's cool, clean air. Spurred by George Vanderbilt's construction of the Biltmore Estate, Asheville became a haven for northern transplants in the 1890s, and Ambler followed the crowd, moving into a house on Merrimon Avenue. A member of the city's elite, active in high society, and one of the driving forces behind the creation of the Great Smoky Mountains National Park, Ambler had three live-in servants, two of whom were African American. In 1904, he finished construction on Rattlesnake Lodge, his elegant summer home in the Craggy Mountains northeast of the city. After the state's ginseng law was passed in 1905, his children, the eldest of whom was eleven, began a ginseng garden "far from the haunts of man . . . , perched on a mountain top."[119] Initially investing $150 in nursery stock and fence material, the Amblers tended to their garden when they visited their summer home, building up a crop that promised to earn the Ambler children some $400. However, when they arrived at their garden that summer, they found a ginseng gardener's worst nightmare: overturned earth and thousands of holes in the ground.[120] Ambler immediately published a reward offer of $100 in local newspapers for information leading to the arrest of the thieves. This recourse had previously been unavailable to people like Anderson Amick.

Evidently someone came forth with information, for within days, two white men, Ive Ingle and Tom Hodge, were charged with violating North Carolina's 1905 law. Ingle and Hodge lived in the Reems Creek area, a rural watershed north of Asheville that drains the western side of the Craggy Mountains. The hardwood forests on the Craggies had long been a de facto commons area where the residents of Reems Creek hunted, fished, ran livestock, and foraged, providing even the poorest and most dependent residents with a means of subsistence. And Hodge and Ingle were some of the poorest. Ingle was a twenty-three-year-old native of Buncombe County, married just two years earlier.[121] He may still have been working as a farmhand on his widowed mother's tenant farm, as he did in 1900. That year, the twenty-five-year-old Hodge was living in a rented home and working as a day laborer for half the year, probably in the nearby Reems Creek Woolen Mills, constructed in 1875 by Dr. Abraham Jobe from Cades Cove, Tennessee.[122] Hodge had recently faced tragedy when he accidentally killed one of his friends on a hunting trip in the mountains surrounding Reems Creek.[123]

Ingle and Hodge knew the forests well, for when sheriff's deputies came to arrest them for the ginseng theft, they disappeared into the mountains, leading the four officers on a twelve-hour search that ultimately proved fruitless.[124] After several more searches through some of the roughest and least accessible stretches of the mountains, deputies finally captured the two men in late July. Ingle told them that since the theft, over two months, he had been camping out in the mountains, changing locations every night to avoid capture.[125]

The reasons Hodge and Ingle robbed the ginseng patch are unclear. During the trial, they did not make a political statement about commons rights. Ingle pled guilty and then testified against Hodge, who maintained that he was a victim of circumstance. The jury found him guilty anyway, and he received a four-year sentence, while Ingle received only three. We can only speculate what the two were thinking. They were not hardened criminals. They had never before been convicted of a crime.[126] Ingle's statement that he had avoided sleeping at home since the burglary suggests he was aware he was breaking the law. More than likely, he simply did not see those laws as just. Like the commons users in Pocahontas County, Hodge and Ingle may have felt that their rights were under attack by landowners and city elites like Ambler, who were arrogant enough to think they could fence off part of the mountain and exclude everyone from it.

Indeed, the world of commons users like Hodge and Ingle was under assault, and they could feel it. In 1907, two years before Hodge and Ingle waded into the Amblers' ginseng patch, the North Carolina legislature passed a bill that regulated the taking of fish and game in Buncombe County. The law set seasons for and bag limits on game birds in the county, and it forbade hunting anything on anyone else's land without written permission from the landowner. The law targeted the Reems Creek mill workers specifically, banning fishing in the creek upstream from the mills for three years, presumably to give fish populations a chance to rebound. The law ignited passions on both sides, aggravating social tensions over the commons. In a 1910 letter to the editor of the *Asheville Gazette* supporting the game law, James Baird, a farmer in the Beaverdam section of the county, hinted at the general discord over the commons.

> No posting of lands or protests of the owners thereof has any avail in keeping off the bands of marauders that daily scour our fields and forests, killing everything that comes in sight—sometimes even our domestic fowls. They will tear down your "posters" and declare they never saw them. If you order them off your premises they will sometimes insult you and if at a safe distance often curse you—some men who claim to be GENTLEMEN set this example of trespassing and no wonder the dirty, worthless crowds follow it.
>
> Our farmers generally are fond of having their friends come out occasionally and have a day's shooting with them, but when it comes to daily raids by marauding thieves, black and white, they are going to ask for laws that will protect them. . . .

Game of every kind is becoming very scarce in Buncombe any way, and it would be well to give a rest of several years to all but that which is predatory or migratory.[127]

As Baird suggests, commons users, perhaps realizing that times had changed, did not mount any public protests against the regime. They protested with their actions, tearing up "posted" signs, burning fences, and digging up ginseng. Thus, when Hodge and Ingle broke into the Amblers' ginseng patch, they may well have been making a political statement.

It is perhaps ironic, then, that Hodge and Ingle's actions helped hasten the changes they sought to resist. The *Asheville Gazette News* believed that the case, which did much to publicize the new law, would effectively deter future thieves. "The result of the Ingle-Hodge trial, it is believed, will have a salutary effect upon the would-be ginseng thieves in this neck o' the woods," it declared in 1909, "and the next time someone has a notion of entering a seng patch to steal therefrom he will probably think first of the undoing of Ingle and Hodge."[128] In all likelihood, however, the law was not nearly as much of a deterrent as was the arms race that followed. Alarmed by the brazen theft, growers across Western North Carolina took their own steps to deter thieves. Several, including John W. McElroy of West Asheville, set bear traps in their gardens.[129] Growers in Swain County discussed burying nitroglycerin beneath theirs.[130] The trial and its coverage by the local press undoubtedly influenced the tide of public opinion. Hodge and Ingle were vilified by the *Asheville Citizen*. One of the roughly twelve articles covering the case cast the culprits as biblical beasts in the garden. They "watched the growth of that garden, as the wolf or panther watches its prey . . . and the Beast, like Satan of old, despoiled the garden."[131] Public opinion in Buncombe County had changed since the 1870s. Ginseng was a privatized commodity, and sang diggers were "beasts in the garden."

Hodge and Ingle worked on county roads for almost a year before they were pardoned by North Carolina governor William Kitchin. In a statement, the governor cited good prison behavior and a lack of prior convictions as reasons for his pardon. Furthermore, Dr. Ambler, the judge, the county prosecutor, and "many citizens" had recommended the pardon.[132] The governor's action may have been a recognition that the punishment did not fit the crime. Or it may have been a gesture of magnanimity offered by a modernizing victor to those embracing a declining way of life. Ambler and his progressive, middle-class allies had won private property rights to ginseng.

The controversies surrounding the privatization of ginseng exposed fault lines within rural communities that would only widen over subsequent decades. Throughout southern and Central Appalachia, as competition for an increasingly scarce root reached all-time highs in the 1880s and 1890s, ongoing concerns over the depletion of ginseng populations prompted countless farmers and other landowners to renew attempts to privatize the plant. Only by removing the ginseng on their property from the commons, they came to realize, could they effectively conserve the plant for their own long-term interests and that of their progeny. Doing so, however, was not easy. It required a reorientation of nature and culture that involved settling many factors, including ginseng agroecology, Chinese markets, and social custom. As sang diggers continued to treat the plant as a commons resource, privatization only exacerbated already heated tensions between them and the landowners, eventually prompting a new wave of legislation that effectively and finally redefined ginseng as a private commodity. Yet, as the cases of Hodge, Ingle, Collins, and countless others reveal, this shift in the commodification of ginseng had sometimes dramatic impacts on rural mountain people. To be clear, this renegotiation of common rights was ultimately incomplete. Some mountain communities continued to acknowledge such rights well into the twentieth century, but doing so would prove increasingly controversial.

7 | Progress and Ginseng
The Growth of the
Sang Digger Stereotype

SOMETIME IN THE EARLY 1870S, SURVEYING AND ENGINEERING CREWS for the West Virginia Central and Pittsburgh Railroad entering the Greenbrier River basin made a remarkable "discovery." There, amid the "high mountains, the deep ravines, the impenetrable forests and the thick undergrowth of laurel [that] have for years repulsed the advance of the engineer and his compass," they found "a primitive people, whose lack of the conveniences and comforts of civilization and general ignorance of the outside world increased as they pushed their way through the forest."[1] These peculiar people, according to the *Baltimore Sun,* knew nothing of politics, owned no clocks or watches, and were unaware that newspapers were printed. They slept on piles of straw in one-room cabins and wore homespun and animal skins. They spent their time hunting bear and deer, and in the summer and fall they wandered the hills in search of ginseng. "Their only contact with civilization before the railroad," the anonymous writer asserted, "was an occasional visit to the general merchandise stores, sometimes 50 and 100 miles distant, where they exchanged deer and bear skins and ginseng for powder, shot, coffee, and tobacco."[2]

The *Baltimore Sun* described the meeting of the two groups as a culture clash of epic proportions. Indeed, these sang diggers could not have been more different than the engineers who found them. The railroad men, imbued with "intelligence, culture, refinement, and progressive spirit," were the "advanced guard of capitalists" who would bring this "undeveloped land into communication with the outside world." According to the article, they were personally led through the mountains by Henry Gassaway Davis, the railroad and coal baron who became West Virginia's US senator in 1871. Civilization dripped from their coattails as they tromped through the mountains in search of coal and timber. The sang diggers, on the other hand, knew nothing of the use of coal and cared nothing for culture or refinement. But they were happy in their ignorance, "not much given to musing upon the whys and wherefores which disturb [their] more cultured brother[s]."[3]

This advanced corps of "civilization" had "discovered" the sang diggers of Appalachia. Of course, it was not really a discovery. Like so many other mountaineer stereotypes, the sang digger was an invention, a caricature created by biased writers that reveals as much about the authors as the subjects.[4] From the 1870s through the 1920s, the "sang digger," or occasionally "sanger," was the subject of dozens, if not hundreds, of newspaper and magazine articles, novels, and short stories. These writers drew on perceptions of sang diggers held by mountain residents themselves, typically town elites and local landowners reacting to the changing dynamics of the mountain commons. In the writing of imaginative reporters and authors from more urban areas inside and outside the region, the sang digger became something of a myth. Based on a kernel of truth, it was nurtured by ignorance, cognitive dissonance, and capitalist goals until it grew to the point of pure fantasy. This chapter explores the origins and life of the sang-digger myth to understand how it informed popular perceptions of the region and the meaning it held for modernizing America. Indeed, the sang digger did important cultural work for these authors and the increasingly progressive consumers of middle-class publications. A cautionary tale for those who would turn their backs on the responsibilities necessary to advance civilization, the image served as a metaphorical commentary on the dichotomy between savagery and civilization, the proper relationship between communities and their environment, and the correlation between nature and culture. These writers drew on the racialized and gendered discourse of civilization to declare sang diggers the ultimate "other." In doing so, they reinforced a modern conception of nature and culture that aimed for a rationalized, orderly landscape in which commons areas, if they continued to exist, were regulated and delineated by law.

From Local to National Context

The term *sang digger* predates the Civil War, but perhaps not by much. One of the earliest references to it appears in a journal of travels through Southern Appalachia by an itinerant Methodist preacher, William C. Daily, who wrote of a friendly encounter with "sang diggers" in the mountains of Watauga County, North Carolina, in 1859.[5] It was during the Civil War that the term entered widespread usage. At least two different companies of Confederate soldiers from the mountains were nicknamed the Sang Diggers or, as the Auburn Company of the Second Tennessee Cavalry preferred, the Sangs.[6] According to one commentator, the nickname was "applied by the Federals to all Southern soldiers who were a little scant in their clothing."[7] However, it was also applied by Confederates to their mountain comrades. Confederate regiments from the Bluegrass region of Kentucky dubbed the Fifth Kentucky, whose members were from the mountainous east, the Sang Diggers because "there were jokes about their hurting themselves with army rifles and bayonets." The Fifth Kentucky performed so effectively at the battle of Chickamauga, however, that its members embraced the name and "made it an honorable title."[8] In all other cases, however, the name was a point of derision, a way to poke fun at the mountaineers that probably had little to do with whether or not they actually dug ginseng. Thus the Civil War strengthened the term in the national lexicon as a byword for the poor and ignorant southern mountaineer.

Much of what later readers would learn about Appalachian sang diggers originated within mountain communities among the wealthier class of farmers and town elites in the context of economic modernization.[9] "These semi-nomads are not regarded with much favor by the farming people near whose corn fields they often make it convenient to camp," the *Wheeling Register* remarked in 1883.[10] John McElroy, the editor of the *National Tribune* who grew up in the ginseng country of eastern Kentucky along its border with West Virginia, divided Civil War–era mountain society into two classes: sang diggers and valley farmers. "The two classes hate each other consumedly," he wrote. Sang diggers are as "incurably lazy, shiftless, and immoral as the other class are upright, industrious, and manly."[11] As the gospel of modernization was carried into the more remote and isolated stretches of the mountains by railroads and their promoters, the epithet "sang digger" was deployed as a rhetorical weapon to denigrate opponents of economic development. One pro-development writer accused sang diggers of being "shiftless, roving people, wholly incapable of keeping up with the march of modern progress."[12] When construction of a section of the B & O Railroad from Wheeling to Parkersburg along the Ohio River was held up in 1882, for example, the *Ohio Valley News* blamed it on the "sang diggers" for refusing to yield the right-of-way.[13] "Sang digger" was also used in political campaigns to paint opponents as backward. During the run-up to the 1877 vote for the location of West Virginia's capital—a choice between Charleston and Clarksburg—the *Weekly Register* in Point Pleasant and the *Clarksburg Telegraph* engaged in a war of words that often deployed the term to attack their opponents.[14] Thus, the rift that opened up between landowners and forest commons users (discussed in chapters 5 and 6) contributed directly to the development of the sang-digger stereotype.

Many northern readers were introduced to real sang diggers immediately after the war, as northern journalists, streaming into the South to report on life during Reconstruction, tapped into the perceptions of local elites. A correspondent from northern Virginia traveling through Western North Carolina in 1867 explained, with the help of a "local informant," the conditions facing the people there for the *New York Herald*. "The wretched class known as the 'poor whites' abound in the mountains, and are met by the way side at every turn," he wrote. "Collecting ginseng is the favorite occupation. Sang, as they call it, is found at certain seasons in large quantities, and the whole community of mountaineers turn sang diggers and hunt the mountain side, through every loamy nook and 'cove.'" Reflecting local divisions over the ginseng commons, his informant called it "a nice business for lazy people."[15] In 1868, a resident of Logan Court House, West Virginia, told a *Springfield (MA) Republican* reporter about "a people living seventy years behind the age" who made their money trading fox skins, tobacco, and ginseng. "So many of the poor people depend in part or wholly upon the business [ginseng] that all other interests are neglected and no improvement or progress is made," he was quoted as saying.[16] Thus, information provided by locals helped craft the reputation of sang diggers among readers of northern newspapers immediately after the war.

The myth of the sang digger began to assume fantastical proportions following a Lynchburg, Virginia, man's journey into the mountains of West Virginia in the fall of 1877. He clearly arrived with his own set of prejudices. "I was warned to look out for a singular race of beings called 'Saugers,'" he misspelled in the *Martinsburg (WV) Statesman*.

> They are found among the mountains in sparsely settled tracts, and are certainly great curiosities. I had heard of them when a boy living in the Roanoke district, but supposed their existence purely problematical. They were represented as a race of Tom Thumbs, and many nursery stories were told concerning them. Plantation hands said that they had seen them lurking in the spurs of the Alleghenies and the Blue Ridge. Their achievements were said to rival those of Beanstalk Jack, and my young blood was curdled by tales of their cruelty. Darkey infants were broiled at their feasts, and the bodies shared with enormous eagles that hovered above them and awaited a division of the spoils. They were described as chunky little rascals who lived in the crevices of the rocks, fed on roots, berries, and babies, and roamed over the mountains like foxes and weasels.[17]

Available sources do not confirm the circulation of any folktales about sang diggers or sangers in western Virginia. This anonymous author may have invented that part of the story for dramatic flair, to add literary weight to a myth that had only recently developed in his mind. While he did not exactly find a race of Tom Thumbs, he did find a "genuine tribe" of sangers living "on the wooded slopes" and "mountain gorges" in Nicholas, Greenbriar, Pocahontas, and Webster Counties. "There are scattering communities in other parts of the State, but in these four counties they seem to attain absolute perfection."[18]

According to the writer's compelling and entirely fantastic story of this peculiar people, sangers existed before the war, but their ranks swelled from the deserters and camp followers of the Confederate army. Now they lived "by themselves and are a law unto themselves." Marriage was unknown among them, lawyers were forbidden, and they "have never heard of Reform or the Constitution." When they could not trap raccoons, opossums, groundhogs, or squirrels, they ate snakes, owls, eaglets, crows, and polecats. The "specimens" he had observed "had a starved, stunted appearance, and were clad, or half clad, in grotesque rags." They lived in one-room log huts with mud chimneys, "apparently happy in their squalor and poverty, without a thought of the outside world." They were not an agricultural people. Indeed, "they seem to have an antipathy to farming and gardening. A few attempt to raise a little corn, but twenty-nine out of thirty trade ginseng roots for cornmeal and never touch a hoe."[19]

After the publication of this article, the sang-digger myth spread rapidly across the country, varying slightly with each iteration. Within the year, the *Wheeling Intelligencer,* the *New York Sun,* the *Springfield (MA) Republican,* the *Democratic Advocate* (Westminster, MD), and the *Indianapolis Sentinel* published articles that were either identical to the one by the Lynchburg man or heavily paraphrased.[20] The myth grew steadily over the next three decades, spread by newspapers and magazines, local-color writers and missionaries. None of them cited the Lynchburg man, instead describing the sangers' extravagant traits as if they were settled fact, occasionally adopting the same misspelling, "Saugers." They repeated the same assertions about the sangers' simple dwellings, exotic fare, unusual occupation, lawlessness, and distaste for marriage. They emphasized their veritable frontier existence, how they lived off the "spontaneous productions of nature," hunting, fishing, and digging ginseng to scrape by. No fewer than twenty articles were printed in major newspapers from 1878 to 1910 describing this curious tribe of mountaineers. Stories about sang diggers appeared in such newspapers as the *Chicago Times,* the *Chicago Tribune,* the *Cincinnati Commercial Tribune,* the *Louisville Courier-Journal,* the *Baltimore Sun,* the *New York Sun,* and the *Atlanta Constitution* as well as in news and literary magazines like *Harper's Weekly Magazine, Frank Leslie's Popular Monthly,* the *Christian Union,* and the *National Tribune.*[21] These articles were all slightly different but drew on the same tropes established by the Lynchburg writer.

The initial reports of sang diggers were always extremely derogatory. "When a man or woman goes 'a sanging,'" one quipped, "it is considered a step beyond taking to drink or thieving, or going to the poor house."[22] They were idle and shiftless and loathed work. The *New York Herald* reported that "they are lazy and idle just to be lazy and idle, having not enough nobleness of feeling left to make an excuse for their mode of life."[23] Perhaps their biggest sin was that they had no respect for private property. "Having no property of his own, real or personal, he has but little respect for that of others," one newspaper remarked.[24] Puzzled by their existence and unsure exactly what to make of this strange group of people, newspapers obsessed over placing sang diggers within a typology of poor types. The *Chicago Times* called them a "cross between a ku-klux and a moonshiner."[25] The *Democratic Advocate* asserted that they "are an order of people somewhat lower than gypsies or tramps," although, according to another source, they were "physically and mentally far above the Digger Indian."[26] Several writers stereotyped all mountaineers as diggers of ginseng.[27]

This barrage of criticism of mountain people touched a nerve among many West Virginians, some of whom sought to correct the record regarding sang diggers and mountain people in general. The *Weston Democrat,* a Lewis County newspaper, castigated the Lynchburg author for "willfully and maliciously exercising his disordered imagination to cast foul aspersions upon four of the finest counties in the State and the State at large."[28] The newspaper suspected the author was "imported from a superstitious corner of Massachusetts with a carpet bag and a few wooden nutmegs and was cheated out of both by his ideal 'Sauger.'"[29] Another longtime resident of West Virginia now living in Massachusetts wrote to the editor of a newspaper in which the description was printed, accusing the author of spreading the "most abominable lies." "The native Virginians themselves exaggerate shamefully when talking about their more humble neighbors in the mountains," he wrote.

> Lawful marriage is known among them, and they are not a distinct class of population. . . . They are simply the shiftless and unthrifty few scattered over the State, in nearly but not all counties. Back from the main highways and water-courses the most of them live, and they are types of the most shiftless in any State. The difference between them and the same kind here in Massachusetts is that they are more isolated and can more easily live without suffering in the mountains of West Virginia than human beings could here. They have plenty of game: deer, bears, coons, opossums, rabbits, squirrels and ducks, quail and partridges are all plenty. . . .

> Every farmer in the State will get ginseng to take to the
> store to sell, if there is any near him. . . . The citizens who have
> acquired the name of sang-diggers or sangers live away from
> the watercourses, and cannot get a chance to cut sawlogs, or
> stave timber or railroad ties without going a long distance, so
> they hunt and haul firewood, and for about a month in the
> year help the children gather ginseng. They usually live in log
> cabins of one room, but they have fireplaces that will take in
> nearly a quarter of a cord of wood at a time, and never suffer
> from cold weather when at home. But this kind of population
> is changing all the time. They go to the railroads or to the riv-
> ers and get work and move their families from the mountains
> to the valleys, send their children to public schools, and make
> rapid improvements.[30]

According to this writer, then, sang diggers were not so different from
other mountain people. They simply relied more heavily on ginseng and
other commons commodities for subsistence. Yet this was not the image
that resonated with the American public.

Around the same time that mountaineers fascinated the public
with their knowledge of Elizabethan ballads, sang diggers aroused interest for their ancient superstitions regarding ginseng. Clifford Smyth was
probably the first to record it.[31] A veteran journalist with a flair for dramatic—and likely exaggerated—storytelling, he was working for the
Atlanta Constitution in 1903 when he ventured into the mountains to
report on the "sang diggers and witches of old Kentucky." Trading in
many of the mountain stereotypes that had earlier helped him frame
Appalachia as the "Land of Feuds," Smyth "discovered" a people so thoroughly behind the times that they applied the same ancient superstitions
regarding the mandrake plant to ginseng.[32] Specifically, they believed
that if ginseng was pulled from the earth in the evening under a new
moon, it made a moaning cry and left traces of blood on the ground. For
Smyth, this was an "old world tradition that their descendants have localized in their isolated environment, thus preserving and bringing down to
the present time a genuine legend, a fairy garland, unwithered by the
breath of the modern spirit."[33] This specific legend of the mandrake actually dates to at least the first century AD, when the Roman physician and

historian Dioscorides first recorded the story of the screaming man-drake.[34] In the 1730s, William Byrd also suspected that ginseng was the same as the mandrake, although he did not share any associated lore.[35] Whether or not the mandrake legends persisted into twentieth-century Appalachia and came to apply to ginseng is difficult to confirm, but Smyth's claim certainly reinforced the common perception of the moun-tains as a repository of Old World traditions.[36]

Newspapers, more so than literature, helped bring sang diggers national attention. In general, sangers were not the primary literary tar-gets of local-color writers, who did so much to create the idea of Appala-chia as a "strange land inhabited by peculiar people." Indeed, novelists and short-story writers like Mary Noalles Murfree, James Lane Allen, John Fox Jr., and even Rebecca Harding Davis—authors who have attracted the most scholarly attention—did not describe sang diggers to their middle-class readership. Part of this can be attributed to the fact that, as Allen Batteau has argued, these writers wanted to portray Appa-lachia as a domestic haven.[37] They wanted to sympathize with a group of family-oriented frontiersmen who had escaped the social disintegration and the environmental destruction of industrial capitalism. Cabins—simple yet quaint and comfortable, complete with handlooms and spin-ning wheels—were central to the setting. In his famous article, "Through the Cumberland Gap on Horseback," which appeared in *Harper's Monthly* in 1886, James Lane Allen was careful to suggest that digging ginseng and other roots and herbs was "formerly . . . a general occupation" and even then only the women and children took part. He acknowledged that "entire families may still be seen 'out sanging,'" in the "wildest parts of the country," but these were not his people.[38] Similarly, William Goodell Frost, the Berea College president who did so much to influence the mountain uplift movement, was not talking about sang diggers when he described mountain people, whom he wanted to cast as the worthy poor. "The mountain men were not the poor whites because they were land-owners," he asserted in an article for the *Independent*. They also main-tained a "code of honor" and a certain "moral standard." This depiction clearly contrasted with the sang-digger myth.[39]

One of the few exceptions, John McElroy wrote extensively about sang diggers in his literary work, but in his 1897 serialized novel, *Where the Laurel Blooms and Men and Women Live Near Nature's Heart,* they served as the "other" mountain folk in contradistinction to the upstanding mountain yeomanry. McElroy, himself a native of the ginseng country of eastern Kentucky, had served in the Union army and spent time in Andersonville. After the war, he became a writer of fiction and nonfiction about the Civil War, an active member of the Grand Army of the Republic (GAR), and eventually editor and publisher of the GAR organ, the *National Tribune.* In McElroy's telling, sang diggers served as a secessionist element in the otherwise Unionist stronghold of East Tennessee. He began his novel, set in East Tennessee during the war, by dividing mountain society into two classes, "as different from one another as if belonging to separate races." One class, descended from the "hardy men who penetrated the mountains," were independent farmers who lived in "rude but comfortable homesteads, which supplied them with substantially everything they ate, used, or wore." The other class consisted of sang diggers, descended from English convicts and paupers.[40] The heroes of the story were mountain Unionists who despised slaveowners as lazy parasites who "eat bread that has not been airned by the sweat o' their own brows, as the Bible orders." They remained loyal to the old flag when the South seceded, but the sang diggers followed the slaveowners into war and did their bidding to persecute the mountain Unionists.[41] McElroy's casting of sang diggers as universally secessionist contributed to the perception that they were fundamentally different from the "true mountaineers."

Missionaries proved to be more sensitive to the class dynamics in mountain society than many local colorists, and the sang-digger myth informed many of their depictions of mountain society. One of the first to incorporate components of the myth was Marion G. Rambo, a former resident of East Tennessee who became a Methodist minister in Iowa. The typical mountaineer, Rambo wrote in 1905, was a hardworking farmer who turned the bounty of nature into a comfortable, if Spartan, living. However, he argued that there was a poorer class of mountaineers, "denizens of the most inaccessible portions of the habitable parts of the mountains," that comprised roughly 10 percent of the mountain population. This "submerged tenth" lived from hand to mouth and "were shiftless and lazy, utterly worthless as farm laborers." They were squatters who moved through the forests after they used up the soil fertility. They "know the mountains and the forests well" and "are acquainted with the haunts and habits of the wild beasts." Because they lacked self-respect and self-reliance, they were "given to small pilfering."[42] Rambo's "submerged tenth" bore a remarkable similarity to the sang diggers of Appalachia. The cleavage of mountain society into classes caught on with other missionaries, who used Rambo's class distinctions to identify the populations that missionaries would target.[43]

In parts of Western North Carolina, missionaries referred to this same class as "galax gatherers," although these depictions were not nearly as fantastic. In the winter of 1901, the influential Presbyterian missionary Edward O. Guerrant toured the backwoods of East Tennessee and Western North Carolina, where he observed that many mountain families resorted to gathering galax leaves from the forests to sell to local dealers. The bronze leaves were in demand as Christmas decorations. "It is a hard way to make a living," he wrote.[44] Guerrant would base the title of his 1910 book, *The Galax Gatherers: The Gospel among the Highlanders,* on this encounter with the residents of Western North Carolina.[45]

Guerrant and other missionaries used the image of the galax gatherer to raise public—and financial—support for their education initiatives in the mountains. Edgar Tufts, a Presbyterian minister and educator who founded what would become Lees-McRae College in Banner Elk, North Carolina, as a school for women, was appalled at the conditions of the galax gatherers, which he believed would stunt mountain society in three ways. First, he said, the women and children "are exposed in pulling the leaves to all sorts of weather," leading to sickness and sometimes death. Second, the children were kept out of school to pull leaves, which caused them to "grow up in ignorance and the homes left in filth and disorder." And finally, according to Tufts, dependence on galax gathering caused "the spendthrift habit [to be] abnormally developed," as people traded the leaves for goods at the stores and thus have no opportunity to save money. However, Tufts admitted that such work "in some respects [has] been a great blessing to the mountain people."[46] A good galax puller could make $1.25 to $1.75 per day, selling leaves for 25 cents per one thousand. Thus, the galax gatherers served the same function for these missionaries as the sang digger did for Rambo and others. While they were most fixated on the social traits exhibited by mountaineers, such writers defined the mountain classes according to the way they used the forests. Sang diggers, galax gatherers, or the submerged tenth—however writers defined them—essentially lived on the commons, scavenging the forest to make a living.

The only novel to feature an Appalachian sang digger as the main character was Amelie Rives's *Tanis, the Sang Digger,* which perhaps did more to popularize the myth than all the newspaper articles and missionary scribblings combined. Rives became a thirty-year-old sensation among the New York literati when she wrote the novel in 1893.[47] Set in the growing western Virginia vacation destination of Warm Springs, *Tanis* tells the story of a "primitive princess," Tanis, who lives in the forest as an outcast from mountain society. George Gilman, a railroad engineer who has come south to help punch a track through the western Virginia wilderness, encounters Tanis half naked and ornery. Lacking houses, Tanis and her fellow diggers make their homes in nature itself, a fact that Alice Gilman, George's wife, finds both worrisome and intriguing. Their manners and speech are crude. They live by the whims of their passions, frequent witch doctors, believe in strange superstitions, and know the woods and its biota intimately. Gilman, captivated by Tanis, brings her to visit Alice, a sickly city woman who hopes that being in the mountains will cure her neuralgia. Seemingly dissatisfied with sang-digger life, Tanis persuades Alice to hire her to perform some "honest work" around the house, and the experience changes her. She learns about love, work, kindness, manners, and God. But the pull of the mountains is strong and comes in the form of an unconventional romance with Sam Rose, a hulking, hardheaded, passionate, and violent man. *Tanis* is a story about a young woman's attempt to reconcile two very different worlds. In the end, Tanis cannot do it, and she eventually returns to her carefree life in the mountains. "A wuz bawn i' the mountains. We b'longs tuh each other," she tells herself. "Seems like that thar house 'll kill me, sometimes. A wan't meant tuh live in a house, no more'n that deer wuz meant to wear a shell like a snail."[48]

First published serially in the New York–based magazine *Town Topics,* Rives's book was praised by reviewers. *Book Chat,* for example, called it a "savage poetry of untutored nature."[49] Some believed it revealed a "people as ignorant and wretched as in the worst hovels of the Czar's domain."[50] Others saw the mountain characters as creatures of "intense fascination and remarkable characteristics."[51] They called Tanis a "devoted and noble savage."[52] By 1893, if anyone among the reading public had not heard of sang diggers earlier, they had now.

Civilization, Savagery, and the Sang Digger

As the sang-digger myth reached national audiences, it was abstracted from its local context, evolving into a more philosophical commentary on progress and civilization and the proper relationship between nature and culture. Indeed, the "discovery" of sang diggers in the wilds of Appalachia activated powerful cultural symbols with a long history in Western civilization. To understand the popularity of the sang-digger myth and its meaning for industrializing America, we must return to a familiar discussion in American cultural history.

In 1893, Frederick Jackson Turner laid out his theory of frontier development in which he described how successive waves of pioneers, beginning with hunters and proceeding to farmers and planters, subdued the forests, spread democracy, and amalgamated the different European ethnicities into one American race.[53] Turner's ideas tapped a deep vein in American thought. According to Turner, the earliest pioneers lived by hunting, fishing, and gathering the natural growth of vegetation. The progress of civilization depended on the displacement of the hunter-gatherer in both its Indian and white forms. It required replacing a culture that lived in the landscape with a culture that controlled and dominated it, supplanting one that used nature with one that owned it and improved it. This was the Lockean version of progress adapted by American thinkers like Thomas Jefferson.[54] Even though ginseng diggers were directly engaged in global commodity chains, the appearance of a seemingly nomadic group of hunter-gatherers punctured America's pretensions to advanced civilization.

The firmness with which Turner and his progressive contemporaries carried the gospel of civilization forward belied an unease about the porosity of the boundary between civilization and savagery. This boundary had to be constantly policed because, quite simply, some people found savagery too attractive. Edmund Morgan has shown that when the earliest settlers of Virginia arrived at Jamestown and first contrasted the European commitment to fixed agriculture with the Native American lifestyle based on hunting and gathering, many preferred the Indian way, finding in it much more freedom. Some even left Jamestown "to live idle among the Salvages," much to the chagrin of colony leaders.[55] Perceiving the same tendency 150 years later, Benjamin Rush mobilized the discourse of civilization to both condemn such tendencies and build a nationalism on Jeffersonian ideas of agriculture. In his 1774 speech to the American Philosophical Society, Rush divided nations into savage, barbarous, and civilized. "The savage live by fishing and hunting, the barbarous by pasturage or cattle, and the civilized, by agriculture," he posited, lamenting that "even the manners of the most civilized nations partake of those of the savage. It would seem as if liberty and indolence were the highest pursuits of man; and these are enjoyed in their greatest perfection by savages, or in the practice of customs which resemble those of savages."[56]

Perhaps the most ardent and sustained attack against this way of life came from J. Hector de St. John de Crèvecoeur, who dedicated part of his famous 1782 essay, "What Is an American?" to denigrating the "wild inhabitant of these venerable woods." In remote districts far from the seats of government, he wrote, there were men who "appear to be no better than carnivorous animals of a superior rank, living on the flesh of wild animals when they can catch them." According to Crèvecoeur, these "back-settlers" did not move into the backcountry out of a preference for the freedom it enabled—for such an admission would cast doubt on the civilizing agricultural project he sought to promote—rather, they were driven there by misfortune, idleness, ancient debts, and "frequent want of economy." Once there, they were unlikely to leave. "In a little time their success in the woods makes them neglect their tillage. They trust to the natural fecundity of the earth, and therefore do little." Their property "no longer conveys to their minds the same pleasure and pride," and they fall into degeneracy. "Their wives and children live in sloth and inactivity. . . . Their tender minds have nothing else to contemplate but the example of their parents; like them they grow up a mongrel breed, half civilized, half savage."[57] Crèvecoeur upheld the agrarian standard not as the antithesis to manufacturing, finance, or centralized government, as later agrarians would, but rather as the antithesis to these backwoodsmen.

Indeed, those who depended on the "natural fecundity of the earth" were even more stigmatized in the late nineteenth century. In the minds of self-designated champions of civilization, digging roots and gathering herbs made one a savage. As a result, virtually no one touted the roots and herbs as important commodities moving forward. Local historians who wrote county-level histories in the nineteenth century were obsessed with documenting the "progress" of their counties—railroads, schools, industries, agriculture—and any who did happen to mention ginseng were careful to consign it to a distant frontier past. Occasionally one might suggest that the root was still being dug, but only by women and children in their spare time.

Perhaps aware of this stigma, William Holland Thomas, the white Cherokee chief, Confederate colonel, and ginseng dealer (see chapter 2), never publicly discussed Cherokee involvement in the ginseng trade. Throughout his life, Thomas was a vocal promoter of the Cherokee in Western North Carolina and played an instrumental role in negotiating for some Cherokee communities to remain in the mountains. In attempting to secure recognition of the Cherokee as worthy citizens of North Carolina in the 1830s and 1840s, he constantly tried to convince state and federal officials of the "progress" they had made. As John Finger has noted, this typically meant extolling their agricultural accomplishments and portraying them as an "idealized Jeffersonian stereotype."[58] Ginseng, too tinged with savage symbolism to discuss publicly, never appeared in Thomas's voluminous correspondence with government officials, despite his heavy involvement in the trade. It conflicted too much with the dominant narrative of civilization.

Critics of such a life also drew on the discourse of civilization as it intersected with race and gender to perpetuate the sang-digger myth and distance themselves from such "savage" habits. Cultural historian Gail Bederman, among others, has shown that the discourse of civilization was used extensively around the turn of the twentieth century to both defend and attack racial and gender hierarchies. According to the hegemonic American theory of civilization in the 1890s, Anglo-Saxons stood at the pinnacle of civilization, and nonwhite peoples were lower down on the evolutionary scale. Gender distinctions became more pronounced the higher a race ascended the scale. Civilized (Anglo-Saxon) men were chivalrous, worked hard, and protected their women. Women, for their part, mastered the domestic arts and focused on raising children in refinement and culture. Savage (nonwhite) men, on the other hand, avoided labor, lacked a protective instinct, and their women were forced to perform exhaustive labor in the fields and forests.[59] Because they were often characterized as white, sang diggers offered a glaring and intensely problematic exception to these rules. These were, after all, part of "the purest Anglo-Saxon stock in the United States," or so claimed geographer Ellen Semple in 1901.[60]

Unsure of how to deal with these embarrassments to the race, some perpetuators of the sang-digger myth lumped their subjects in with "swarthy gypsies" and "wild Africans." One newspaper described their skin not as white but as "yellow as parchment."[61] Marion Rambo claimed sang diggers had a "mixture of the aboriginal Indian blood."[62] Tellingly, when Ive Ingle and Tom Hodge were arrested for robbing a ginseng patch near Asheville (discussed in chapter 6), the *Asheville Weekly Citizen* mistakenly labeled them "colored."[63] "There is absolutely no glamor or romance around the people or their history," one especially brutal critic wrote, asserting that they were "as savage in instinct as those who roam the impenetrable wilds of Zululand and . . . seem even more impervious to the softening influences of civilization than do the benighted blacks of darkest Africa."[64] Thus, some mythologizers simply excised sang diggers from the white race in order to maintain their uncomplicated views of race, civilization, and savagery.

In addition to race, assumptions about gender also helped frame negative perceptions of sang diggers in the minds of middle-class Americans. Critics asserted that sang diggers lacked any gender distinctions. Both men and women hunted and gathered ginseng, and they disavowed any commitment to marriage. Women exhibited "no trace of womanly grace."[65] In her novel *Tanis, the Sang Digger*, Amelie Rives frames the dichotomy between civilization and savagery primarily as two competing conceptions of love, highlighting the role of gender in maintaining it. Tanis has deep feelings for Sam, but she knows he is a "bad man" (although we never know exactly how he earned this reputation) and wants to remain living with the Gilmans, "respectable" people. Unfamiliar with her emotions for Sam but increasingly captivated by them, Tanis seeks advice from both the Gilmans, who teach her about love, marriage, and commitment, and her Aunt Libby, another sang digger, who tells the young woman that marriage unnecessarily complicates life. Tanis, who initially bragged about her bulging muscles and crude manners, comes closer to the Gilmans' idea of femininity as she learns about love.[66] Tanis and Alice find common interests in their love of the mountains, their appreciation for nature, and, after Tanis learns about love and commitment, their femininity. Tanis ultimately decides that Sam cannot really *love* her. He only *wants* her, and she fears that he could not provide the commitment she desires. Rives portrays Sam as the primitive masculine antagonist to George Gilman, the railroad engineer and model of progressive manhood. Thus, conventional assumptions about race, gender, and civilization established sang diggers as the ultimate "other" mountaineers.

The Sang Digger Romanticized

It is important to note, however, that the sang-digger myth was not always negative. Emerging as it did during a time in which the lessons of savagery and civilization were being remade, there was a romantic side to it. Bederman has argued that a crisis of American manhood precipitated this remaking. Challenges to Victorian ideals of manhood seemed to come from all corners in the 1890s: the rise of the working class, women's rights, and racial advocacy; the proliferation of desk jobs and managerial positions; the erosion of small businesses; the dearth of wars; and the closing of that great proving ground of American masculinity, the frontier. Men were, in effect, becoming too civilized, too separated from nature. Concerned about the way society was positioning them in this new order, some American men in the burgeoning middle class believed that some savagery would do a male's character good. Around the 1890s, "back to nature" became a rallying cry. Psychologists like G. Stanley Hall began preaching that American boys and men needed to return to "the primitive" to restore virility to American manhood.[67] They formed clubs like the Boy Scouts and fraternal orders. They hunted big game and moved west to become ranchers. They took up boxing. The manly self-restraint held up as the Victorian ideal no longer seemed applicable to modern problems, and so millions of American men turned to a more primitive form of masculinity to help men feel like men. This impulse initiated a widespread movement that, as Roderick Nash and others have demonstrated, helped pave the way for greater protections of wilderness and natural resources as well as greater emphases on nature study and naturalist writing.[68] It was this context that gave rise to more sympa-

211

thetic accounts of the Appalachian sang diggers and a romantic version of the sang-digger myth.

Sang diggers found able defenders among proponents of the "back-to-nature" movement that was gaining steam in the 1880s. One of the earliest was Guy LaTourette, a New Jersey insurance salesman who moved to Fayette County, West Virginia, to manage a fire insurance company after the Civil War and remained there the rest of his life. In his 1882 article in the *Pharmaceutical Journal,* he portrayed the sang diggers as happy-go-lucky creatures who may have disliked work but were content and even admirable in some ways. "The sang digger is called lazy and shiftless," he wrote, "but I confess that wandering among the mazes of the wild hills and mountains, by the side of rocky, foaming trout streams, and through the cool wind-swept forests in pursuit of one's livelihood is far more agreeable to one's senses and feelings than hoeing corn on a blistering hillside during the dog days, and even for those who do not have to dig ginseng for a living, there is a strange fascination in the search for the plant that cannot be fully understood except by those who have experienced it."[69] From his descriptions, it seems likely that LaTourette engaged in some ginseng digging himself, no doubt a welcome distraction from his desk job. Other writers praised sang diggers as students of nature. "The digger is a pretty shrewd fellow about nature," one writer observed of Tennessee herb diggers. "He was a weather prophet, a woodsman, and a natural astronomer from infancy, and the encouraging pay of the pharmacists made him a mixture of businessman, herb doctor, and botanist."[70]

One of the most prominent back-to-nature writers to embrace sang diggers was the naturalist Maurice Thompson.[71] He was born in Indiana in 1844, but in 1853 his family moved to the hills of North Georgia, where he "grew up a mountaineer boy."[72] Wandering the hills with bow and arrow, browsing and nibbling at the luxuriant flora that surrounded him, he developed an "unlimited love of savage, absolute freedom."[73] After fighting for the Confederacy, he returned to North Georgia and continued his "savage" life, but he also studied law, literature, and mathematics and became a traveling naturalist, studying the flora and fauna across the Southeast. In the late 1870s, he embarked on a literary career and became a well-known writer and naturalist, championing a return to nature as an antidote to excessive civilization. In an 1884 article for the popular magazine *Outing and the Wheelman,* which was published the following year as part of his book, *By-ways and Bird Notes,* he recounted a summer spent with sang diggers in the mountains of North Carolina. Finding their ways alluring, he described them as a "queer folk; very interesting in a way, ignorant, superstitious, strong, stingy, and honest—a sort of mountain tribe to themselves." But he admitted that "I really had grown to like their careless, nomadic life, with its flavor of chestnuts and ginseng."[74] Thus, while Thompson still saw them as a unique "tribe," he appreciated their closeness to nature, their wild, "savage" freedom. Indeed, Thompson believed that the future of civilization depended on the back-to-nature movement. "There must be a safety-valve to any high-pressure system, social, moral, or intellectual," he wrote in the same article, exhorting the reader, "Let us go out occasionally to browse and nibble, and gather the savage sweets of primeval things; to revel in the crude materials of creation; to get the essential oils, the spices, the fragrance, the pungent elements of originality."[75] From his primitivistic perspective, sang diggers were romantic figures, living off the fruits of nature as denizens of the wilderness.

The sang-digger myth exhibited characteristics similar to those Anthony Harkins has identified in the broader hillbilly stereotype. According to Harkins, the hillbilly image served a dual purpose in modern society. While some used it to "define the benefits of advanced civilization through negative counterexample," others employed it to "challenge the generally unquestioned acceptance and legitimacy of 'modernity' and 'progress.'"[76] These contrary portrayals were often in dialogue with one another, as purveyors of the myths used them to debate the relative merits of "advanced civilization." Yet they ultimately served the same end: making modern life acceptable and, indeed, attractive to nonrural, middle-class, white Americans. White males like Theodore Roosevelt were obsessed with carrying the torch of civilization forward in time and space, and while a temporary return to savagery could help invigorate American civilization, a life of idle hedonism such as that in which savages ostensibly engaged posed a threat to progress.

At the same time they were preaching a virile manhood rooted in nature, Roosevelt and others advocated what historian Daniel T. Rodgers has called the "cult of strenuosity" which, in essence, meant that white American men should embrace their responsibilities of building a better and ever-expanding civilization. They should become excellent managers, factory workers, businessmen, imperialists—all to achieve the good of progress. And when they engaged in recreation, they should do it for a purpose. "A life of slothful ease, a life of that peace which springs merely from lack either of desire or of power to strive after great things," Roosevelt told the Hamilton Club in a famous speech in 1899, "is as little worthy of a nation as of an individual."[77] The ideas embodied in the cult of strenuosity had deep roots in Western history, stretching back to Puritanism and beyond, and they found fertile ground primarily in northern, middle-class, Protestant society through the nineteenth century. Rodgers argues that the cult of strenuosity that emerged in the late nineteenth century was, in part, a way to legitimize the factory-based economy and ennoble factory labor in the face of increasing criticism over the degradation of such work.[78] But the idea that strenuosity was the only way to advance civilization had implications for the sang diggers of Appalachia.

The romantic portrayal of sang diggers posed a problem for those concerned that primitive masculinity promoted too much "natural freedom." Sang diggers provided a cautionary tale for those who might be seduced by a primitive life on the commons. James Lane Allen called them "lotos-eaters," and it was an apt symbol to use.[79] Alfred Lord Tennyson's 1833 poem, "The Lotos-Eaters," based on an Odyssean legend, tells the story of Greek mariners who land on a mysterious island, lush and covered with delicious and possibly narcotic lotus flowers that grow in the forest. The natives, "mild-eyed lotos-eaters," live lives of indolence and pleasure off of nature's abundance in a "land where all things always seem'd the same." When the mariners eat the lotus, they lose all worry, ambition, and care for other humans, including their wives, and they drift into a perpetual dreamlike state. In this condition, they realize that their previous lives of constant labor and strife were worthless, and they give up on the "ill-used race of men that cleave the soil / sow the seed, and reap the harvest with enduring toil." The poem became a commentary on epicureanism, on the life of ease and pleasure, limited ambitions, and simple contentment.[80] By linking sang diggers to lotus eaters, Allen and others were providing a commentary on their lives. They posed a similar philosophical conundrum. By all accounts, sang diggers avoided labor and lacked ambition, but they seemed content with their lot. Even their most critical observers occasionally remarked, "They seem to enjoy this nomadic life hugely."[81] Indeed, the sang digger was "a happy fellow."[82] Yet these were people who had turned their backs on society and on the civilizing project of the United States. They had no interest in wealth, time, property, or any kind of social commitment. In short, they disavowed every value necessary for civilization to progress. In Progressive Era America, sang diggers became a symbol of this epicurean philosophy, even as the myth served to undermine it.

Thus, like the broader mountaineer/hillbilly stereotype, the sang-digger myth was Janus-faced: one face the benighted sang digger, the other the romantic sang digger. As they emerged in the national consciousness, these two sides were in tension with one another. The benighted sang digger reinforced a progressive vision of the countryside that saw economic rationalization and liberal developmentalism as the only real future for the nation's poorest people. The romantic sang digger myth, on the other hand, was a product of middle-class anxieties regarding race, labor strife, and other consequences of the industrial transformation of American life. It was deployed, among other ways, as a critique of the "overcivilization" that was suffocating American manhood. Beneath the layers of fantastic assertions, a debate over the lessons of savagery and civilization was occurring that reflected a general sense of unease with the industrialization of America. And this unease often existed in tension within the same progressive minds.

Another novel about an herb gatherer published in 1911 offered a way out of this seeming paradox. Gene Stratton-Porter's 1911 novel, *The Harvester,* laid out a vision of nature and culture that reconciled the tensions between the romantic and the benighted sang-digger myth and between the conflicting lessons they seemed to teach. It was not set in Appalachia but in Stratton-Porter's native eastern Indiana near the fictional town of Onabasha. Its hero, David Langston, lives the life of a hermit with his dog on a piece of property he named Medicine Woods where he very conscientiously cultivates literally hundreds—Stratton-Porter names them all throughout the book—of medicinal roots, barks, leaves, herbs, seeds, and fruits. Langston, the consummate nature lover, harvests them and sells them to the doctors and the hospital in Onabasha. At first he is content with his bachelor life, but after having a dream of the perfect woman—beautiful, innocent, virginal—he decides to dedicate his life to attracting this woman to Medicine Woods rather than leaving his hermitage for the city. In Thoreauesque fashion, he single-handedly builds a luxurious new cabin by Loon Lake on his property with this woman in mind, paying close attention to everything she might need. Then, after several months of waiting, he finds his "dream girl" in Onabasha. Ruth Jameson, a sickly girl, had come from Chicago to live with her uncle Henry after her mother died. David marries her to protect her from her violent and vengeful uncle and then works hard to "earn her love" for the remainder of the novel, pampering her, buying her things, and teaching her how to commune with nature. Sober, industrious, moral, and environmentally responsible, Langston is Stratton-Porter's model of manhood.[83]

In the character of Langston, Stratton-Porter provides a masculine ideal for a new era of responsible stewardship of nature. He is a reformed commoner, but he is no commercial farmer. Rather than clear his six hundred acres of woodland and plant corn, as his neighbors do, he keeps his land in forest, harvesting the wild-growing medicinal herbs on his and his neighbors' woodlots. But this commons practice faces pressure from both overharvesting and deforestation for agricultural purposes. Growing scarcity of roots and herbs forces him to rethink the commons idea. As he tells Ruth, "When medicinal herbs, roots, and barks became so scarce that some of the most important were almost extinct, it occurred to me that it would be a good idea to stop travelling miles and poaching on the woods of other people, and turn our land into an herb garden."[84] So he begins transplanting medicinal plants from other peoples' property to his own, building a garden that rivals the best in the country. Some of his neighbors ridicule him for refusing to drain his lake and swamp, fell the trees, and plant corn.[85] Others greedily eye his ginseng beds, forcing him to take elaborate precautions to prevent theft. Langston remains something of an outcast from the rest of rural society, having closer ties to the town intelligentsia.

Indeed, Langston presents a different land ethic than both the city dwellers and the rural farmers. Here is a man who demonstrates how to blend an ascetic life with a worldly one, an epicurean life with a strenuous one, a life of commercial success, ambition, and intelligence with an admiration and respect for nature. As a means of improving society, Langston manipulates and controls the landscape, and although not to the same extent as his farming neighbors, it is measurably more than the

sang diggers. He is, in essence, a small-scale land manager. The sang diggers of Appalachia, representatives of disorder, exploitation, and social
irresponsibility, have no place in this progressive vision of order on the
landscape. Thus, Stratton-Porter displayed a way to reconcile progress
and simplicity, the cultural refinement of civilization and the moral lessons of the woods, the lotus eaters and the cult of strenuosity. *The Harvester* can be read as an attempt by Stratton-Porter to legitimize this new
standard of manliness by incorporating a little more femininity to create
a cooperative relationship to nature rather than an imperialistic one.[86]

Undoubtedly, sang diggers continued to be a topic of conversation around
hearths and campfires well into the twentieth century, but by the 1920s,
the myth had largely dissipated among the literati. Parts of it had been
absorbed into more general mountaineer, or hillbilly, stereotypes, but
ginseng stopped being the defining point for an entire class of people.
Ginseng digging, if it was still part of the conversation, became merely
one of the many peculiar habits of what Cratis Williams called the
"branchwater mountaineers."[87] One reason for this is likely the fact that
the realities of mountain life had shifted. As the forests were cleared, the
plants overharvested, and population increases brought more property
boundaries and property laws, people found fewer opportunities to make
money from the forest commons, and so they turned to other sources of
income. The myth also disappeared because it no longer spoke to the
needs of twentieth-century Americans. Changes to the American landscape rendered common rights increasingly anachronistic, unsustainable, and backward, even in the New South, even in Appalachia. People
who insisted on them were seen at best as quixotic and at worst as criminals. From its origins in West Virginia politics, the sang-digger myth
grew to national proportions because newspaper reporters, missionaries,
local colorists, and novelists wanted to distance themselves culturally
from such commons users, and the need to do so disappeared with the
commons users. Indeed, perpetuators of the sang-digger myth advanced
a relationship between nature and culture that embraced property rights
and a rationalized landscape. It was, in essence, the cultural supplement
to the renegotiation of the commons.

Epilogue

The Decline of Root and Herb Gathering and the Fate of the Commons

As World War I stimulated a resurgence of the botanical drug trade, Appalachia's root diggers and herb gatherers became the romantic protagonists in a peculiar new national drama. After traveling to Western North Carolina in 1916, Edward Lansing Cowles (no relationship to Calvin J. Cowles), a producer for the American Film Company, was surprised to find that "the war in Europe has . . . revive[d] the occupations of our forefathers . . . , that of gathering herbs." Cowles called the mountaineer "a natural student of nature and all her marvelous products. He knows where to dig for flagroot, where to find the wild cherry trees, the root of the sassafras, the leaf of wild lettuce, and he's more fully aware of the highest market valuation per pound of more than 100 such herbs and roots and the products of the mountains and valleys than you would possibly imagine."[1] In 1920, one herb dealer in West Jefferson, North Carolina, reported that his diggers revived harvesting strategies reminiscent of fifty years earlier. "Some of these families live in tents and move from place to place as the supplies of valuable herbs are exhausted. Choosing a good camping spot, where some herb or root is present in abundance, the tent is pitched and here it remains until the stuff, which will later be compounded in various medicines, is gathered and prepared for the dealer. Then a new location is sought."[2] This dealer, who conducted roughly $75,000 worth of business in roots and herbs per year, asserted that these gatherers "get back to nature, and they learn to love it. . . . The gath-

219

ering of crude drugs . . . is much more profitable than laboring for wages in these parts."[3]

Hoping to capitalize on public interest in pharmaceutical geography stimulated by World War I, Henry Fuller, a pharmaceutical chemist and drug industry consultant, published *The Story of Drugs* in 1922. He noted that interest in the drug supply became "almost universal" during the war. "It possessed a certain element of romance, made excellent dinner conversation, and was discussed at almost any gathering where two or more people were assembled," he wrote, "much the same as prohibition later became the popular topic."[4] Fuller shared Cowles's romantic imagery of Appalachian drug collectors. "To follow the seasons in a region where the medicinal flora exists in its virgin state is a privilege that must be experienced in order to be appreciated," Fuller wrote, "and as the years go by the opportunity to do so is passing. Outside of the comparatively inaccessible mountainous country where drug-collecting forms the chief remunerative occupation of the inhabitants, there are very few localities in which one can observe an array of medicinal flora growing undisturbed."[5] Yet, sounding a note of optimism, he wrote that "the natural supplies of drugs yielded by this producing area in our Southern mountains will be adequate for the demands of the medicine-maker for many years to come."[6]

Despite the ecological and economic changes that took place across Appalachia around the turn of the twentieth century, root digging and herb gathering did continue to form an important component of rural life through World War I and beyond. Ginseng was not entirely exterminated, and the strength of the botanical drug trade in the wake of the war maintained markets for other roots and herbs through the 1930s.

Roots and herbs helped some mountain families get through the Great Depression. Oral histories from northwestern North Carolina reveal that participation in the trade was integral to the family budget. Council Main, who grew up in the Pottertown community in Watauga County in the 1930s, remembered that "there was always somebody who would buy roots and herbs."[7] Children used medicinal herbs as well as galax, chestnuts, and other commons commodities to purchase clothes, shoes, school supplies, candy, and, according to Bessie Greer, "whatever we wanted" at the nearest store.[8] Anne Mains Potter, another Watauga County native, depended heavily on the sale of roots and herbs in the

1930s and 1940s for survival. "You had to dig yourself a sack of roots like ginseng to buy bread and stuff," she told an interviewer in 2000. "We'd dig just anything that they bought. Any kind of black cohosh, burdock root. We traded with the roots. It's what I got my eating with. See, my husband worked . . . so I had to get out and dig roots in the wintertime. There was a store down there in the fork of the road. If I had roots to sell them, we bought things. I'd walk down to the store to get something to eat."[9]

Thus, just as they had done in the nineteenth, throughout the first half of the twentieth century, roots and herbs continued to provide a safety net for some mountain people. It was one of their many strategies for maintaining a livelihood in the mountains, and many of them enjoyed it. Main remembers his root-digging days fondly. "I could make more money and easier digging roots and herbs than I could make in the corn-field," he declared, "and you could work in the woods. It was a lot cooler in hot weather. I learned all the roots and herbs." Main also relied on the commons for other resources, such as maple syrup, rabbits, galax, and chestnuts.[10] Root digging and herb gathering continued to blur the line between work and leisure, and many people chose to spend their spare time doing it. Donald McCourry, who grew up in Dog Flat Hollow in Yancey County, North Carolina, in the 1920s and 1930s, claimed, "Hunting sang is one of the only ways of making money in the mountains that is more fun than hard work. [A] sang digging excursion was something I enjoyed every minute of. I could have a good time roaming the woods because I was doing something that would bring in money."[11] Thus, just as they had done in the wake of the Civil War, mountain people fell back on the commons to make ends meet during the depths of the Great Depression.

However, Fuller's prediction that Appalachia could supply drug markets for "many years to come" did not exactly come true. Over the latter half of the twentieth century, gathering medicinal roots and herbs became less and less important to local communities. There were many reasons—economic, ecological, and social—for this shift. Perhaps the most important had to do with changes in drug markets. Another therapeutic revolution over the first half of the century saw the rise of antibiotics and synthetically created drugs. By the 1950s, Americans had all but abandoned botanical medicine. Pharmacists and physicians, many of whom maintained a prejudice against botanical medicine dating back to the heyday of patent medicines, eagerly embraced the new class of drugs, discarding botanicals.[12] The lack of profitability of botanical drug making also played a role. According to Purdue professor of pharmacognosy Varro Tyler, pharmaceutical companies moved away from botanicals in part because they were more difficult to patent. S. B. Penick Jr., son of the founder of Asheville-based S. B. Penick & Co., discussed in chapter 4, admitted as much to him in the 1970s.[13] By 1960, virtually all native American plants, including lobelia, bloodroot, sarsaparilla, sassafras, Seneca snakeroot, Virginia snakeroot, pinkroot, and hellebore were dropped from the official US *Pharmacopoeia*. Mayapple was the only one to remain.[14] Pharmaceutical botany was removed from the curricula of many pharmacy schools, and botanical drugs seemed to be on the verge of irrelevancy.[15]

The crude botanical drug houses in Appalachia either moved away from botanicals or got out of the business altogether. R. T. Greer's business declined precipitously after World War II. In 1945, the company closed its Brownwood, North Carolina, herb warehouse, and the building eventually became a feed-and-seed store. Greer continued to operate the main warehouse in Marion, Virginia, until it, too, was sold in 1968.[16] S. B. Penick & Co. acquired New York Quinine and Chemical Works in 1947, which signaled its move away from botanicals. It subsequently started manufacturing antibiotics, specifically Tyrothricin, Bacitracin, and Neomycin. However, financial troubles soon engulfed the company, and in 1967, it was sold to a large conglomerate, Corn Products Company.[17] The Wallace Brothers Company continued to operate in a diminished capacity throughout the 1920s and 1930s, but after World War II, it met the same fate. In 1944, the company razed its botanic depot in Statesville, and in 1950, the last of the Wallaces in the business, Sigmond Wallace, closed shop.[18] The Boone, North Carolina–based Wilcox Drug Company proved the longest lasting of the region's crude-drug companies. It survived long enough to benefit from a renewed interest in herbal medicine in the 1960s and 1970s. The folk revivals of that era and the popularity of "natural medicine" among some circles gave Wilcox a boost that sustained it until 1982, when it was sold to a Swiss company and reorganized under the name Wilcox Natural Products, which lasted until 2000.[19]

Changing drug markets were not the only threat to root digging and herb gathering in the mountains. Habitat destruction and overharvesting continued to contribute to a general decline in the practices. Deforestation for agricultural purposes as well as for homebuilding and other building construction altered prime ginseng habitats, particularly in areas like Western North Carolina. In West Virginia and other parts of Central Appalachia, invasive surface coal mining was even more destructive, physically removing the mountaintops that had served as commons areas and deforesting large swaths of land around the mining sites. In addition to endangering human health and contaminating ecosystems for generations to come, mountaintop removal has been a severe threat to mountain people's way of life, which has historically been dependent on the forest.

As harvests have steadily declined, prices for ginseng have skyrocketed. In 2001, prices paid to diggers ranged from $180 to $300 per pound in North Carolina, and by 2014, prices got as high as $1,000 per pound.[20] In 2001, just 46,000 pounds of wild ginseng were sold in the United States, generating more than $12 million.[21] As a point of comparison, in 1876, at the height of the postwar boom, 550,000 pounds were exported, generating $646,000 (somewhere near $16 million today).

Indeed, wild ginseng has remained scarce in most of Appalachia since at least World War II. A complex web of state and federal laws and international treaties that emerged after the war further restricted common rights to medicinal plants. It is now a common requirement across the region for harvesters to obtain and keep on their person written permission from landowners to harvest a wide variety of plants. Driven by international pressures under the Convention on International Trade in Endangered Species of Wild Flora and Fauna (CITES) treaty, ginseng harvesting has become heavily regulated. Diggers can harvest only during the season, which typically runs from September to December, depending on the state, and they cannot harvest plants less than five years old. In West Virginia, diggers are also forbidden to remove the seeds from a collection site and are required to replant them.[22]

In addition to ecological changes, the social renegotiation of common rights that began in the late nineteenth century continued well into the twentieth with the arrival of a wave of second-home buyers and migrants who held different values and attitudes toward private property. One study by the Appalachian Land Ownership Task Force found that between 1968 and 1973, ten counties in Western North Carolina experienced a 26 percent increase in the number of nonlocal landowners. The same study also found that native North Carolinians' landownership declined, while out-of-state landowners increased by 50 percent.[23] Many mountain natives began to feel as though the commons had disappeared. Leonard Greer, a native of Meat Camp, Watauga County, told an interviewer in 2010 that prior to these newcomers' arrival, "there was somewhat of a feeling that those things that the land provided were intended to benefit everyone. Only those things built or cultivated were owned in total. It was shocking to the natives that newcomers would post land or prosecute trespassers."[24] Juanita Jones lamented that the forest was being "closed off and their houses are going to be going up and I hate to see it. . . . When they come into an area, the first thing they do is put up a No Trespassing sign and they don't want anything to do with the community."[25] George Washington Main, a Pottertown native, believed that the population growth spurred by in-migrants brought about a general philosophical change in attitudes toward the land.

> Many years ago, commons were common. Anybody who owned land, they didn't mind you going across it, if you didn't destroy it. They took a more philosophical view of it. It doesn't really belong to anybody, no matter how possessive you are. Because you're living much more close together, the attitudes change about land use and land access—and not for the better. I couldn't believe it, for example, in Watauga County, the first time I saw a gated farm. And people are now taking the attitude that "I want mine, and you stay away from it," but I feel free to share yours. I'm sorry, but that's the way it is, and we have a lot of people in Watauga County.[26]

Indeed, the forest commons was central to natives' community identity, and many felt that newcomers' enclosure of the commons was a threat to that sense of community.

The changes that have taken place over the past century have reduced the insulating power that roots and herbs—and the commons economy in general—once had. When hard times return, as they have repeatedly since World War II, people no longer have the same ability to retreat to the forests as they did after the Civil War. Roots and herbs are not the only resources affected by these changes. Beginning in the 1920s, the Asian chestnut blight destroyed that valuable tree. Hunting and fishing cost money and are subject to a wide range of regulations. Little by little, the shrinking and fragmentation of the commons have made it more difficult for mountain people to make ends meet.

Yet root digging and herb gathering persists. Despite the gradual shrinking of markets, commons spaces, and herb populations as well as changing economic opportunities Appalachian residents, both old and new, continue to exhibit a remarkable tendency to piece together livelihoods, and the forest still plays an important role. In her book, *The Livelihood of Kin*, anthropologist Rhoda Halperin has found that people in eastern Kentucky employ what she calls "multiple livelihood strategies" for making ends meet in order to remain in their communities. These strategies include hunting, fishing, gathering, subsistence gardening, temporary wage work, labor exchanges within kin networks, and the buying and selling of secondhand goods in local periodic marketplaces (flea markets). She argues that these strategies should be understood as "forms of resistance to capitalism and to dependence upon the state."[27] Anthropologist Shannon McBride has found that natives in the more rural Graham County, North Carolina, continue to dig roots and herbs as part of their multiple livelihood strategies, although far less than they once did.[28] As one longtime resident of Graham County, North Carolina, put it: "[Graham Countians] learnt how to live here by diversifying their income, by being flexible in so many different things that they found to do. From cutting timber, logging, splitting posts and rails, to gathering the log moss, catching spring lizards, to digging the herbs and selling rock. Just doing whatever they could find to do, you know, working on the farm, working in the plants and mechanicing—whatever they could find to do. And as you visit around you find a lot of people that's not really dependent on one occupation."[29]

Ginseng digging remains an important component of some mountain people's identities, although it has diminished since the nineteenth century.[30] Through her interviews with ginseng diggers in the Coal River region of central West Virginia, folklorist Mary Hufford has found that ginseng digging is still bound up in mountain identity, shaping the way people interact with the landscape and with one another. Place names such as Seng Run, Seng Camp Creek, and Three-Prong Holler testify to

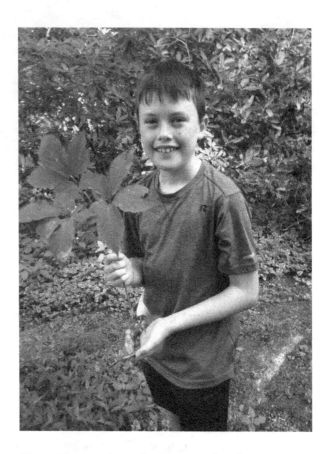

Henry Manget, the author's son, with a three-pronged ginseng plant. (Photo by author.)

the long cultural history of the plant in West Virginia. Before the Coal Valley's Sundial Tavern closed down in the late 1990s, a six-pronged ginseng top pressed in glass occupied a prominent place behind the bar, where tales of large patches and giant roots were still regularly swapped.[31]

Markets continue to exist for some Appalachian plants. The emergence of the herbal dietary supplement industry since the 1970s helped sustain a limited trade in some Appalachian plants, including bloodroot and black cohosh. Today, bloodroot is marketed primarily in Europe, where it is used as an anti-parasitic animal feed additive and appetite enhancer. Black cohosh is generating interest from some pharmaceutical companies for its value in treating menopausal symptoms. Other non-timber forest products, such as ramps (*Allium tricoccum*), morel mushrooms, and chanterelle mushrooms, have found niches in the recent "foodie" movement, while others—log moss, azaleas, mountain laurel, galax, and trilliums—make their way to markets for floral décor and ornamental nursery plants.[32]

While the commons has been heavily fragmented in parts of Appalachia, in other parts, such as interior West Virginia, where patterns of corporate ownership of the mountaintops continue, it persists with some strength. A 1983 survey by the Appalachian Land Ownership Task Force of landownership patterns in eighty Appalachian counties found that nearly half of the 20 million acres surveyed were owned by absentee individuals and corporations.[33] In his interviews with ginseng diggers of southwestern West Virginia in the late 1990s, Brent Bailey found that they hunt sang primarily on company lands, although they sometimes admitted not knowing who owned the land. "We just call it 'the mountain,'" one woman replied when asked where she hunted ginseng. "Nobody lives up there, and my cousin's first wife's brother always used to tell us nobody'd mind if we went there. 'Course they'd never know, either."[34] Indeed, many still regard sang digging as a "birth right" and remain defiant of any attempts to curtail their rights, whether perpetrated by the government or by corporate landowners. In the Upper Midwest, including Wisconsin and Michigan, intensive ginseng cultivation has all but replaced the digging of wild ginseng, but in the southern mountains, ginseng cultivation remains limited.[35] Root diggers and herb gatherers continue to obtain much of their commodities from private properties, whether their owners consent to it, as the law dictates, or not. A 2003 study found that 66 percent of the wild ginseng, 17 percent of galax, and 83 percent of bloodroot and black cohosh harvested in Western North Carolina came from private lands.[36]

Public lands, including those owned by the US Forest Service (USFS), provide commons access to many mountain families, although unlike the de facto commons of the nineteenth century, this de jure commons is subject to an array of federal, state, and international regulations.[37] The Appalachian Landownership Task Force found that some 8 percent of the total surface land in the surveyed area was owned by state and federal governments, including the USFS. From around 1914 through World War II, the USFS purchased large swaths of mountain

lands from timber companies and individual landowners, and by the end
of the century, it owned nearly 5 million acres of land, mostly forested
mountaintops. The federal government now makes decisions on who can
harvest what resources. While timber has historically been given top priority, the USFS has increasingly accorded equal priority to multiple uses,
including hunting, fishing, hiking, and foraging. As part of its mandate
to manage resources according to conservation guidelines, the USFS
requires plant harvesters to purchase low-cost permits, a constraint that
many locals have found onerous. Ginseng has become so scarce that the
USFS has severely restricted the number of permits it distributes,
recently instituting a lottery in North Carolina to determine who gets
one. Locals have mixed views of the forest service, but there is no question that they use national forests. A 1976 survey revealed that some 90
percent of respondents who lived near national forests used them regularly for multiple purposes, including hunting, fishing, firewood collecting, and herb gathering.[38] As they have done for generations, mountain
people continue to turn to the commons—whether it is the de jure commons of national forests or private property still treated as commons—
as a way to squeeze a livelihood out of rural areas that lack stable,
dependable sources of income.

Areas characterized by poverty and unstable wage work rely more
heavily on non-timber forest resources, specifically ginseng. In 2019,
researchers at the University of Georgia found that poverty and high
levels of unemployment were the most important indicators of high ginseng harvest rates.[39] This confirms what Brent Bailey found twenty years
earlier in his study of West Virginia ginseng diggers. In 1994, some 61
percent of West Virginia's ginseng came from an eight-county region in
southwestern West Virginia that produces most of the state's coal.
Boone County, which includes the Coal River valley, topped the list at
eighteen hundred pounds sold that year. It was also the second leading
coal-producing county in the state. The valley sits on top of the state's largest coalfield—the Kanawha—and several large mining companies across
the valley have been engaged in mountaintop removal since the 1970s.
Increased mechanization and the vagaries of global markets make coal
mining an unstable livelihood, and, as they have done throughout their
history when hard times descended upon them, mountain people turn to
the commons, or what is left of it. Coal River Mountain is the only intact

mountain remaining in the Coal River valley. It stands as both a figurative and literal battleground between the forces of modern capitalism engaged in mountaintop removal and a way of life built around the forest commons. Thus, the commons custom continues in Appalachia today in areas of high economic distress, although it faces new enemies—social, cultural, economic, and ecological forces—that make it increasingly tenuous.

Appalachia has changed tremendously over the past hundred years, and the decline of botanical drug markets is just one more adjustment that mountain people have had to make, one more instance in which they were forced to reckon with global market forces that were beyond their control. For generations, they have pieced together livelihoods from whatever resources were available. In the early nineteenth century, those resources came from the farm and the forest, and ginseng was the most important income-producing forest product. As markets for botanical drugs expanded in the late nineteenth century, they could find more marketable commodities in the forest. Some became entirely dependent on them. Most continued to use them to supplement their farm production. With the arrival of large-scale industry and the proliferation of wage work over the course of the twentieth century, some used roots and herbs to insulate themselves from destructive fluctuations in the global economy. Yet these commodities too were creations of global markets, and when these markets declined, people turned to other income-producing activities. And when global demands change and other markets for non-timber forest products expand or open in the future, they will find ways to supply them—if, that is, there are forest commons left.

The story of roots and herbs directs our attention to the peripheries of capitalism, where alternative forms of economy have developed and persisted. On a fundamental level, it points to ways of understanding capitalism and its evolution without assuming the inevitability of progress and efficiency. As Anna Tsing has pointed out, these assumptions have been baked into many analyses of capitalism, from Adam Smith to Karl Marx. The commonly accepted narrative tends to portray the transformation of nature into commodities as a process that always leads to the rationalization of nature and labor. As natural objects are abstracted from their ecological communities, capital is concentrated, the landscape is homogenized, and labor is regimented and commoditized. What would the history of capitalism look like, Tsing asks, without these assumptions?[40] The story of roots and herbs injects contingency back into the narrative of capitalism. In displaying one alternative form of production, it sheds light on how ideas of progress, with its attendant commitment to ever-greater levels of efficiency, have to a large extent shaped the process of commodification as we know it. But there is another story.

A new narrative could go something like this: commodification often leads to rationalization, but not always. It often leads to the enclosure of commons, but it does not have to. When efficiency cannot or will not be maximized—for whatever cultural or ecological reason—labor and nature are free to interact in other ways. Ecological communities may be altered, but they needn't be entirely reshuffled. In this form of salvage capitalism, laborers can occupy a position somewhat akin to independent contractors, utilizing the market in ways that maintain their autonomy and allow them to dictate the terms of their own labor. They can, to a large extent, determine their own parameters for how they engage with the system. Access to commons—either de facto or de jure— is a critical component of this relationship. Commons can provide people many things, including community identity and access to markets, but this access is often precarious and unpredictable. To make it work, the commons must be managed for sustainable use, whether that means using statutes and regulations or creating exclusive commons accessible only to a group of trusted users. If—and it is a big if—we can ensure that the forces of exploitation do not destroy the commons, the social benefits would be great.

The human forces of efficiency are pervasive, however, and they exploit the precarity of commons commodities by offering a "gospel of efficiency" as a stable and superior alternative. They continue to apply pressure to impose organization and order on the landscape. These pressures can be economic (profit motives), cultural (stereotypes), and social (alienation). And thus far, they have been extremely successful. By making it seem like present arrangements were inevitable from the start, development theorists have naturalized the current system. One of the biggest environmental challenges facing the world today is a crisis of imagination, a failure to envision alternatives to the existing structure. In providing a different perspective on capitalism from the bottom up, the root and herb trade—at the very least—fuels the imagination.

Acknowledgments

THIS BOOK, WHICH STARTED AS A GRADUATE SCHOOL SEMINAR PAPER and then a dissertation, would not have been possible without the help of countless individuals along the way. First and foremost, I'd like to thank my wonderful wife, Natalie, without whose support for my education—not to mention her love and unceasing dedication to raising our three boys, Henry, Charlie, and Jack—I would never even have started this project. I have benefited from having some great kin. I would also like to thank my parents, Tom and Debbie Manget, and my sister, Helen, who provided much-needed funds, babysitting, and moral support. I also have to thank my brother, Daniel, who has heard more than he cares to know about ginseng and the commons but who nevertheless continues to indulge me and encourage me, and the rest of my extended family, who helped us survive and enjoy graduate school by ensuring that we had support and enjoyable times. David Martinez, Matt Williams, and my other neighbors at Brandon Oaks Apartments also deserve credit for their regular conversations, encouragement, and friendship.

I have benefited from some excellent mentors along the way. John Inscoe, my major professor, advisor, and friend, deserves more credit than I can say. A one-of-a-kind scholar and mentor, he read anything and everything I put on his desk, from dissertation chapters to articles and seminar papers, and despite his busy schedule, he gave me insightful feedback and encouragement, often over lunch or in the car as he drove me home from campus. At Western Carolina University, I was fortunate to have the guidance of Richard Starnes, who advised my thesis, helped me decide to pursue a PhD, and has remained a friend and advisor ever since. It was Dr. Starnes who read a first-semester graduate student's seminar paper on ginseng and said, "You should try to publish this," sending me on a life-changing road. I want to thank the rest of my dissertation committee as well. Shane Hamilton always provided me with penetrating analysis and provoking questions on my work, and Tim Cleaveland gave me very helpful comments as well as career guidance. Dave Hsiung also provided invaluable support and feedback on early drafts of this manuscript

I could not have written this book without the pioneering scholarship of Kathryn Newfont on the Appalachian commons. I cannot thank her enough for her support and encouragement throughout this process and the many conversations we have had on the commons idea. Many other professors at the University of Georgia, especially Stephen Mihm, Stephen Berry, Brian Drake, Dan Rood, Jamie Kreiner, Cindy Hahamovitch, Scott Nelson, and Jim Cobb, have also provided valuable feedback at different times during my graduate career. Additionally, without the help of the excellent history faculty at Western Carolina University, including Alex Macaulay, Libby McRae, Gael Graham, Andy Denson, and Jessie Swigger, I probably would not have pursued a PhD.

I have been a beneficiary of an excellent community of graduate students at the University of Georgia. My Appalachian history cohorts— Sam McGuire, Kevin Young, James Owen, Kate Dahlstrand, and Robby Poister—have given me countless hours of good conversations, friendship, and comradery that made graduate school enjoyable, not to mention helped me locate sources, attend conferences, and refine arguments. Additionally, I want to thank Kaylynn Washnock, Katie Brackett-Fialka, Ashton Ellett, Kurt Windisch, Trae Welborn, James Wall, Tim Johnson, and Andrew Fialka for helping make LeConte Hall a supportive and congenial place to spend five years.

I would like to thank the many colleagues who have shaped my understanding of Appalachian and environmental history through countless conversations at conferences. These include Steven Nash, Tom Lee, Ron Eller, Dan Pierce, Donald Davis, Brian McKnight, Paul Sutter, Mark Fiege, Lisa Brady, Michael Weeks, Mark Hersey, Bert Way, Tom Okie, and many more.

I literally could not have accomplished this first book without the librarians and archivists who provided advice, and the organizations that supplied financial support. Specifically, the archivists of the W. L. Eury Collection at Appalachian State University, the Wilson Library at University of North Carolina, the North Carolina State Archives, the West Virginia and Regional History Center, and the numerous small county museums like the Ashe County Historical Museum and the Cherokee County Historical Museum were all very helpful in my research. I have to thank Amanda and Greg Gregory, whose fund at the University of Georgia has helped countless graduate students, including myself, conduct research all over the world. The North Caroliniana Society, the Willson Center at the University of Georgia, the Hagley Museum, and the Winterthur Museum, Gardens, and Library have also contributed financially to seeing this project through. Their dedication to learning and research made this book possible.

Notes

Introduction

1. See entries for Henry Webb in Taylor and Moore Store Ledger, 1853–1917, W. L. Eury Appalachian Collection, Special Collections, Belk Library, Appalachian State University, Boone, NC.

2. US Bureau of the Census, *Population Schedules of the 7th Census of the United States, 1850, North Carolina* (Washington, DC: National Archives and Records Service, 1851); US Bureau of the Census, *Population Schedules of the 8th Census of the United States, 1860, North Carolina* (Washington, DC: National Archives and Records Service, 1861); US Bureau of the Census, *Population Schedules of the 9th Census of the United States, 1870, North Carolina* (Washington, DC: National Archives and Records Service, 1871); Taylor and Moore Ledger

3. Details were compiled from Gardner S. Cheney in the US Civil War Soldier Records and Profiles, 1861–1865, Historical Data Systems, Inc., Duxbury, MA 02331, American Civil War Research Database, https://www.ancestrylibrary.com/Discoveryuni-content/view/1587017:1555?tid=&pid=&queryId=736293531402c8dd10545c6a489c3672&phsrc=vek181&_phstart=successSource]; Account Ledger, 1868–1870, Harper Family Account Books, Southern Historical Collection, Wilson Library, University of North Carolina, Chapel Hill; G. W. F. Harper Diary, 1866–1883, G. W. F. Harper Papers, Southern Historical Collection, Wilson Library.

4. See "A Singular Southern Industry," *Atlanta Constitution,* 9 December 1886. This source claimed that an agent for Wallace Brothers, a botanical drug firm in Statesville, North Carolina, purchased roots and herbs from that many people, and that there were a half dozen other firms engaged in the trade.

5. Clare Ewing and Ernest Stanford, "Botanicals of the Blue Ridge," *Journal of the American Pharmaceutical Association* 8, no. 1 (January 1919): 20.

6. Scholars have long known that rural Appalachian people engaged in root digging and herb gathering. See, for example, Ina Yoakley, "Wild Plant Industry of the Southern Appalachians," *Economic Geography* 8, no. 3 (July 1932): 311–

17; Edward T. Price, "Root Digging in the Appalachians: The Geography of Botanical Drugs," *Geographical Review* 50, no. 1 (January 1960): 1–20; Arnold Krochmal, "Medicinal Plants in Appalachia," *Economic Botany* 22, no. 4 (December 1968): 332–37; Alice Henkel, *Wild Medicinal Plants of the United States*, USDA Bureau of Plant Industry Bulletin 89 (Washington, DC: Government Printing Office, 1906); Gary R. Freeze, "Roots, Barks, Berries, and Jews: The Herb Trade in Gilded-Age North Carolina," *Essays in Economic and Business History* 13 (1995): 107–27; Donald Davis, "Medicinal and Cultural Uses of Plants in the Southern Appalachians," in *Homeplace Geography: Essays for Appalachia* (Macon, GA: Mercer University Press, 2006), 165–76; Kathryn Newfont, *Blue Ridge Commons: Environmental Activism and Forest History in Western North Carolina*, Environmental History and the American South (Athens: University of Georgia Press, 2012). The harvesting of what land managers call non-timber forest products in Appalachia today has received in-depth attention from some anthropologists and folklorists. See Mary Hufford, "Knowing Ginseng: The Social Life of an Appalachian Root," *Cahiers de litterature orale* 53–54 (2003): 265–92; Mary Hufford, "Reclaiming the Commons: Narratives of Progress, Preservation, and Ginseng," in *Culture, Environment, and Conservation in the Appalachian South*, ed. Benita J. Howell (Urbana: University of Illinois Press, 2002), 100–120. More recently, two popular books on the ginseng trade, although not focused exclusively on Appalachia, have contributed to a growth in popular interest in the subject: Kristin Johannsen, *Ginseng Dreams: The Secret World of America's Most Valuable Plant* (Lexington: University Press of Kentucky, 2006); David A. Taylor, *Ginseng, the Divine Root* (Chapel Hill, NC: Algonquin Books, 2006). See also David Cozzo, "Herb Gatherers and Root Diggers of Northwestern North Carolina" (MA thesis: Appalachian State University, 1999).

7. The botanical drug trade involved hundreds of different species of plants, each with its own market and each subject to its own ecological and cultural dynamics. Thus this book tries to be sensitive to the uniqueness of each commodity. Ginseng, for example, was unique among the roots and herbs analyzed here because the market for it was in China and was, thus, subject to its own peculiarities. The markets for most other roots and herbs were created by particular cultural and material developments in the United States and Europe in the nineteenth century. But all of these roots and herbs can be analyzed here together as a distinct species of commodity because in the Southern Highlands they were treated as such. At the level of production, they were subject to similar social, cultural, and ecological dynamics.

8. The term *commons* is not a perfect description. Some natural and social scientists may object to the use of the term in this context, as it has come to mean something more specific in these circles. Due to critiques of Garrett Hardin's "Tragedy of the Commons" thesis, most notably by Elinor Ostrom, many scholars have sought to distinguish between true commons, which are managed collectively, and "open-access resources," which are simply naturally occurring

resources that anyone can harvest. While this is a meaningful debate, this book uses "commons" in a more expansive way to acknowledge a variety of competing claims and rights on property and to recognize that some economic activities did not take place on one's own property. This is the way contemporary Americans used the term, or sometimes the singular "common." For more on this debate, see Garrett Hardin, "The Tragedy of the Commons," *Science*, n.s., 162, no. 3859 (December 13, 1968): 1243–48; Elinor Ostrom, *Governing the Commons: The Evolution of Institutions for Collective Action* (New York: Cambridge University Press, 1990); Bryan E. Burke, "Hardin Revisited: A Critical Look at Perception and the Logic of the Commons," *Human Ecology* 29, no. 4 (December 2001): 449–76.

9. Patricia Beaver, Sandra Ballard, and Brittany Hicks, eds., *Voices from the Headwaters: Stories from Meat Camp, Tamarack (Pottertown) & Sutherland, North Carolina* (Boone, NC: Center for Appalachian Studies, 2013), 200–201.

10. The literature on commodities is vast and growing. For more on the intersections of environmental history and capitalism, see Theodore Steinberg, *Nature Incorporated: Industrialization and the Waters of New England* (Amherst: University of Massachusetts Press, 1994); Theodore Steinberg, *Down to Earth: Nature's Role in American History* (Oxford: Oxford University Press, 2002); Mark Kurlansky, *Salt: A World History* (New York: Penguin Books, 2003); John Soluri, *Banana Cultures: Agriculture, Consumption, and Environmental Change in Honduras and the United States* (Austin: University of Texas Press, 2006); Sven Beckert, *Empire of Cotton: A Global History* (repr., New York: Vintage, 2015); Giorgio Riello, *Cotton: The Fabric That Made the Modern World* (repr., Cambridge: Cambridge University Press, 2015); Richard Follett et al., *Plantation Kingdom: The American South and Its Global Commodities* (Baltimore: Johns Hopkins University Press, 2016); Thomas Okie, *The Georgia Peach: Culture, Agriculture, and Environment in the American South,* Cambridge Studies on the American South (New York: Cambridge University Press, 2016); Barbara Hahn, *Making Tobacco Bright: Creating an American Commodity, 1617–1937,* Johns Hopkins Studies in the History of Technology (Baltimore: Johns Hopkins University Press, 2011); Drew A. Swanson, *Beyond the Mountains: Commodifying Appalachian Environments,* Environmental History and the American South (Athens: University of Georgia Press, 2018).

11. Anna Lowenhaupt Tsing, *The Mushroom at the End of the World: On the Possibility of Life in Capitalist Ruins* (Princeton: Princeton University Press, 2015), 5–6, 63–66.

12. Harry M. Caudill, *Night Comes to the Cumberlands: A Biography of a Depressed Area.* (Boston: Little, Brown, 1963); Robert D. Mitchell, *Commercialism and Frontier: Perspectives on the Early Shenandoah Valley* (Charlottesville: University Press of Virginia, 1977); Ronald D. Eller, *Miners, Millhands, and Mountaineers: Industrialization of the Appalachian South, 1880–1930* (Knoxville: University of Tennessee Press, 1982); Paul Salstrom, *Appalachia's Path to Dependency: Rethinking a Region's Economic History, 1730–1940* (Lexington: University Press

of Kentucky, 1994); Wilma A. Dunaway, *The First American Frontier: Transition to Capitalism in Southern Appalachia, 1700–1860* (Chapel Hill: University of North Carolina Press, 1996); Ronald Lewis, *Transforming the Appalachian Countryside: Railroads, Deforestation, and Social Change in West Virginia, 1880–1920* (Chapel Hill: University of North Carolina Press, 1998); Steven Stoll, *Ramp Hollow: The Ordeal of Appalachia* (New York: Hill and Wang, 2017).

13. Ronald Eller, for example, argues that this transition to capitalism occurred in the late nineteenth century when coal and timber companies arrived in the region. Wilma Dunaway, on the other hand, contends that the transition happened much earlier, in the eighteenth century, when trade with the Cherokee pulled them into the capitalist orbit. See Eller, *Miners, Millhands, and Mountaineers;* Dunaway, *The First American Frontier.*

14. Stoll, *Ramp Hollow,* 32–34.

15. Steven Hahn, *The Roots of Southern Populism: Yeoman Farmers and the Transformation of the Georgia Upcountry, 1850–1890* (New York: Oxford University Press, 1983); Crawford King, "The Closing of the Southern Range: An Exploratory Study," *Journal of Southern History* 48, no. 1 (February 1982): 53–70; Shawn Kantor and J. Morgan Kousser, "Common Sense of Commonwealth? The Fence Law and Institutional Change in the Postbellum South," *Journal of Southern History* 59, no. 2 (May 1993): 201–42; Shawn Everett Kantor, *Politics and Property Rights: The Closing of the Open Range in the Postbellum South,* Studies in Law and Economics (Chicago: University of Chicago Press, 1998); Brian Sawers, "Property Law as Labor Control in the Postbellum South," *Law and History Review* 33, no. 2 (May 2015): 351–76.

16. Harry Watson, "'The Common Rights of Mankind': Subsistence, Shad, and Commerce in the Early Republican South," in *Environmental History and the American South: A Reader,* ed. Paul Sutter and Christopher J. Manganiello (Athens: University of Georgia Press, 2009), 131–67; Jack Temple Kirby, *Poquosin: A Study of Rural Landscape & Society* (Chapel Hill: University of North Carolina Press, 1995); Hahn, *The Roots of Southern Populism;* Karl Jacoby, *Crimes against Nature: Squatters, Poachers, Thieves, and the Hidden History of American Conservation* (Berkeley: University of California Press, 2001); Gary Kulik, "Dams, Fish, and Farmers: Defense of Public Rights in Eighteenth-Century Rhode Island," in *The Countryside in the Age of Capitalist Transformation: Essays in the Social History of Rural America,* ed. Steven Hahn and Jonathan Prude (Chapel Hill: University of North Carolina Press, 1985), 25–50; Newfont, *Blue Ridge Commons,* 22.

17. Stephen Aron, *How the West Was Lost: The Transformation of Kentucky from Daniel Boone to Henry Clay* (Baltimore: Johns Hopkins University Press, 1999), 102–23.

18. Christine Keiner, *The Oyster Question: Scientists, Watermen, and the Maryland Chesapeake Bay since 1880* (Athens: University of Georgia Press, 2009).

19. Newfont, *Blue Ridge Commons;* Hufford, "Reclaiming the Commons."

20. Hardin, "The Tragedy of the Commons," 1244.

21. Bonnie J. McCay and James M. Acheson, eds., *The Question of the Commons: The Culture and Ecology of Communal Resources,* Arizona Studies in Human Ecology (Tucson: University of Arizona Press, 1987); Michael Goldman, "'Customs in Common': The Epistemic World of the Commons Scholars," *Theory and Society* 26, no. 1 (February 1997): 1–37; David Feeny et al., "The Tragedy of the Commons: Twenty-Two Years Later," *Human Ecology* 18, no. 1 (1990): 1–19; Bryan E. Burke, "Hardin Revisited: A Critical Look at Perception and the Logic of the Commons," *Human Ecology* 29, no. 4 (December 2001): 449–76; Aletta Biersack and James B. Greenberg, eds., *Reimagining Political Ecology* (Durham: Duke University Press, 2006), 3–40.

22. Ostrom, *Governing the Commons.*

23. The literature on Appalachian stereotypes is vast. A good beginning is Henry D. Shapiro, *Appalachia on Our Mind: The Southern Mountains and Mountaineers in the American Consciousness, 1870–1920* (Chapel Hill: University of North Carolina Press, 1978); Anthony Harkins, *Hillbilly: A Cultural History of an American Icon* (New York: Oxford University Press, 2004); Bruce E. Stewart, *Moonshiners and Prohibitionists: The Battle over Alcohol in Southern Appalachia* (Lexington: University Press of Kentucky, 2011); Altina Waller, *Feud: Hatfields, McCoys, and Social Change in Appalachia, 1860–1900* (Chapel Hill: University of North Carolina Press, 1988); Dwight Billings, Gurney Norman, and Kathryn Ledford, eds., *Confronting Appalachian Stereotypes: Back Talk from an American Region* (Lexington: University Press of Kentucky, 1999); David Hsuing, *Two Worlds in the Tennessee Mountains: Exploring the Origins of Appalachian Stereotypes* (Lexington: University Press of Kentucky, 1997). As Steven Stoll and others have shown, the agents of modernization wielded these stereotypes to justify the modernizing project and effectively excise commons users from the body politic. It was a form of disenfranchisement. Stoll, *Ramp Hollow.*

1. The Journey of Ewing's Roots

1. Unidentified Private Account Book, 1783–1785 [microfilm], Monroe County Court Records, West Virginia History Center, West Virginia University, Morgantown, WV.

2. Pehr Kalm and Adolph B. Benson, *Peter Kalm's Travels in North America: The English Version of 1770* (New York: Dover, 1987).

3. James Mooney, *James Mooney's History, Myths, and Sacred Formulas of the Cherokees: Containing the Full Texts of "Myths of the Cherokee" (1900) and "The Sacred Formulas of the Cherokees" (1891) as Published by the Bureau of American Ethnology; With a New Biographical Introduction* (Asheville, NC: Historical Images, 1992), 425.

4. William Byrd, "Letters of William Byrd II, and Sir Hans Sloane Relative to Plants and Minerals of Virginia," *William and Mary Quarterly,* 2nd ser., 1, no. 3 (July 1921): 199; Kalm and Benson, *Peter Kalm's Travels in North America,* 435.

5. Stephen Fulder, *The Tao of Medicine: Ginseng, Oriental Remedies and the Pharmacology of Harmony* (New York: Destiny Books, 1982), 88–89.

6. James Adair, *History of the American Indians; Particularly Those Nations Adjoining to the Mississippi, East and West Florida, Georgia, South and North Carolina, and Virginia* (London: Edward and Charles Dilly, 1775), 362.

7. William Byrd to William Mayo, 26 August 1731, in William Byrd, William Byrd II, and William Byrd III, *The Correspondence of the Three William Byrds of Westover, Virginia, 1684–1776*, ed. Marion Tining (Richmond: Virginia Historical Society, 1977).

8. It must be noted that while many ginseng diggers, past and present, believe that ginseng grows best on north-facing slopes, modern studies have shown that the plant grows just as well in other places. See James B. McGraw et al., "Ecology and Conservation of Ginseng (Panax Quinquefolius) in a Changing World," *Annals of the New York Academy of Sciences* 1286 (2013): 80.

9. Philip Chadwick Foster Smith, *The Empress of China* (Philadelphia: Philadelphia Maritime Museum, 1984), 41–42.

10. Jun Wen and Elizabeth A. Zimmer, "Phylogeny and Biogeography of PanaxL. (the Ginseng Genus, Araliaceae): Inferences from ITS Sequences of Nuclear Ribosomal DNA," *Molecular Phylogenetics and Evolution* 6, no. 2 (October 1996): 167–77.

11. Qiu-Yun Xiang et al., "Timing the Eastern Asian–Eastern North American Floristic Disjunction: Molecular Clock Corroborates Paleontological Estimates," *Molecular Phylogenetics and Evolution* 15, no. 3 (June 2000): 462–72. Naturalist George Constantz, however, disagrees with the assertion that Asian flora arrived in the New World via Asia, claiming that the migration patterns occurred via Europe. He argues that many of the disjunct species date back further than the era of Beringia. See George Constantz, *Hollows, Peepers, and Highlanders: An Appalachian Mountain Ecology* (Missoula, MT: Mountain, 1994), 43–45.

12. Qiu-Yun Xiang, Douglas E. Soltis, and Pamela S. Soltis, "The Eastern Asian and Eastern and Western North American Floristic Disjunction: Congruent Phylogenetic Patterns in Seven Diverse Genera," *Molecular Phylogenetics and Evolution* 10, no. 2 (October 1998): 178–90.

13. Xiang, Soltis, and Soltis, "Eastern Asian and Eastern and Western North American Floristic Disjunction."

14. This account is largely apocryphal. While there are references to this earlier work in the third and fourth centuries AD, the earliest surviving work, called *Shen-nung pen-ts'ao ching* (Shen Nung's Book of Herbs), was written in the sixth century AD. According to medical historian Paul Unschuld, it is unlikely that the Chinese developed practices of drug therapy until the arrival of Taoism in roughly the fourth century BC. Taoism challenged both the belief in "demonic medicine" of the pre-Confucian era and the medical theories of Confucianism by emphasizing the role of the natural world in human health. Whereas Confucian

thought had held that illness was the result of humans failing to conform to social customs, Taoism asserted that ill health was the consequence of humans failing to live according to the laws of nature. They believed that studying nature could reveal the secrets of human health, and the development of a pragmatic drug therapy based on the study of medicinal herbs was the outgrowth of this cultural development. See Paul U. Unschuld, *Medicine in China: A History of Ideas* (Berkeley: University of California Press, 1985), 101–16; Fulder, *The Tao of Medicine,* 69–70.

15. Fulder, *The Tao of Medicine,* 107–13.

16. John Berthrong, "Motifs for a New Confucian Ecological Vision," in *The Oxford Handbook of Religion and Ecology,* ed. Roger S. Gottlieb (Oxford: Oxford University Press, 2010), 236–65.

17. Fulder, *The Tao of Medicine,* 108–17.

18. In her analysis of the case studies written by sixteenth-century physician Wang Ji, Joanna Grant states that ginseng was Wang's most frequently prescribed herb, used to treat a variety of illnesses. She also suggests that his prescriptions of ginseng were somewhat controversial, which could mean that ginseng was gaining importance. See Joanna Grant, "Medical Practice in the Ming Dynasty—A Practitioner's View: Evidence from Wang Ji's 'Shishan Hi'an,'" *Chinese Science* 15 (1998): 37–80.

19. McGraw et al., "Ecology and Conservation of Ginseng."

20. Morris Rossabi, *Blackwell History of the World: History of China* (Somerset, NJ: John Wiley and Sons, 2013), 265, http://site.ebrary.com/lib/alltitles/docDetail.action?docID=10738690; Gang Zhao, *Perspectives on the Global Past: Qing Opening to the Ocean; Chinese Maritime Policies, 1684–1757* (Honolulu: University of Hawaii Press, 2013), 64–65.

21. [Pierre] Jartoux, "The Description of a Tartarian Plant, Call'd Gin-Seng; with an Account of Its Virtues. In a Letter from Father Jartoux, to the Procurator General of the Missions of India and China. Taken from the Tenth Volume of Letters of the Missionary Jesuits, Printed at Paris in Octavo, 1713," *Philosophical Transactions of the Royal Society of London* 28 (1713), 238, http://archive.org/details/philtrans05305296.

22. Jartoux, "Description of a Tartarian Plant," 241–42.

23. Jartoux, "Description of a Tartarian Plant," 240.

24. James Reardon-Anderson, "Land Use and Society in Manchuria and Inner Mongolia during the Quing Dynasty," *Environmental History* 5, no. 4 (October 2000): 505–7.

25. Because there are few written sources on Native American medicine that predate the advent of the transpacific ginseng trade, it is hard to determine how far back these relationships with ginseng actually go. Some tribes seem to have learned about the plant through native cross-cultural exchanges starting in the nineteenth century; others apparently knew about it only from European traders. It is possible that many native tribes focused more medical attention on the

root because traders paid such a high price for it. The Mikasuki Seminole of Florida incorporated the root into their pharmacopoeia as late as the 1920s after receiving roots from Oklahoma (which were themselves brought from elsewhere). See William Sturtevant, *The Mikasuki Seminole: Medical Beliefs and Practices* (Ann Arbor: University Microfilms International, 1955), 158. The ethnobotanist Huron Smith suggested in 1932 that the Ojibwa's name for the plant, *jissens,* was an attempt to pronounce "ginseng," the traders' term for it. Huron H. Smith, *Ethnobotany of the Ojibwe Indians* (Milwaukee: Public Museum of the City of Milwaukee, 1932), 356.

The Delaware (Lenni Lenape) referred to ginseng as either "Grandmother" or "Grandfather," depending on whether the root was shaped like a man or a woman. They believed it was the most potent of all medicinal herbs and used it both as a general tonic and as a cure-all when other herbs had failed. The Fox tribe (Meskwaki) similarly used it as a love medicine, a "universal remedy" for all ailments, and as a "seasoner" to increase the potency of other medicines. The Mohegan and Menominee tribes also viewed the plant as a panacea. Huron H. Smith, *Ethnobotany of the Meskwaki Indians* (Milwaukee: Public Museum of the City of Milwaukee, 1928), 204; Gladys Tantaquidgeon, *A Study of Delaware Indian Medicine Practice and Folk Beliefs* (Harrisburg: Pennsylvania Historical Commission, 1942), 27; Huron H. Smith, *Ethnobotany of the Menominee* (Milwaukee: Public Museum of the City of Milwaukee, 1923), 24; Gladys Tantaquidgeon, *Folk Medicine of the Delaware and Related Algonkian Indians* (Harrisburg: Pennsylvania Historical and Museum Commission, 1972), 174.

26. Quoted in David N. Cozzo, "Ethnobotanical Classification System and Medical Ethnobotany of the Eastern Band of the Cherokee Indians" (PhD diss., University of Georgia, 2004), 211. Henry Timberlake commented in the 1760s that the Cherokee used it to treat venereal diseases, "which, however, they never had occasion for . . . before the arrival of Europeans among them." Henry Timberlake, *Lieut. Henry Timberlake's Memoirs, 1756–1765,* ed. Samuel Cole Williams (Marietta, GA: Continental, 1948), 70–71.

27. Cozzo, "Ethnobotanical Classification System"; Mooney, *James Mooney's History, Myths, and Sacred Formulas of the Cherokees,* 326.

28. James Mooney, an ethnologist who lived among the Cherokee in the 1880s, hinted that the high prices paid by traders had "doubtless increased their idea of its importance," but prehistoric Cherokee already valued ginseng. Mooney, *James Mooney's History, Myths, and Sacred Formulas of the Cherokees,* 326.

29. Cozzo, "Ethnobotanical Classification System," 136, 209–10; David Cozzo, lecture given 4 October 2010, Western Carolina University, Cullowhee, NC.

30. Adair, *History of the American Indians,* 362.

31. Scholars, specifically anthropologists, have warned against generalizing native cultures to promote an image of an "ecological Indian," but as Annie Booth has argued, Native American tribes did share some common conceptions

of their relationship to nature that can serve as a useful analytical framework for comparing their ecological worldviews with those of Euro-Americans. See Annie L. Booth, "We Are the Land: Native American Views of Nature," in *Nature across Cultures,* ed. Helaine Selin and Arne Kalland (New York: Springer, 2003), 329–30.

32. Booth, "We Are the Land," 332.

33. Heidi M. Altman and Thomas Belt, "Tohi: The Cherokee Concept of Well-being," in *Under the Rattlesnake: Cherokee Health and Resiliency,* ed. Lisa J. Lefler and Susan Foz (Tuscaloosa: University of Alabama Press, 2009), 13–14, http://site.ebrary.com/lib/alltitles/docDetail.action?docID=10387673.

34. The myth of the origins of disease is described in Mooney, *James Mooney's History, Myths, and Sacred Formulas of the Cherokees,* 319–22.

35. Gary Goodwin estimates that eight hundred species were used by the Cherokee. Gary C. Goodwin, *Cherokees in Transition: A Study of Changing Culture and Environment Prior to 1775* (Chicago: University of Chicago Press, 1977), 60.

36. Cozzo, "Ethnobotanical Classification System."

37. Mooney, *James Mooney's History, Myths, and Sacred Formulas of the Cherokees,* 420.

38. John Howard Payne et al., *The Payne-Butrick Papers,* Indians of the Southeast (Lincoln: University of Nebraska Press, 2010), 46, 161.

39. Mooney, *James Mooney's History, Myths, and Sacred Formulas of the Cherokees,* 339.

40. Jartoux, "Description of a Tartarian Plant."

41. Jartoux, "Description of a Tartarian Plant," 238.

42. John Appleby, "Ginseng and the Royal Society," *Notes and Records of the Royal Society of London* 37, no. 2 (March 1983): 121–45.

43. Christopher Parsons, "The Natural History of Colonial Science: Joseph-François Lafitau's Discovery of Ginseng and Its Afterlives," *William and Mary Quarterly* 73, no. 1 (January 2016): 38–51.

44. Kalm and Benson, *Peter Kalm's Travels in North America,* 436.

45. Kalm and Benson, *Peter Kalm's Travels in North America,* 436.

46. Parsons, "The Natural History of Colonial Science," 39.

47. Kalm and Benson, *Peter Kalm's Travels in North America,* 437. Lafitau also warned that "the plant will soon be destroyed near the French habitations." Parsons, "The Natural History of Colonial Science," 68.

48. Kalm and Benson, *Peter Kalm's Travels in North America,* 437.

49. Parsons, "The Natural History of Colonial Science," 67.

50. David L. Preston, *The Texture of Contact: European and Indian Settler Communities on the Frontiers of Iroquoia, 1667–1783,* The Iroquoians and Their World (Lincoln: University of Nebraska Press, 2009), 210.

51. William Byrd II, "The History of the Dividing Line betwixt Virginia and North Carolina Run in the Year of Our Lord 1728," in *The Prose Works of William Byrd of Westover,* ed. Louis B. Wright (Cambridge, MA: Belknap Press of Harvard University Press, 1966), 161.

52. William Byrd to John Perceval, 20 August 1730, in Byrd, Byrd, and Byrd, *Correspondence*.

53. William Byrd to Hans Sloane, 20 August 1738, in Byrd, Byrd, and Byrd, *Correspondence*, 528.

54. William Byrd to Charles Boyle, 18 June 1730, in Byrd, Byrd, and Byrd, *Correspondence*, 431.

55. William Byrd to Peter Collinson, 5 July 1737, in Byrd, Byrd, and Byrd, *Correspondence*, 523.

56. Peter Collinson to John Bartram, 16 September 1741, in John Bartram and Humphry Marshall, *Memorials of John Bartram and Humphry Marshall*, ed. William Darlington (Philadelphia: Lindsay and Blakiston, 1849), 146.

57. *Pennsylvania Gazette*, 27 July 1738.

58. Appleby, "Ginseng and the Royal Society," 133.

59. John Fothergill to John Bartram, 5 January 1769, in Bartram and Marshall, *Memorials*, 339.

60. Peter Collinson to John Bartram, 24 February 1738, in Bartram and Marshall, *Memorials*, 127.

61. Hans Sloane, the king's physician, held some thirteen specimens of the plant in his collection and frequently referred to Du Halde's account. Appleby, "Ginseng and the Royal Society," 126.

62. Kavita Philip, "Imperial Science Rescues a Tree: Global Botanic Networks, Local Knowledge, and the Transcontinental Transplantation of Cinchona," *Environment and History* 1, no. 2 (June 1995): 173–200.

63. William Byrd to Charles Boyle, 18 June 1730, in Byrd, Byrd, and Byrd, *Correspondence*.

64. Joseph Banks to Humphry Marshall, 5 April 1786, in Bartram and Marshall, *Memorials*, 559–60.

65. Humphry Marshall to Joseph Banks, 14 November 1786, in Bartram and Marshall, *Memorials*, 560–61.

66. Without the availability of any systematic study of the ginseng trade, several scholars have implied that the Cherokee engaged in the trade throughout the eighteenth century, but they seem to have based their claim on one source by John Drayton. However, this source was written in 1802 and therefore is referring to the post-Revolution boom. See Wilma A. Dunaway, *The First American Frontier: Transition to Capitalism in Southern Appalachia, 1700–1860* (Chapel Hill: University of North Carolina Press, 1996), 46; Timothy Silver, *A New Face on the Countryside: Indians, Colonists, and Slaves in South Atlantic Forests, 1500–1800*, Studies in Environment and History (Cambridge: Cambridge University Press, 1990), 101.

67. Rather than publicize Beverley's discovery of ginseng in 1729 or promote the economic benefits that the plant could bring to Virginia, he attempted to maintain strict secrecy. Tellingly, when he instructed a surveyor working for him to keep an eye out for ginseng, he made him promise to "tell the secret to no

mortal." While Byrd did attempt to raise his scientific stature by sending roots back to Europe, he did not promote its wild gathering as an economic solution. See William Byrd to William Mayo, 26 August 1731, in Byrd, Byrd, and Byrd, *Correspondence.*

68. Adair, *History of the American Indians,* 362.

69. "Exported from the Upper District of James River between the 25th of October 1765 and the 25th of October 1766," *New York Gazette,* 23 March 1767.

70. Harry Handley, "The Mathews Trading Post," *Journal of the Greenbrier Historical Society* 1, no. 1 (August 1963): 8–14.

71. Kalm and Benson, *Peter Kalm's Travels in North America,* 436; François Michaux, *Michaux's Travels to the West of the Alleghany Mountains* (Carlisle, MA: Applewood Books, 2012), 232.

72. Johann Schoepf, *Travels in the Confederation, 1783–1784,* trans. Alfred Morrison, vol. 1 (Philadelphia: William J. Campbell, 1911), 236. In 1784, on a surveying trip to the Cheat River area in western Virginia, General George Washington similarly encountered "numbers of Persons & Pack horses going in with Ginsang; & salt & other articles at the Markets below." See Donald Jackson and Dorothy Twohig, eds., *The Diaries of George Washington,* vol. 4, *The Papers of George Washington* (Charlottesville: University Press of Virginia, 1978), 20.

73. Smith, *The Empress of China,* 9–12.

74. Smith, *The Empress of China,* 28–34.

75. John Rogers Haddad, *America's First Adventure in China: Trade, Treaties, Opium, and Salvation* (Philadelphia: Temple University Press, 2013), 11–13; Kendall Johnson, "A Question of Character: The Romance of Early Sino-American Commerce in the Journals of Major Samuel Shaw, the First American Consul at Canton (1847)," in *Narratives of Free Trade: The Commercial Cultures of Early US-China Relations,* ed. Kendall Johnson Global Connections (Hong Kong: Hong Kong University Press, 2012), 40–43.

76. Smith, *The Empress of China,* 31.

77. Smith, *The Empress of China,* 38.

78. Smith, *The Empress of China,* 40.

79. Smith, *The Empress of China,* 42.

80. As historian John Haddad has pointed out, ginseng held great symbolic value for many Americans who viewed the root through a brand-new nationalistic lens. If it could help establish a lucrative trade relationship with China independent of European intermediaries, the American dream of economic and political independence might become a reality. See Haddad, *America's First Adventure in China,* 11–14.

81. *Columbia Herald,* 19 January 1786, 2.

82. Samuel Shaw, "Remarks on the Commerce of America with China," *City Gazette,* 30 June 1790.

83. [Repubesco], *City Gazette,* 20 December 1797.

84. Schoepf, *Travels in the Confederation,* 236.

2. Appalachia's First Ginseng Boom and the Evolution of Commons Culture

1. A member of the Massachusetts militia during the Revolution who participated in the Boston Tea Party, May was appointed agent of the Boston-based Ohio Company around 1786 and put in charge of purchasing land for company shareholders under the Land Ordinance of 1785. Among his many land acquisitions in 1786–1787 were areas along the Ohio River at the mouth of Muskingham Creek and Limestone Creek that would, within three years, become sites of the emerging commercial hubs of Marietta (Ohio) and Maysville (Kentucky), respectively. See John May, *The Western Journals of John May, Ohio Company Agent and Business Adventurer* ([Cincinnati]: Historical and Philosophical Society of Ohio, 1961), 3–5, http://archive.org/details/westernjournals000mayj; John May, "Journal of Col. John May, of Boston, Relative to a Journey to the Ohio Country, 1789," *Pennsylvania Magazine of History and Biography* 45, no. 2 (1921).

2. May, "Journal of Col. John May, " 139.

3. May, "Journal of Col. John May," 153. The reason for this depreciation is unclear. In his study of early US-Chinese trade relations, John Haddad claims that the *Empress of China* flooded the market, and by 1786, unbeknownst to many in the backcountry, prices for ginseng in Canton had dropped from $32 a pound to 32 cents per pound. However, the performance of the ginseng market throughout the rest of the eighteenth and nineteenth centuries indicates that the market was virtually impervious to glut. Thus the depreciation in 1789 may have had more to do with the poor quality of the roots on board the *Empress* and the conservative tastes of Chinese consumers. John Rogers Haddad, *America's First Adventure in China: Trade, Treaties, Opium, and Salvation* (Philadelphia: Temple University Press, 2013), 26–27.

4. May, "Journal of Col. John May," 133.

5. May, "Journal of Col. John May," 145.

6. May, "Journal of Col. John May," 161–65.

7. Robert Beverley, *The History and Present State of Virginia, in Four Parts* (London: R. Parker, 1705), 1.

8. Stephen Aron, *How the West Was Lost: The Transformation of Kentucky from Daniel Boone to Henry Clay* (Baltimore: Johns Hopkins University Press, 1996), 103–6.

9. Allan Greer, "Commons and Enclosure in the Colonization of North America," *American Historical Review,* April 2012.

10. François Michaux, *Michaux's Travels to the West of the Alleghany Mountains* (Carlisle, MA: Applewood Books, 2012), 204.

11. Aron explains this best in *How the West Was Lost.*

12. Johann Schoepf, *Travels in the Confederation, 1783–1784,* trans. Alfred Morrison, vol. 1 (Philadelphia: William J. Campbell, 1911), 236, http://hdl.handle.net/2027/uc1.10061306742?urlappend=%3Bseq=259.

13. John Preston, who owned a store in Abingdon, Virginia, as part of his commercial enterprise, became a leading ginseng trader in subsequent decades. In one season in 1826, for instance, he sold 147 barrels of ginseng totaling more than thirteen thousand pounds to a Philadelphia merchant. "Invoice for 147 Barrells of Ginseng," Robert A. Taylor Business Papers, Special Collections, Virginia Tech, Blacksburg.

14. Anonymous Diary, undated folder, John Preston Papers, Virginia Historical Society, Richmond.

15. May, *Western Journals,* 149.

16. There has been some debate about how much ginseng Boone hauled. Nathan Boone told Lyman Draper that they had collected some "twelve or fifteen tons," but recent scholars have challenged this. Believing it is impossible that Boone could have collected and transported thirty thousand pounds of roots upriver, Robert Morgan argues that Boone used the term *tuns,* or barrels, instead of *tons,* as Draper recorded. While this is a definite possibility, it is also possible that Boone, with skilled help over two seasons, could have collected thirty thousand pounds of roots. Writing during a time in which the largely untouched populations of ginseng still covered the ground, two observers in the 1780s estimated that a good digger could harvest sixty in a day. Given 120 days to harvest over a two-year period and assuming that eight diggers averaged around twenty-five pounds a day, they could have reached twelve tons. Nathan Boone et al., *My Father, Daniel Boone: The Draper Interviews with Nathan Boone* (Lexington: University Press of Kentucky, 1999), 81–83.

17. Mathews's father-in-law was Rufus Putnam, a shareholder in the Ohio Company who was instrumental in founding the town of Marietta in 1788. Andrew Clayton, "Marietta and the Ohio Company," in *Appalachian Frontiers: Settlement, Society & Development in the Preindustrial Era,* ed. Robert D. Mitchell, Shenandoah Valley Historical Institute, and American Frontier Culture Foundation (Lexington: University Press of Kentucky, 1991), 187.

18. Joseph Buell and John Mathews, "The Journals of Joseph Buell and John Mathews," in *Pioneer History: Being an Account of the First Examinations of the Ohio Valley, and the Early Settlement of the Northwest Territory, Chiefly from Original Manuscripts,* ed. Samuel P. Hildreth (Cincinnati: H. W. Derby, 1848), 187.

19. Buell and Mathews, "Journals," 188.

20. May, "Journal of Col. John May," 119.

21. Greer, "Commons and Enclosure"; Virginia DeJohn Anderson, *Creatures of Empire: How Domestic Animals Transformed Early America* (Oxford: Oxford University Press, 2006).

22. Kenneth D. Swope, "Ginseng," *Journal of the Greenbrier Historical Society* (1982): 107.

23. Oren Frederic Morton, *A History of Monroe County, West Virginia* (Dayton, VA: Ruebush-Elkins, 1916), 191–94.

24. Unidentified Private Account Book, 1783–1785 [microfilm], Monroe

County Court Records, West Virginia History Center, West Virginia University, Morgantown.

25. List of voters and patentees are found in Morton, *A History of Monroe County*, 80–101, 472–73.

26. Morton, *A History of Monroe County*, 191–93.

27. Edward T. White, "Andrew and Oliver Beirne of Monroe County," *West Virginia History* 20, no. 1 (October 1958): 16–23.

28. Anne Royall, *Sketches of History, Life, and Manners in the United States* (New Haven, CT: Anne Royall, 1826), 36–38.

29. White, "Andrew and Oliver Beirne of Monroe County," 16–23.

30. Michaux, *Michaux's Travels*, 233.

31. This statistic was compiled by the author using export statistics from letters from the secretary of the treasury Alexander Hamilton to the House of Representatives, American State Papers, Commerce and Navigation, 1st–10th Congresses, Library of Congress, Washington, DC, https://memory.loc.gov/cgi-bin/ampage?collId=llsp&fileName=014/llsp014.db&recNum=4.

32. The entire process of ginseng manufacturing is laid out in an 1802 letter from John Rhea to Smithfield, Virginia, planter John Preston. See John Rhea to John Preston, September 1802, box e8-422, Preston Family Papers, 1769–1864, Virginia Historical Society, Richmond.

33. Lian-Wen Qi, Chong-Zhi Wang, and Chun-Su Yuan, "Ginsenosides from American Ginseng: Chemical and Pharmacological Diversity," *Phytochemistry* 72, no. 8 (June 2011): 693, https://doi.org/10.1016/j.phytochem.2011.02.012.

34. John Rhea to John Preston, September 1802, box e8-422, Preston Family Papers, 1769–1864, Virginia Historical Society.

35. John Rhea to John Preston, September 1802, box e8-422, Preston Family Papers, 1769–1864, Virginia Historical Society.

36. Michaux, *Michaux's Travels*, 233.

37. Robert Wellford Diary, 3 June–14 October 1801, Virginia Historical Society, Richmond.

38. Southern Tribes, Communicated to Congress, 12 January 1790, American State Papers, Indian Affairs, vol. 1, 1st Cong., 2nd Sess., no. 9, Library of Congress, Washington DC, https://memory.loc.gov/cgi-bin/ampage?collId=llsp&fileName=007/llsp007.db&recNum=4.

39. John Drayton, *A View of South Carolina, as Respects Her Natural and Civil Concerns* (Charleston: W. P. Young, 1802), 83, http://archive.org/details/viewofsouthcar0100dray.

40. By "Alleghenies," Michaux was referring to the portions of the Appalachian Mountain chain that extend from Pennsylvania down to Georgia. This was a common term used for this geographical region prior to the late nineteenth century, when it was referred to as Appalachia. Michaux, *Michaux's Travels*, 231.

41. Tyler Blethen and Curtis Wood, "A Trader on the Carolina Frontier," in Mitchell, *Appalachian Frontiers*, 150–65.

42. "Ginseng," *Wilmington Daily Herald,* 6 March 1860. This article asserts that Heylin traveled to China but places the date at 1807, which does not make sense given his involvement with the trade at an earlier date.

43. George Hunter, "The Western Journals of Dr. George Hunter, 1796–1805," ed. John Francis McDermott, *Transactions of the American Philosophical Society,* n.s., 53, no. 4 (1963): 42.

44. Moore Family Tree, Ancestry Family Trees, accessed 2 December 2015, ancestry.com.

45. John Lyon, Joseph Ewan, and Nesta Ewan, "John Lyon, Nurseryman and Planter Hunter, and His Journal, 1799–1814," *Transactions of the American Philosophical Society* 53, no. 2 (1963): 39.

46. A. T. Davidson, "Reminiscences of Western North Carolina," *Lyceum,* January 1891, 5–6. For another good source on Smith, see his obituary in "The Late Bacchus Smith," *Asheville Citizen,* 6 August 1886.

47. Conaro Drayton Smith, "Autobiography of Dr. Conaro Drayton Smith VI," in *A History of the Methodist Church in the Toe River Valley,* ed. Lloyd Bailey (Burnsville, NC: Self-published, 1986), 328.

48. Mary Kite, "A Visit to North Carolina," *Friend,* 7 September 1869.

49. Walter H. Lewis and Vincent E. Zenger, "Population Dynamics of the American Ginseng *Panax Quinquefolium* (Araliaceae)," *American Journal of Botany* 69, no. 9 (October 1982): 1483–90.

50. Buell and Mathews, "Journals," 187; Schoepf, *Travels in the Confederation,* 236–37.

51. Michaux, *Michaux's Travels,* 231.

52. Michaux, *Michaux's Travels,* 231.

53. Humphrey Marshall to Joseph Banks, 14 November 1786, in John Bartram and Humphry Marshall, *Memorials of John Bartram and Humphry Marshall,* ed. William Darlington (Philadelphia: Lindsay and Blakiston, 1849).

54. James B. McGraw et al., "Ecology and Conservation of Ginseng (*Panax Quinquefolius*) in a Changing World," *Annals of the New York Academy of Sciences* 1286 (2013): 62–91.

55. McGraw et al., "Ecology and Conservation of Ginseng," 69.

56. Schoepf, *Travels in the Confederation,* 239.

57. Aron, *How the West Was Lost,* 55–57.

58. Michaux, *Michaux's Travels,* 233.

59. May, *Western Journals,* 115.

60. It must be noted that the census category includes the value for "ginseng, and all other productions of the forest." It is unclear what other productions are referred to, and it is impossible to know how much of the sum totals was for ginseng alone. There were separate categories for timber, tar, pitch, turpentine, pot ashes, skins, and furs. US Census Office, *Compendium of the Enumeration of the Inhabitants of the United States of the Sixth Census, 1840* (Washington, DC: Thomas Allen, 1841).

61. In Kentucky, the leading ginseng counties were Perry, Lawrence, Breathitt, Pike, Harlan, Clay, and Knox, all clustered in the mountainous eastern portion of the state. In West Virginia, large amounts of ginseng came from Logan, Cabell, and Jackson Counties, located on the eastern bank of the Tug Fork.

62. US Census Office, *Compendium of the Enumeration of the Inhabitants of the United States, 1840.*

63. US Census Office, *Compendium of the Enumeration of the Inhabitants of the United States, 1840.*

64. US Census Office, *Compendium of the Enumeration of the Inhabitants of the United States, 1840.*

65. Determined from manuscript census records. Ancestry.com, *1850 United States Federal Census* (Provo, UT: Ancestry.com Operations, 2009).

66. Ronald L. Lewis, *Transforming the Appalachian Countryside: Railroads, Deforestation, and Social Change in West Virginia, 1880–1920* (Chapel Hill: University of North Carolina Press, 1998), 85.

67. Thomas Miller and Hu Maxwell, *West Virginia and Its People,* vol. 2 (New York: Lewis Historical Publishing, 1913), 157.

68. The economic impact of the forest commons was greater than these numbers would suggest, however. First of all, rural people drew heavily on many resources from the forest commons, including fish, game, livestock forage, and berries, that did not register as a market transaction, as households used these resources at home. Furthermore, much of the cash used by customers likely came from hogs, of which some $13,000 worth were owned by Randolph County farmers in 1850. Most farmers, as elsewhere in Appalachia, relied on the forest commons to raise them. Marking their hogs' ears to identify them, they turned them out into the forests for most of the year to feed on mast such as acorns and chestnuts before rounding them up in the fall to slaughter or drive to overland markets. Additionally, sheep were frequently herded along the mountaintops to graze on native grasses. Ely Butcher Store Account Books, Randolph County, 1841–1883, West Virginia State Archives, Charleston. US Census Bureau, *Statistical View of the United States . . . , Being a Compendium of the Seventh Census* (Washington, DC: Government Printing Office, 1854), 321–23.

69. John Davison Sutton, *History of Braxton County and Central West Virginia* (Sutton, WV, 1919), 213, http://archive.org/details/historyofbraxton00sutt.

70. Sutton, *History of Braxton County,* 213.

71. This can be seen in US Census Office, *Compendium of the Enumeration of the Inhabitants of the United States, 1840.* In the fifty-two counties of western Virginia (now West Virginia), $35,000 worth of ginseng was sold, whereas only $22,000 of skins and furs were sold in 1841. Moreover, exports from 1790 to 1820, as conveyed in letters from the treasury secretary to the House of Representatives in the American State Papers, indicates a steady decline in skins and furs.

72. Sutton, *History of Braxton County*, 214.

73. "Diary of James B. Hamilton," in *History of Fayette County, West Virginia*, ed. J. T. Peters and H. B. Carden (Charleston, WV: Jarrett, 1926), 200–212.

74. Ancestry.com, *1860 United States Federal Census*.

75. Ely Butcher Store Account Books.

76. "Ginseng," *People's Press* (Winston-Salem, NC), 23 February 1860.

77. Buell and Mathews, "Journals," 183.

78. Hunter, "Western Journals," 38–39.

79. Barbara Rasmussen, *Absentee Landowning and Exploitation in West Virginia, 1760–1920* (Lexington: University Press of Kentucky, 1994), 29–31; Wilma A. Dunaway, *The First American Frontier: Transition to Capitalism in Southern Appalachia, 1700–1860* (Chapel Hill: University of North Carolina Press, 1996), 52–57; Aron, *How the West Was Lost*, 60–63.

80. This conflict between commons users and landowners is more fully explained in chapter 6.

81. Arthur Spaulding, *Men of the Mountains: The Story of the Southern Mountaineer and His Kin of the Piedmont; with an Account of Some of the Agencies of Progress among Them* (Nashville: Southern Publishing Association, 1915), 171.

82. See, for example, Kathryn Newfont, *Blue Ridge Commons: Environmental Activism and Forest History in Western North Carolina*, Environmental History and the American South (Athens: University of Georgia Press, 2012), 22–35.

83. John Nuttall, *Trees Above with Coal Below* (San Diego: Neyenesch, 1961), 18.

84. Royall, *Sketches of History, Life, and Manners*, 56.

85. John Sherwood Lewis, "Becoming Appalachia: The Emergence of an American Subculture, 1840–1860" (PhD diss., University of Kentucky, 2000).

86. "The Mountains of West Virginia," *Forest and Stream*, 19 August 1875.

87. Davidson, "Reminiscences," 5–6.

88. See, for example, Dunaway, *The First American Frontier*, 185–86.

89. Pehr Kalm and Adolph B. Benson, *Peter Kalm's Travels in North America: The English Version of 1770* (New York: Dover, 1987), 437.

90. Jonathan Edwards to William McCulloch, 24 November 1752, quoted in "Ginseng," *Fur-Fish-Game Magazine* 5–6 (Summerville, NJ, 1907): 56.

91. William Holland Thomas to H. P. King, 9 August 1839, Southeastern Native American Documents, 1730–1842, Galileo, Digital Library of Georgia, https://dlg.usg.edu/.

92. William Holland Thomas to Isaac Heylin, 22 November 1839, Southeastern Native American Documents, 1730–1842.

93. US Census Office, *Compendium of the Enumeration of the Inhabitants of the United States, 1840*.

94. See, for example, Ledger and Indian Accounts, 1840–1858, Quallatown, Haywood County, NC, William H. Thomas Papers, Rubenstein Rare Book and

Manuscript Collection, Duke University, Durham, NC. See also Ledger [New Firm], 1839–1843, William H. Thomas Papers.

95. Thomas Green, for example, bought $5 worth of chestnuts in 1839. See Ledger [New Firm], 1839–1843, William H. Thomas Papers.

96. The Siler store ledger can be found at the Macon County Historical Museum, Franklin, NC. There are two ledgers from William Walker's store that have survived the ages. One is located at the Cherokee County Historical Museum, Murphy, NC. The other, while it is not identified as Walker's ledger, can be found labeled North Carolina Store Account Book, 1850–1871, North Carolina Department of Archives and History, Raleigh. A. R. S. Hunter's store ledger is located in the Cherokee County Historical Museum.

97. He instructed his manager in Qualla Town to give 1 cent per pound more for it than his competitor, Nimrod S. Jarrett, offered. See William Holland Thomas to H. P. King, 9 August 1839, Southeastern Native American Documents, 1730–1842.

98. See US Census Office, *Agriculture of the United States in 1860; Compiled from the Original Returns of the Eighth Census, under the Direction of the Secretary of the Interior* (Washington, DC: Government Printing Office, 1864).

99. John R. Finger, *The Eastern Band of Cherokees, 1819–1900* (Knoxville: University of Tennessee Press, 1984), 13–15.

100. Johnson W. King, Affidavit, 21 August 1843, box 2, William H. Thomas Papers.

101. Ely Butcher Store Account Books.

102. Henry Colton, *The Scenery of the Mountains of Western North Carolina and Northwestern South Carolina* (Raleigh, NC: W. L. Pomeroy, 1859), 97.

103. J. Q. A. Clowes, "Ginseng Planting, Medial Properties and Experiences, Etc.," *Special Crops* 5, no. 43 (March 1906): 44–45.

104. Ely Butcher Store Account Books.

105. Michaux, *Michaux's Travels*.

106. W. Scott Persons, *American Ginseng: Green Gold*, rev. ed (Asheville, NC: Bright Mountain Books, 1994), 9.

3. Marketing the Mountain Commons

1. Calvin J. Cowles to Martha Cowles, 28 October 1850, Calvin J. Cowles Papers, Southern Historical Collection, University of North Carolina, Chapel Hill.

2. Ellen McGrew, "Calvin Josiah Cowles," in *Dictionary of North Carolina Biography*, ed. William Powell (Chapel Hill: University of North Carolina Press, 1979), NCPedia, https://www.ncpedia.org/biography/cowles-calvin-josiah.

3. "Dr. Carter wants a pound of Seneka Snake Root," his father informed Calvin Cowles after the 1848 season. See Josiah Cowles to Calvin J. Cowles, 21 January 1849, and "A List of Produce Sent to Alva Spears," 9 December 1848,

both in Calvin J. Cowles Papers, North Carolina Department of Archives and History, Raleigh.

4. "A History of the Worth Family in Ashe County," David Worth Family Papers, W. L. Eury Appalachian Collection, Special Collections, Belk Library, Appalachian State University, Boone, NC.

5. Josiah Cowles to Calvin J. Cowles, 29 October 1849, Calvin J. Cowles Papers, North Carolina Department of Archives and History.

6. Discussions of this schism can be found in John S. Haller, *Medical Protestants: The Eclectics in American Medicine, 1825–1939* (Carbondale: Southern Illinois University Press, 1994), 24–27; Richard H. Shryock, *Medicine and Society in America, 1660–1860* (New York: New York University Press, 1960), 49–50; Barbara Van der Zee, *Green Pharmacy: A History of Herbal Medicine* (New York: Viking, 1982), 132–53.

7. Shryock, *Medicine and Society,* 49–75; Haller, *Medical Protestants,* x–27.

8. Van der Zee, *Green Pharmacy,* 133–66.

9. Quoted in Van der Zee, *Green Pharmacy,* 138.

10. Haller, *Medical Protestants,* 5.

11. A good primer on Euro-American settlers and their perceptions of health and the environment is Conevery Bolton Valenčius, *The Health of the Country: How American Settlers Understood Themselves and Their Land* (New York: Basic Books, 2004).

12. Virgil Vogel, *American Indian Medicine* (Norman: University of Oklahoma Press, 1970), 129; Anthony P. Cavender, *Folk Medicine in Southern Appalachia* (Chapel Hill: University of North Carolina Press, 2003).

13. John Lawson, *A New Voyage to Carolina: Containing the Exact Description and Natural History of That Country, Together with the Present State Thereof. And a Journal of a Thousand Miles, Traveled through Several Nations of Indians, Giving a Particular Account of Their Customs, Manners, &c.* (London, 1709), 10–11.

14. James Adair, *History of the American Indians; Particularly Those Nations Adjoining to the Mississippi, East and West Florida, Georgia, South and North Carolina, and Virginia* (London: Edward and Charles Dilly, 1775), 234; Thomas Ashe, *Travels in America, Performed in 1806, for the Purposes of Exploring the Rivers Alleghany, Monongahela, Ohio, and Mississippi, and Ascertaining the Produce and Condition of Their Banks and Vicinity* (London: William Sawyer, 1808), 5.

15. Van der Zee, *Green Pharmacy,* 132–34.

16. Esther Louise Larson and Peter Kalm, "Peter Kalm's Short Account of the Natural Position, Use, and Care of Some Plants, of Which the Seeds Were Recently Brought Home from North America for the Service of Those Who Take Pleasure in Experimenting with the Cultivation of the Same in Our Climate," *Agricultural History* 13, no. 1 (January 1939): 33–64; Christopher Hobbs, "The Medical Botany of John Bartram," *Pharmacy in History* 33, no. 4 (1991): 181–89; Laura E. Ray, "Podophyllum Peltatum and Observations on the Creek and Cher-

okee Indians: William Bartram's Preservation of Native American Pharmacology," *Yale Journal of Biology and Medicine* 82, no. 1 (March 2009): 25–36.

17. Van der Zee, *Green Pharmacy*, 134.

18. Van der Zee, *Green Pharmacy*, 152.

19. The best account of this is Richard William Judd, *The Untilled Garden: Natural History and the Spirit of Conservation in America, 1740–1840* (Cambridge: Cambridge University Press, 2009), 94–109.

20. Haller, *Medical Protestants*, 14–17, xv.

21. Quoted in Haller, *Medical Protestants*, 10.

22. Leonard Warren, *Constantine Samuel Rafinesque: A Voice in the American Wilderness* (Lexington: University Press of Kentucky, 2004).

23. *The Pharmacopoeia of the United States of America* (Philadelphia: John Grigg, 1831), 1–38.

24. J. W. Cooper, *The Experienced Botanist; or, Indian Physician* (Lancaster, PA: J. W. Cooper, 1840), vi.

25. Samuel Thomson, *New Guide to Health; or, Botanic Family Physician: Containing a Complete System of Practice, upon a Plan Entirely New; With a Description of the Vegetables Made Use of, and Directions for Preparing and Administering Them to Cure Disease* (Boston: J. Q. Adams, 1835), 6.

26. The best account of Thomson and Thomsonism is in John S. Haller, *The People's Doctors: Samuel Thomson and the American Botanical Movement, 1790–1860* (Carbondale: Southern Illinois University Press, 2000). See also Alex Berman and Michael A. Flannery, *America's Botanico-Medical Movements: Vox Populi* (New York: Pharmaceutical Products, 2001).

27. Haller, *Medical Protestants*, 46–51.

28. Haller, *Medical Protestants*, 51.

29. John C. Gunn, *Gunn's Domestic Medicine; or, Poor Man's Friend: Describing in Plain Language, the Diseases, of Men, Women, and Children, and the Latest and Most Approved Means Used in Their Cure; Designed Especially for the Use of Families*, 13th ed. (Pittsburgh: J. Edwards and J. J. Newman, 1839), 13, 17.

30. Ben H. McClary, "Introducing a Classic: *Gunn's Domestic Medicine*," *Tennessee Historical Quarterly* 45, no. 3 (Fall 1986): 210–16.

31. James Harvey Young, *The Toadstool Millionaires: A Social History of Patent Medicines in America before Federal Regulation* (Princeton: Princeton University Press, 1961), 34–37.

32. See, for example, the advertisement in the *Louisville Daily Courier*, 22 February 1859.

33. Young, *Toadstool Millionaires*, 60–68.

34. The best historical account of the patent medicine industry remains Young, *Toadstool Millionaires*, 52–75.

35. Thomson, *New Guide to Health*, 38.

36. Haller, *The People's Doctors*, 14–17.

37. C. S. Rafinesque, *Medical Flora; or, Manual of the Medical Botany of the United States of North America* (Philadelphia: Atkinson and Alexander, 1828), 60.

38. John U. Lloyd, "Resin of Podophyllum and Podophyllin," *American Journal of Pharmacy,* December 1890, 606.

39. John King, *The American Eclectic Dispensatory* (Cincinnati: Moore, Wilstach, Keys, 1856), 843–44, http://archive.org/details/americaneclectic00kinguoft.

40. Rafinesque, *Medical Flora,* 79.

41. See, for example, William Tully, "An Essay, Pharmacological and Therapeutical, on Sanguinaria-Canadensis, with a Plate. Sanguinaria-Canadensis," *American Medical Recorder* 13, no. 1 (January 1828): 1.

42. Gunn, *Gunn's Domestic Medicine,* 454; King, *The American Eclectic Dispensatory,* 704.

43. Jacob Bigelow, *American Medical Botany: Being a Collection of the Native Medicinal Plants of the United States, Containing Their Botanical History and Chemical Analysis, and Properties and Uses in Medicine, Diet and the Arts, with Coloured Engravings* (Boston: Cummings and Hilliard, 1817), 94.

44. See Rafinesque, *Medical Flora,* 56.

45. Bigelow, *American Medical Botany,* 94.

46. William P. C. Barton, *Vegetable Materia Medica of the United States; or, Medical Botany* (Philadelphia: M. Carey and Son, 1818), 200.

47. Gunn, *Gunn's Domestic Medicine,* 453.

48. The following discuss important developments in the rise of botanical pharmacy, although none discuss the supply of crude drugs: Berman and Flannery, *America's Botanico-Medical Movements,* 115–47; John P. Swann, "The Evolution of the American Pharmaceutical Industry," *Pharmacy in History* 37, no. 2 (1995): 76–86; John Uri Lloyd, "The Eclectic Alkaloids, Resins, Resinoids, Oleoresins, and Concentrated Principles," *Bulletin of the Lloyd Library of Botany, Pharmacy, and Materia Medica* 12, no. 2 (1910): 1–54; Amy Bess Williams Miller, *Shaker Herbs: A History and a Compendium* (New York: C. N. Potter, 1976); Michael A. Flannery, *Civil War Pharmacy: A History of Drugs, Drug Supply and Provision, and Therapeutics for the Union and Confederacy,* Pharmaceutical Heritage (New York: Pharmaceutical Products, 2004).

49. Miller, *Shaker Herbs;* Edward D. Andrews, *The Community Industries of the Shakers,* New York State Museum Handbook 15 (Albany: University of the State of New York, 1933), 87–95.

50. The Shakers may have been the first to produce and distribute manufactured plant medicines on a wide scale, although the historical record is not clear about it. Based on claims made in the mid-nineteenth century by Shakers, author Amy Miller argues that Shakers had begun their operations shortly after the turn of the nineteenth century, making them the first by several years. However, written records for that period of Shaker history are rare, and there is no mention of

the industry until the early 1820s, at which point New Lebanon became the first to enter the trade. Regardless, it is safe to say that the Shakers were one of the first to mass manufacture plant medicine. See Miller, *Shaker Herbs*, 5–7.

51. Ledger, New Lebanon, 1827–1838, Edward Deming Andrews Shaker Collection, Winterthur Museum, Garden, and Library, Winterthur, DE.

52. Harvard Herb Dept Accounts, 1847–1853, Edward Deming Andrews Shaker Collection.

53. Rafinesque, *Medical Flora*, 17.

54. There is some dispute about the details of the company's founding. Some scholars have cited the date as 1824, when Elam Tilden, the father of future New York governor and Democratic presidential candidate Samuel J. Tilden, purportedly opened a botanical manufacturing establishment. However, several nineteenth-century sources suggest that Henry A. Tilden, a son of Elam, started the business around 1847 with the help of a "seceder" from the New Lebanon Society. In 1838, a former Shaker named Josephus Seeley, who had lived with the New Lebanon Society for twenty years, wrote a deposition in which he laid out details of a conspiracy in which he helped Tilden, who was then owner of a store in New Lebanon, establish himself in the herb business. He confessed that after leaving the society in 1835, he and another "seceder" from the Shakers, Aaron Gilbert, aided Tilden & Co. in purchasing herbs at wholesale prices from a Hancock Shaker named Lewis Wheeler, who was, in turn, pocketing the money. Regardless of the veracity of the details, it is clear that Tilden's business began sometime prior to 1835 amid suspicious circumstances and that it was heavily influenced by, if not a replica of, the Shaker model. See Flannery, *Civil War Pharmacy*, 30–33; "Tilden & Co. and the Medical Journals," *American Journal of Pharmacy*, January 1859, 86: Josephus Seeley, Letter Regarding the Illegal Sale of Herbs, 1838, Edward Deming Andrews Shaker Collection.

55. "The Valley of New Lebanon (N.Y.) as a Source of Medicinal Plants," *American Journal of Pharmacy*, November 1855, 567A.

56. "The Valley of New Lebanon (N.Y.) as a Source of Medicinal Plants," 567A; "New Lebanon: Its Physic Gardens and Their Products," *American Journal of Pharmacy*, October 1851, 386.

57. The Shakers actually claimed that they should be credited with the development of vacuum evaporation, but Tilden & Co. vigorously denied this. The *American Journal of Pharmacy* sided with Tilden in this debate. See "Tilden & Co. and the Medical Journals," 86; "Extracts Prepared in Vacuo," *American Journal of Pharmacy*, April 1852, 187.

58. See Account Books, New Lebanon, NY, 1855–1871, Edward Deming Andrews Shaker Collection.

59. Samuel Thomson, "Caution! Caution," *Boston Thomsonian Manual*, December 1840; B. O. Wilson and G. C. Wilson, *Botanic Materia Medica; or, The Physician's Guide to the Remedies of the Botanic Kingdom* (Boston: John Putnam,

1850); Tom Mahoney, *Merchants of Life: An Account of the American Pharmaceutical Industry* (New York: Harper and Brothers, 1959), 1–9.

60. "Death of Dr. Ayer," *Farmer's Cabinet*, 9 July 1878.

61. In 1828, Rafinesque encouraged pharmacists to more thoroughly investigate the chemical properties of plants. "The active principles of medical plants may be obtained in a concentrated form by chemical operations," he wrote. Quoted in Edward Kremers, George Urdang, and Glenn Sonnedecker, *Kremers and Urdang's History of Pharmacy*, 4th ed. (Philadelphia: Lippincott, 1976), 175.

62. Berman and Flannery, *America's Botanico-Medical Movements*, 126–28; Lloyd, "The Eclectic Alkaloids, Resins, Resinoids, Oleoresins, and Concentrated Principles," 20.

63. King, *The American Eclectic Dispensatory*, ix, 441, 596, 749.

64. "New Lebanon: Its Physic Gardens and Their Products," 88.

65. "Report on the Drug Market," *Proceedings of the American Pharmaceutical Association at the Ninth Annual Meeting, Held in the City of New York, September 1860* (Philadelphia: Merrihew and Thompson, 1860), 86.

66. B .O. and G. C. Wilson to Calvin J. Cowles, 1 March 1850, folder 9, Calvin J. Cowles Papers, Southern Historical Collection.

67. Calvin J. Cowles to Tilden & Co., 25 January 1851, folder 111.25.1, Calvin J. Cowles Papers, North Carolina Department of Archives and History.

68. Root Accounts, 1851–1858, J and C. J. Cowles, vol. 59, Calvin J. Cowles Papers, Southern Historical Collection.

69. For pricing, see Root Accounts, 1851–1858, J and C. J. Cowles, Calvin J. Cowles Papers, Southern Historical Collection.

70. Barter Book, 1853–1856, vol. 73, Calvin J. Cowles Papers, Southern Historical Collection.

71. While ascending the mountains en route from Charleston in 1775, Bartram remarked that the soil was "of an excellent quality for the production of every vegetable suited to the climate" not only of the southern uplands but also of "Pennsylvania, New York and even Canada." William Bartram, *Travels of William Bartram*, ed. Francis Harper (Athens: University of Georgia Press, 1997), 213; André Michaux, "Journal of André Michaux, 1793–1796," in *Travels West of the Alleghenies: Made in 1793–96 by André Michaux; in 1802 by F. A. Michaux; and in 1803 by Thaddeus Mason Harris, M.A.*, ed. Reuben Gold Thwaites (Cleveland: Arthur Clark, 1904), 288.

72. Charles F. Jenkins, "Asa Gray and His Quest for Shortia Galacifolia," *Arnoldia* 2, nos. 3–4 (1946): 18–28.

73. Ronald H. Peterson, "Moses Ashley Curtis's 1839 Expedition into the North Carolina Mountains," *Castanea* (*Southern Appalachian Botanical Society*) 53, no. 2 (June 1988): 110–21.

74. Asa Gray, "Notes of a Botanical Excursion to North Carolina," in *Scien-*

tific Papers of Asa Gray, vol. 2: *Essays, Biographical Sketches,* ed. Charles Sprague Sargent (Boston: Houghton Mifflin, 1889), 34.

75. Gray, "Notes of a Botanical Excursion," 53–54.

76. A good biography of Gray is A. Hunter Dupree, *Asa Gray: American Botanist, Friend of Darwin* (Baltimore: Johns Hopkins University Press, 1988).

77. Gray, "Characteristics of the North American Flora," in *Scientific Papers of Asa Gray,* vol. 2: *Essays, Biographical Sketches,* 276.

78. D. E. Boufford and S. A. Spongberg, "Eastern Asian–Eastern North American Phytogeographical Relationships: A History from the Time of Linnaeus to the Twentieth Century," *Annals of the Missouri Botanical Garden* 70 (1983): 423–39.

79. S. B. Buckley, "Notes of a Botanical Tour," *Southern Agriculturist, Horticulturist, and Register of Rural Affairs,* July 1846; S. B. Buckley, "Notes of a Botanical Tour, No. II," *Cultivator,* July 1845; S. B. Buckley, "Notes of a Botanical Tour, No. III," *Cultivator,* September 1845; S. B. Buckley, "Botanical Tour, No. IV," *Cultivator,* November 1845; S. B. Buckley, "Notes of a Botanical Tour, No. V," *Cultivator,* June 1846.

80. Peterson, "Moses Ashley Curtis's 1839 Expedition," 117.

81. S. B. Buckley, "Botanical Tour, No. IV," 339.

82. Drew A. Swanson, *Beyond the Mountains: Commodifying Appalachian Environments,* Environmental History and the American South (Athens: University of Georgia Press, 2018), 33–52.

83. Calvin J. Cowles to B. O. and G. C. Wilson, 15 March 1851, Calvin J. Cowles Papers, North Carolina Department of Archives and History.

84. Calvin J. Cowles to Mr. Arthur, 6 July 1852, Calvin J. Cowles Papers, North Carolina Department of Archives and History.

85. Accounts of Cowles's botanical drug customers can be found in Root Accounts, 1851–1860, Calvin J. Cowles Papers, Southern Historical Collection.

86. Cavender, *Folk Medicine,* 55.

87. Cavender, *Folk Medicine,* 25.

88. Cavender, *Folk Medicine,* 25.

89. Cavender, *Folk Medicine,* 24–25.

90. Florence Cope Bush, *Dorie: Woman of the Mountains* (Knoxville: University of Tennessee Press, 1992), 25.

91. Cavender, *Folk Medicine,* 33.

92. Bush, *Dorie,* 25.

93. Cavender, *Folk Medicine,* 197–201; Judith Bolyard, *Medicinal Plants and Home Remedies of Appalachia* (Springfield, IL: Charles C. Thomas, 1981).

94. Josiah Cowles to Calvin J. Cowles, 19 March 1849, Calvin J. Cowles Papers, North Carolina Department of Archives and History.

95. Josiah Cowles to Calvin J. Cowles, 11 May 1849, Calvin J. Cowles Papers, North Carolina Department of Archives and History.

96. Calvin J. Cowles to James Kaime, 24 May 1855, folder 111.26, Calvin J. Cowles Papers, North Carolina Department of Archives and History.

97. Calvin J. Cowles to Mr. McAllister, 15 July 1852, folder 111.25.3, Calvin J. Cowles Papers, North Carolina Department of Archives and History.

98. See Adelaide Fries, ed., *Records of the Moravians in North Carolina*, vol. 2: *1752–1775* (Raleigh: Edwards and Broughton, 1925), 571.

99. Gray, "Notes of a Botanical Excursion," 47.

100. Gray, "Notes of a Botanical Excursion," 66.

101. For a great discussion of Appalachian plant communities, see Timothy P. Spira, *Wildflowers & Plant Communities of the Southern Appalachian Mountains & Piedmont: A Naturalist's Guide to the Carolinas, Virginia, Tennessee, & Georgia*, A Southern Gateways Guide (Chapel Hill: University of North Carolina Press, 2011), 345–46, 388–89, 417, 445–46.

102. See, for example, Bush, *Dorie.*

103. The clearest evidence for this comes from the ginseng trade in West Virginia. See Ely Butcher Store Account Books, Randolph County, 1841–1883, West Virginia State Archives, Charleston.

104. 1850 census, accessed through University of Virginia's Historical Census Browser, http://mapserver.lib.virginia.edu/.

105. Calvin J. Cowle to Mr. Arthur, 6 July 1852, folder 111.25.3, Calvin J. Cowles Papers, North Carolina Department of Archives and History.

106. W. C. Norwood, "Veratrum Viride, or American Hellebore," *New Jersey Medical Reporter and Transactions of the New Jersey Medical Society*, February 1853, 154.

107. See Calvin J. Cowles to Larkin Maxwell, 24 May 1855, folder 111.26, Calvin J. Cowles Papers, North Carolina Department of Archives and History.

4. Mountain Entrepreneurs

1. James R. Troyer, "The Hyams Family, Father and Sons, Contributors to North Carolina Botany," *Journal of the Elisha Mitchell Scientific Society* 117, no. 4 (2001): 240.

2. See, for example, entry on p. 55 of Day Book, 1867–1868, vol. 99, Calvin J. Cowles Papers, Southern Historical Collection, University of North Carolina, Chapel Hill; M. E. Hyams to Calvin J. Cowles, 29 January 1863, folder 111.6, Calvin J. Cowles Papers, North Carolina Department of Archives and History, Raleigh. At least one scholar has asserted that he formed a partnership with Cowles, but Cowles's records do not indicate that this was the case. See Troyer, "The Hyams Family," 241. Although Troyer does not attribute this claim, he undoubtedly relied on William S. Powell, "Mordecai E. Hyams," in *Dictionary of North Carolina Biography*, vol. 3, ed. William S. Powell (Chapel Hill: University of North Carolina Press, 1988), 246. Primary sources disagree on this topic. In 1891, the *Wilkesboro Chron-*

icle asserted that Hyams had received "training and experience while with Mr. Cowles in this county," but Charles Hyams, Mordecai's son, rebutted this claim in the *Statesville Landmark,* saying that Hyams received no training or experience from him. See Charles Hyams, "Historical Facts," *Statesville Record and Landmark,* 17 September 1891.

3. Hyams, "Historical Facts"; see also Gary R. Freeze, "Roots, Barks, Berries, and Jews: The Herb Trade in Gilded-Age North Carolina," *Essays in Economic and Business History* 13 (1995): 112–13.

4. The entrance of Wallace Brothers into the root and herb business is obscured by history. According to historian Gary Freeze, one local tradition claims that the brothers began by selling herbs from their Statesville store to the Confederate government. Another asserts that the New York drug firm Olcott, McKesson, & Co. induced the Wallaces to sell them herbs. Freeze, "Roots, Barks, Berries, and Jews," 112–13. Hyams himself took credit for convincing the Jewish merchants to enter the trade. See Hyams, "Historical Facts."

5. See "The Herb Depot," *Charlotte Observer,* 19 December 1888.

6. "The Valley of New Lebanon (N.Y.) as a Source of Medicinal Plants," *American Journal of Pharmacy,* November 1855; "New Lebanon: Its Physic Gardens and Their Products," *American Journal of Pharmacy,* October 1851, 386–88.

7. John Maisch, "Report on the Drug Market," in *Proceedings of the American Pharmaceutical Association at Its Twelfth Annual Meeting Held in Cincinnati, O., September 1864* (Philadelphia: Merrihew and Son, 1864), 197–98.

8. This can be seen most readily in Inventory of the Money and Stock Held at the Beginning of Each Year, 1839–1864, vol., 38, Shaker Manuscripts, Case Western Reserve University, Cleveland, OH. It can also be observed in the daybook kept at the New Lebanon herb department from 1860 to 1862, which suggests business continued as usual: Account Book, New Lebanon Community, 1860–1862, ASC 839, Edward Deming Andrews Shaker Collection, Winterthur Museum, Garden, and Library, Winterthur, DE. An entry for 25 October 1861: "Received an order from California for over 100 lbs fluids." In June 1861, there was another mention of sending 960 pounds of extracts to Chicago. In the fall of 1860, the Shakers of New Lebanon were producing roughly 500–600 pounds of extracts monthly, and by 1862, the number had risen to 600–700 pounds of solid and fluid extracts.

9. "Union and Confederate Standard Supply Tables," reprinted in Michael A. Flannery, *Civil War Pharmacy: A History of Drugs, Drug Supply and Provision, and Therapeutics for the Union and Confederacy,* Pharmaceutical Heritage (New York: Pharmaceutical Products, 2004), 239–48.

10. Flannery, *Civil War Pharmacy,* 117–18.

11. Flannery, *Civil War Pharmacy,* 150–55.

12. Flannery, *Civil War Pharmacy,* 98–109.

13. Flannery, *Civil War Pharmacy,* 109–14.

14. Flannery, *Civil War Pharmacy,* 192–202; Joseph Jacobs, "Drug Condi-

tions during the War between the States," in *Proceedings of the American Pharmaceutical Association at the Forty-Sixth Annual Meeting, Held at Baltimore, MD, August 1898* (Baltimore: American Pharmaceutical Association, 1898), 198–200.

15. Jacobs, "Drug Conditions during the War between the States," 195.

16. Jacobs, "Drug Conditions during the War between the States," 204.

17. Flannery, *Civil War Pharmacy*, 173.

18. Scott Legan, "Drugs for Louisiana: The Louisiana State Laboratory, 1864–1865," *Louisiana History* 48, no. 2 (Spring 2007): 193–202; Guy Hasegawa, "'Absurd Prejudice': A. Snowden Piggot and the Confederate Medical Laboratory at Lincolnton," *North Carolina Historical Review* 81, no. 3 (July 2004): 313–34; Guy Hasegawa, "The Confederate Medical Laboratories," *Southern Medical Journal* 96, no. 12 (December 2003): 1221–30.

19. Hasegawa, "'Absurd Prejudice,'" 327.

20. Quoted in Norman Franke, "Official and Industrial Aspects of Pharmacy in the Confederacy," *Georgia Historical Quarterly* 37, no. 3 (September 1953): 179.

21. The CSA Supply Table is reprinted in Flannery, *Civil War Pharmacy,* 249–56.

22. F. Peyre Porcher, "A Medico-Botanical Catalogue of the Plants and Ferns of St. John's, Berkeley, South Carolina," *Southern Journal of Medicine and Pharmacy* 2 (1847): 255–417; Allan D. Charles, "The Man with the Microscope," *Sandlapper* (Winter 1997–1998): 33–35.

23. F. Peyre Porcher, "Resources of the Southern Fields and Forests," *De Bow's Review* 6, no. 2 (August 1861): 2.

24. Francis Peyre Porcher, *Resources of the Southern Fields and Forests, Medical, Economical, and Agricultural: Being Also a Medical Botany of the Southern States with Practical Information on the Useful Properties of the Trees, Plants, and Shrubs,* rev. ed. (Charleston, SC: Walker, Evans, and Cogswell, 1869).

25. A good discussion of the influence of slaves on Porcher's medical knowledge can be found in Martia Goodson, "Enslaved Africans and Doctors in South Carolina," *Journal of the National Medical Association* 95, no. 3 (March 2003): 225–33.

26. Porcher, *Resources of the Southern Fields and Forests,* 33–34.

27. The Opinion of Mr. Ravenel as Expressed in a Letter to the Author, and Reviews of F. P. Porcher's *Resources of the Southern Fields and Forests,* Porcher Family Collection, South Carolina Historical Society, Charleston. Many thanks to Dr. Lester Stephens for sending me this file.

28. Porcher, *Resources of the Southern Fields and Forests,* x.

29. William Gilmore Simms, "Porcher's Resources of the South," *Journal of Materia Medica* [1869], undated clipping in Reviews of F. P. Porcher's *Resources of the Southern Fields and Forests.*

30. Moore told Porcher in 1864 that it "has been distributed widely among Medical Officers." Communication from Surgeon General S.P. Moore, CSA, to the author upon completion of the task assigned him, in Reviews of F. P. Porcher's *Resources of the Southern Fields and Forests.*

31. Quoted in Flannery, *Civil War Pharmacy,* 66.

32. A price list can be found in *Carolina Watchman,* 28 July 1862.

33. For example, Porcher identifies the mountains as the primary location of spikenard (*Aralia racemose*), wild sarsaparilla (*Aralia nudicaulis*), ginseng, blue cohosh (*Caulophyllum thalictroides*), willow herb (*Epilobium augustifolium*), Seneca snakeroot (*Polygala senega*), Indian physic (*Gillenia trifolata*), American ipecac (*Gillenia stipulacea*), and many more. See Porcher, *Resources of the Southern Fields and Forests,* 51, 52, 54, 59, 91, 175.

34. M. E. Hyams, "The Botanic Business of Western North Carolina," *Charlotte Democrat,* 23 November 1877.

35. Calvin J. Cowles to James J. Waring, 25 December 1861, Calvin J. Cowles Papers, North Carolina Department of Archives and History.

36. Calvin J. Cowles to James J. Waring, 25 December 1861, Calvin J. Cowles Papers, North Carolina Department of Archives and History.

37. James J. Waring to Calvin J. Cowles, 15 February 1862, Calvin J. Cowles Papers, North Carolina Department of Archives and History.

38. Calvin J. Cowles to Marion Howard, 16 July 1862, Calvin J. Cowles Papers, North Carolina Department of Archives and History

39. Porcher, *Resources of the Southern Fields and Forests,* 606; J. and C. J. Cowles, Contract with Medical Purveyor, 25 November 1862, Calvin J. Cowles Papers, North Carolina Department of Archives and History. For another list of Cowles's orders from Howard, see entry for M. Howard in Root Accounts, 1850–1860, Calvin J. Cowles Papers, Southern Historical Collection, University of North Carolina, Chapel Hill.

40. Calvin J. Cowles to Marion Howard, 7 November 1862, Calvin J. Cowles Papers, North Carolina Department of Archives and History.

41. Samuel P. Moore to Calvin J. Cowles, 6 March 1863, folder 111.6, Calvin J. Cowles Papers, North Carolina Department of Archives and History.

42. See Marion Howard to Calvin Cowles, 4 October 1862, Calvin J. Cowles Papers, North Carolina Department of Archives and History; Calvin J. Cowles to Marion Howard, 10 October 1862, Calvin J. Cowles Papers, North Carolina Department of Archives and History.

43. See Calvin J. Cowles to Marion Howard, 26 September 1862, Calvin J. Cowles Papers, North Carolina Department of Archives and History.

44. Calvin J. Cowles to Marion Howard, 22 January 1863, Calvin J. Cowles Papers, North Carolina Department of Archives and History.

45. Calvin J. Cowles to M. A. Curtis, 5 February 1863, Calvin J. Cowles Papers, North Carolina Department of Archives and History.

46. M. A. Curtis to Calvin J. Cowles, 17 February 1863, Calvin J. Cowles Papers, North Carolina Department of Archives and History.

47. M. A. Curtis to Calvin J. Cowles, 17 February 1863, Calvin J. Cowles Papers, North Carolina Department of Archives and History.

48. Calvin J. Cowles to M. A. Curtis, 26 February 1863, Calvin J. Cowles Papers, North Carolina Department of Archives and History.

49. Calvin J. Cowles to M. A. Curtis, 5 February 1863, Calvin J. Cowles Papers, North Carolina Department of Archives and History.

50. M. A. Curtis to Calvin J. Cowles, 29 December 1862, Calvin J. Cowles Papers, North Carolina Department of Archives and History.

51. "Attention All," *Carolina Watchman,* 28 July 1862.

52. Norman Franke, "Medico-Pharmaceutical Conditions and Drug Supply in the Confederate States of America, 1861–1865" (PhD diss., University of Wisconsin–Madison, 1956).

53. Flannery, *Civil War Pharmacy,* 229.

54. Anthony P. Cavender, *Folk Medicine in Southern Appalachia* (Chapel Hill: University of North Carolina Press, 2003), 70–77.

55. Arthur D. Cowles to Calvin J. Cowles, 4 December 1877, folder 87, Calvin J. Cowles Papers, Southern Historical Collection.

56. Mahlon Kline, "The Origin and History of the National Wholesale Druggists' Association," *American Journal of Pharmacy,* November 1900, 520–30.

57. Edward Kremers, George Urdang, and Glenn Sonnedecker, *Kremers and Urdang's History of Pharmacy,* 4th ed. (Philadelphia: Lippincott, 1976), 327–31.

58. Kremers, Urdang, and Sonnedecker, *Kremers and Urdang's History of Pharmacy,* 330.

59. Charles O. Lee, "Shakers as Pioneers in the American Herb and Drug Industry" (paper presented to the American Pharmaceutical Association, 1959), Edward Deming Andrews Shaker Collection.

60. Flannery, *Civil War Pharmacy,* 235.

61. James Harvey Young, *The Toadstool Millionaires: A Social History of Patent Medicines in America before Federal Regulation* (Princeton: Princeton University Press, 1961), 110.

62. Kremers, Urdang, and Sonnedecker, *Kremers and Urdang's History of Pharmacy,* 325.

63. Young, *The Toadstool Millionaires,* 93–144.

64. See, for example, the advertisement in the *Lenoir (NC) Topic,* 17 February 1881.

65. *Tulsa Daily World,* 8 November 1916.

66. "Report of the Committee on the Drug Market," *Proceedings of the American Pharmaceutical Association at the Twenty-Second Annual Meeting, Held in Louisville, KY, September 1874* (Philadelphia: Sherman, 1875), 617.

67. C. Lewis Diehl, "Indigenous Drugs," *Proceedings of the American Pharmaceutical Association at the Eighteenth Annual Meeting, Held in Baltimore, MD, September 1870* (Philadelphia: Sherman, 1870), 137–38.

68. Diehl, "Indigenous Drugs," 137–38.

69. Andrew A. Scroggs, "A Report to the Agricultural Society of North Caro-

lina on Medicinal Plants, Roots, Etc., Dated October 18, 1871," RG 5029, N.C. Department of Archives and History, Raleigh.

70. "Roots and Herbs," *Farmer's Cabinet,* 20 September 1871.

71. W. C. Kerr, "Communication from the State Geologist to the State of North Carolina," *Legislative Documents,* no. 27, session 1868–69 (Raleigh: State Printer, 1870), 50–51.

72. See, for example, *Branson's North Carolina Business Directory for 1872* (Raleigh: Branson and Jones, 1873).

73. State Board of Agriculture, *North Carolina and its Resources* (Raleigh: M. I. and J. C. Stewart, 1896), 23.

74. Calvin J. Cowles to B. Keith, 30 September 1865, Calvin J. Cowles Papers, North Carolina Department of Archives and History.

75. Calvin J. Cowles to Arthur Cowles, 11 November 1865, Calvin J. Cowles Papers, North Carolina Department of Archives and History.

76. Calvin J. Cowles to Samuel P. Moore, 19 September 1865, Calvin J. Cowles Papers, North Carolina Department of Archives and History.

77. Root and Herb Shipments, 1865–1867, Vol. 96, Calvin J. Cowles Papers, Southern Historical Collection.

78. *Weekly North Carolina Standard,* 7 November 1866; see also Ellen McGrew, "Calvin J. Cowles," in *Dictionary of North Carolina Biography,* vol. 1, ed. William S. Powell (Chapel Hill: University of North Carolina Press, 1979), 444–45.

79. McGrew, "Calvin J. Cowles"; see also Susan Sokol Blosser, "Calvin J. Cowles's Gap Creek Mine: A Case Study in Mine Speculation in the Gilded Age," *North Carolina Historical Review* 51, no. 4 (October 1974): 379–400. A good discussion of Cowles's postwar career can be found in Steven E. Nash, *Reconstruction's Ragged Edge: The Politics of Postwar Life in the Southern Mountains,* Civil War America (Chapel Hill: University of North Carolina Press, 2016).

80. Arthur Lloyd Fletcher, *Ashe County: A History,* Contributions to Southern Appalachian Studies 14 (Jefferson, NC: McFarland, 2006), 233.

81. Unfortunately, I have been unable to locate the records of Arthur D. Cowles, but some of his correspondence has been preserved in the Calvin J. Cowles Papers, Southern Historical Collection. See Messrs Garrison and Murray, Chicago, Ill., in a/c with A. D. Cowles, 10 August 1871, folder 72; see also Price List, 6 June 1870, Calvin J. Cowles Papers, Southern Historical Collection.

82. Scroggs, "A Report to the Agricultural Society of North Carolina."

83. See, for example, Ledger, James Harper, 1856–1858, vol. 18, and Ledger, J. Harper and Son, 1859–1861, vol. 22, Harper Family Account Books, Southern Historical Collection, Wilson Special Collections Library, University of North Carolina, Chapel Hill.

84. Richard A. Shrader, "George Washington Finley Harper," in Powell, *Dictionary of North Carolina Biography,* vol. 3, 37–38.

85. See G. W. F. Harper Diaries, vols. 17–26, G. W. F. Harper Papers, Southern Historical Collection, Wilson Special Collections Library.

86. See Ledger, G. W. and S. F. Harper, 1868–1871, vol. 28, Harper Family Account Books. Also, see Produce Books, 1869–1871, Bernhardt-Seagle Company Records, Southern Historical Collection, Wilson Special Collections Library. Buyers included Coolidge, Adams, and Bond (New York); Cheney, Myrick, and Hobbs (Boston); William Peek & Co. (New York); Wilson and Burns (Baltimore); B. Keith & Co. (New York); and William S. Merrell (Cincinnati).

87. G. W. F. Harper to Joel Curtis, 6 March 1871, folder 54, Bernhardt-Seagle Company Records.

88. See entry for 26 May 1869, G. W. F. Harper Diaries, vol. 19.

89. "Report of the Committee on Exhibition of Specimens," *Proceedings of the American Pharmaceutical Association at the Twenty-First Annual Meeting, Held in Richmond, VA, September 1873* (Philadelphia: Sherman, 1874), 453.

90. M. E. Hyams, "The Botanic Business of Western North Carolina" (paper presented to the North Carolina State Agricultural Society), *Charlotte Democrat,* 23 November 1877.

91. Hyams, "The Botanic Business of Western North Carolina."

92. Asa Gray, "Roots and 'Yarbs'—In the Mountains of North Carolina," *American Agriculturist,* September 1879.

93. William Simpson, "The Names of Medicinal Plants of Commercial Value That Are Gathered in North Carolina: Their Value, and Relative Amount Sold in This Country and Exported," *American Journal of Pharmacy,* October 1894, 488.

94. Freeze, "Roots, Barks, Berries, and Jews," 114–15.

95. Simpson, "The Names of Medicinal Plants," 488.

96. Hyams, "The Botanic Business of Western North Carolina." C. E. Wiley, a resident of North Carolina who worked for the US Treasury Department, visited the Wallaces and reported to the US House of Representatives that "while many of the articles are found in other States, most of them abound chiefly in this, some are peculiar to this region, and no other locality is so favorable to the business as a whole." See C. H. Wiley, "North Carolina," in *The Executive Documents of the House of Representatives for the Second Session of the Forty-Ninth Congress, 1886–87* (Washington, DC: Government Printing Office, 1887), 231.

97. Simpson, "The Names of Medicinal Plants," 488.

98. Scroggs, "A Report to the Agricultural Society of North Carolina."

99. "A Singular Southern Industry," *Atlanta Constitution,* 9 December 1886.

100. Hyams, "The Botanic Business of Western North Carolina."

101. "A Singular Southern Industry."

102. Hyams, "The Botanic Business of Western North Carolina."

103. Freeze, "Roots, Barks, Berries, and Jews," 115.

104. "The Late Prof. M. E. Hyams," *Statesville (NC) Landmark,* 21 May 1891.

105. Charles F. Jenkins, "Asa Gray and His Quest for Shortia Galacifolia," *Arnoldia* 2, nos. 3–4 (1946): 9.

106. Jenkins, "Asa Gray and His Quest for Shortia Galacifolia," 10.

107. J. H. Redfield, "Notes of a Botanical Excursion into North Carolina," *Bulletin of the Torrey Botanical Club* 6, nos. 55–56 (July–August 1879): 333. Gray's description of the Wallace brothers' business can be found in Gray, "Roots and 'Yarbs,'" 337–38.

108. Quotes from Freeze, "Roots, Barks, Berries, and Jews," 121.

109. "A Great Misfortune," *Hickory (NC) Press*, 10 October 1895.

110. Freeze, "Roots, Barks, Berries, and Jews," 121–23.

111. William Connelley and E. M. Coulter, *History of Kentucky*, vol. 5 (Chicago: American Historical Society, 1922), 41. A good history of the R. T. Greer Herb Company can be found at Sherry Joines Wyatt, R. T. Greer and Company Root and Herb Warehouse National Register of Historic Places Nomination, 2003, North Carolina Historic Preservation Office, Raleigh; see also "J. Q. McGuire & Co., Dealers in Crude Botanical Drugs, etc," *Asheville Gazette-News*, 16 August 1909.

112. *Watauga Democrat*, 23 November 1905.

113. See Valle Crucis Company Records, 1907–1952, W. L. Eury Appalachian Collection, Appalachian State University, Boone, NC.

114. "Geography of U.S. Botanical Drugs," *Pharmaceutical Era*, March 1919, 63–66. For a discussion of the impacts of World War I on the drug trade, see Martin Wilbert, "The Source and Supply of Medicines, with Special Reference to the Interference Caused by the Existing European War," *Public Health Reports* 29, no. 41 (October 1914): 2715.

115. Clare Ewing and Ernest Stanford, "Botanicals of the Blue Ridge," *Journal of the American Pharmaceutical Association* 8, no. 1 (January 1919): 16.

116. "Geography of U.S. Botanical Drugs," 65.

117. Ewing and Stanford, "Botanicals of the Blue Ridge," 20.

118. "The Story of S. B. Penick: The House of Botanicals," *Medical Times* (1960): 526–29; J. D. Ratcliff, "From Sandalwood to Ant Eggs," *Saturday Evening Post*, 11 October 1947.

119. Joseph Jacobs, "Southern Herbs in War Hospitals," *Atlanta Constitution*, 1 September 1918.

120. Ratcliff, "From Sandalwood to Ant Eggs."

121. Ratcliff, "From Sandalwood to Ant Eggs."

122. "Penick Elected Drug President," *Asheville Citizen*, 8 May 1929.

123. *Watauga Democrat*, 1 May 1919.

124. Wyatt, R. T. Greer and Company Root and Herb Warehouse National Register of Historic Places Nomination.

125. Wyatt, R. T. Greer and Company Root and Herb Warehouse National Register of Historic Places Nomination, 10.

126. Connelley and Coulter, *History of Kentucky*, 41.

127. This is based on an extrapolation of one month's worth of business. From 16 March to 16 April 1928, the company paid harvesters $8,675. See R. T.

Greer and Co. Check Register, 1928–1929, R. T. Greer Herb Company Records, 1918–1946, State Library of Virginia, Richmond.

128. R. T. Greer and Co. Check Register, 1928–1929.

129. Wyatt, R. T. Greer and Company Root and Herb Warehouse National Register of Historic Places Nomination, 10.

130. August Gattinger, *The Medicinal Plants of Tennessee* (Nashville: Franc M. Paul, State Printer, 1894), xi.

5. Nature's Emporium

1. In 2002, John Inscoe, one of the deans of Appalachian history, commented that the Reconstruction era "remains one of the least examined eras" in the region's history. See John C. Inscoe, "The Discovery of Appalachia: Regional Revisionism as Scholarly Renaissance," in *A Companion to the American South,* ed. John Boles (Malden, MA: Blackwell, 2002), 377–78. Since then, several good works of scholarship have been published on the Reconstruction era, including Andrew L. Slap, ed., *Reconstructing Appalachia: The Civil War's Aftermath* (Lexington: University Press of Kentucky, 2010); Steven E. Nash, *Reconstruction's Ragged Edge: The Politics of Postwar Life in the Southern Mountains,* Civil War America (Chapel Hill: University of North Carolina Press, 2016); T. R. C. Hutton, *Bloody Breathitt: Politics and Violence in the Appalachian South,* New Directions in Southern History (Lexington: University Press of Kentucky, 2013); Bruce E. Stewart, *Moonshiners and Prohibitionists: The Battle over Alcohol in Southern Appalachia* (Lexington: University Press of Kentucky, 2011). The foci of this scholarship remain the politics of Civil War loyalty, violence, and stereotypes.

2. E. B. Olmsted to Lanman and Kemp, 14 September 1870, folder: 12 Letters, WLEAC from a Ginseng Expedition in WNC plus two Pamphlets 1870, W. L. Eury Appalachian Collection, Special Collections, Appalachian State University, Boone, NC (hereafter cited as 12 Letters, WLEAC).

3. A Cherokee man named James Taylor claimed that the lands the state sold Olmsted were actually his, and he spent the next several decades trying to get them back. Although his claim was dismissed by the Treasury Department in 1915, Olmsted's financial reputation casts suspicion over the deal, and Taylor's allegations may well have been accurate. See *Cong. Rec.*, 64th Cong., 1st sess. (1915), 146, 187.

4. His concern for his family is revealed in the following statement he made to Lanman and Kemp on 14 September 1870: "My embarrassed . . . condition gives me great anxiety for my dear family of wife and four boys—and were it not that my eldest son is receiving $1200 as a clerk in the Census Bureau we should be in actual want." Information on Olmstead's arrest and prosecution is patchy, leaving an incomplete picture of the deal he struck with the federal government. James Taylor's (see preceding note) petition to the Treasury Depart-

ment indicates that Olmsted had turned over his lands to the federal government as part of his settlement sometime after his arrest, but questions still remain as to why he was not imprisoned for embezzlement. In his letters to Lanman and Kemp, he referred to "my land" in Cherokee County, suggesting that in 1870, when he made his trip to the county, he had not yet turned over his land to the government. It is possible, therefore, that he was on the lam again. For more information on Olmsted's arrest and his deal with the government, see "The Case of Mr E.B. Olmsted," *Daily National Intelligencer* (Washington, DC), 21 October 1868; *Alexandria Gazette,* 20 October 1868; "Washington Items," *Alexandria Gazette,* 23 September 1868; *Cong. Rec.,* 64th Cong., 1st sess. (1915), 146.

5. Olmsted to Lanman and Kemp, 10 September 1870, 12 Letters, WLEAC.

6. The fact that Lanman and Kemp did not deal in botanic drugs is evident from the company's many orders and price lists in correspondence with various buyers and suppliers. See Lanman and Kemp records, Hagley Museum and Library, Wilmington, DE.

7. *US Census Reports, 1850–1860,* Historical Census Browser, Geospatial and Statistical Data Center, University of Virginia, accessed 26 November 2010, http://fisher.lib.virginia.edu/collections/stats/histcensus/index.html.

8. US Bureau of the Census, *Agriculture of the United States in 1860,* 104; these statistics are noted in Donald Edward Davis, *Where There Are Mountains: An Environmental History of the Southern Appalachians* (Athens: University of Georgia Press, 2000), 131.

9. *US Census Reports, 1860–1870,* Historical Census Browser, Geospatial and Statistical Data Center, University of Virginia, accessed 26 November 2010, http://fisher.lib.virginia.edu/collections/stats/histcensus/index.html.

10. Paul Salstrom, *Appalachia's Path to Dependency: Rethinking a Region's Economic History, 1730–1940* (Lexington: University Press of Kentucky, 1994), 14–15; Robert Tracy McKenzie, "'Oh, Ours Is a Deplorable Condition': The Economic Impact of the Civil War," in *The Civil War in Appalachia: Collected Essays,* ed. Shannon H. Wilson and Kenneth W. Noe (Knoxville: University of Tennessee Press, 2004), 199–226.

11. John Muir, *A Thousand-Mile Walk to the Gulf* (Boston: Houghton Mifflin, 1916), 37.

12. Muir, *Thousand-Mile Walk to the Gulf,* 40–41.

13. Franklin Hough, *A Report upon Forestry, Prepared under the Direction of the Commissioner of Agriculture in Pursuance of an Act of Congress Approved August 15, 1876,* vol. 2 (Washington, DC: Government Printing Office, 1880), 374; Frederick Watts, *Report of the Secretary of Agriculture, United States Department of Agriculture, for the Year 1872* (Washington, DC: Government Printing Office, 1872), 452.

14. US House of Representatives, *The Annual Report of the Chief of the Bureau of Statistics, on the Commerce and Navigation of the United States for the Fiscal Year Ended June 30, 1872,* Ex. Doc. No. 242, 42nd Cong., 3rd sess., 172.

15. According to Olmsted (Letter to Lanman and Kemp, 8 October 1870), the average digger dug two pounds per day. In 1867, North Carolina mandated a ginseng season that began the first of September, giving diggers less than two months to dig ginseng before the leaves fell off. To sustain that level of trade, if everyone adhered to the season (which typically did not happen), would require seven hundred diggers. If two pounds was the average day's production, even if the roots were dug in the summer, it is safe to say that there were hundreds of people around Murphy engaged in digging ginseng. *US Census Reports, 1860–1870.*

16. Depending on how much dealers paid diggers (somewhere between 25 and 27 cents per pound, according to Watts), the ginseng trade generated anywhere from $18,750 to $23,000 in 1871. According to the 1870 Census, Cherokee County residents earned $6,202 in farming wages and $5,429 in manufacturing wages, and they collected $4,853 in orchard products, $90 in forest products, and $80 in garden products. They also produced $14,629 worth of home manufactures, suggesting that ginseng production was second only to the value of total farm production ($203,743). *US Census Reports, 1860–1870.*

17. "North Carolina," *New York Herald,* 29 April 1867.

18. "Letters of Itinerant," *Raleigh Sentinel,* 7 November 1867.

19. Export statistics were culled from annual communications on exports from the treasury secretary to the US Congress. Prior to 1817, these can be found in the American State Papers, Commerce and Navigation, Library of Congress, Washington, DC, accessed 26 November 2010, https://memory.loc.gov/cgi-bin/ampage?collId=llsp&fileName=014/llsp014.db&recNum=4. After 1817, they can be found in the US Congressional Serial Set, Library of Congress, Washington, DC, accessed 26 November 2010, https://memory.loc.gov/ammem/amlaw/lwsslink.html. These statistics are also corroborated by Alvar Carlson, who also used statistics from the US Treasury Department's reports on foreign commerce and navigation. See Alvar Carlson, "Ginseng: America's Drug Connection to the Orient," *Economic Botany* 40, no. 2 (April–June 1986).

20. By the late 1860s, the great Minnesota ginseng boom that began in 1859 appeared to diminish, and other ginseng-producing areas in the North and Midwest, though they still contributed to the trade, suffered more from overharvesting and deforestation. The amount of ginseng exported from Minnesota fell from its peak of 245,434 pounds in 1860 to under 90,000 pounds in 1866. In 1860 and 1861, Minnesota ginseng comprised the great bulk of total US exports, but by 1866, that proportion had dropped to less than one-fifth of the nation's totals. See William E. Lass, "Ginseng Rush in Minnesota," *Minnesota History* 41, no. 6 (Summer 1969): 249–66. One group of scientists has conducted historical surveys of herbarium collections for ginseng and three related plants to determine the extent of ginseng harvesting over the past 150 years across nineteen states, concluding that there were "significant decreases" in the frequency of specimens found in the herbariums of six of the northern states in

ginseng's range, while its southern range, along with Ohio and Illinois, "showed no significant changes." See Martha A. Case, Kathryn M. Flinn, Jean Jancaitis, Ashley Alley, and Amy Paxton, "Declining Abundance of American Ginseng (*Panax quinquefolius L.*) Documented by Herbarium Specimens," *Biological Conservation* 134 (2007): 22–30. Writers of the period consistently refer to the ginseng of northern states becoming scarce and in danger of extinction. See, for example, "Big Profits in Ginseng," *New York Sun,* 17 September 1899; *Third Annual Report of the Pennsylvania Department of Agriculture, Part I* (Harrisburg: William Stanley Ray, State Printer, 1898). One root buyer from Charleston, West Virginia, told Arthur Harding that he consistently traveled through much of the South and Midwest and obtained more of the root from West Virginia, Kentucky, and Tennessee than he did from Ohio or Indiana. See Arthur Robert Harding, *Ginseng and Other Medicinal Plants: A Book of Valuable Information for Growers as Well as Collectors of Medicinal Roots, Barks, Leaves, etc.* (Columbus, OH: AR Harding 1908), 155. Nicholas Pike, who published a widely read article in *Scientific American* in 1891, was "quite surprised" to find poor farmers in "back of the Catskills" who found ginseng in a strip of forest twenty miles long, but he feared that the plants "will soon be exterminated." This anecdote reveals the nature of ginseng digging in the North. It was conducted on a much smaller scale, geographically and demographically, than in the South. Pike, "The Ginseng," *Scientific American,* 10 January 1891.

21. Olmsted to Lanman and Kemp, 22 September 1870, 12 Letters, WLEAC.

22. Olmsted to Lanman and Kemp, 29 September 1870, 12 Letters, WLEAC.

23. Olmsted to Lanman and Kemp, 3 October 1870, 12 Letters, WLEAC.

24. Olmsted to Lanman and Kemp, 29 September 1870, 12 Letters, WLEAC.

25. Olmsted to Lanman and Kemp, 8 October 1870, 12 Letters, WLEAC.

26. Olmsted to Lanman and Kemp, 8 October 1870, 12 Letters, WLEAC.

27. Carlos B. Paseador, *Ginseng: The Crop That's Worth Its Weight in Sterling Silver* (Joplin, MO: Chinese-American Ginseng Co., 1901), 5.

28. Olmsted to Lanman and Kemp, 14 October 1870, 12 Letters, WLEAC.

29. Olmsted to Lanman and Kemp, 8 October 1870, 12 Letters, WLEAC.

30. Thomas's lands would be included in the boundaries of Swain County when it was carved out of Jackson in 1871. The actual number of Cherokee in Cherokee County may have been higher; Olmsted estimated three thousand.

31. James Mooney, *James Mooney's History, Myths, and Sacred Formulas of the Cherokees: Containing the Full Texts of "Myths of the Cherokee" (1900) and "The Sacred Formulas of the Cherokees" (1891) as Published by the Bureau of American Ethnology; With a New Biographical Introduction* (Asheville, NC: Historical Images, 1992), 180–81.

32. See Olmsted to Lanman and Kemp, 8 October 1870, 12 Letters, WLEAC.

33. *Fourth Annual Report of the Bureau of Labor Statistics of the State of North Carolina for the Year 1890* (Raleigh: State Printers, 1890), 254.

34. Olmsted to Lanman and Kemp, 3 October 1870, 12 Letters, WLEAC.

35. Olmsted to Lanman and Kemp, 3 October 1870, 12 Letters, WLEAC.

36. Olmsted to Lanman and Kemp, 8 October 1870, 12 Letters, WLEAC.

37. Olmsted to Lanman and Kemp, 3 October 1870, 12 Letters, WLEAC.

38. Olmsted to Lanman and Kemp, 8 October 1870, 12 Letters, WLEAC.

39. "North Carolina," *New York Herald,* 29 April 1867, 4.

40. *US Census Reports, 1860–1870.*

41. Olmsted to Lanman and Kemp, 29 September 1870, 12 Letters, WLEAC.

42. A complete price list for Wallace Brothers for 1884 is found in "A Descriptive List of Roots, Herbs, Barks, Seeds, Flowers, Mosses, etc.: Collected by Wallace Brothers, Wholesale Dealers in Southern Botanic Crude Drugs," Rubenstein Rare Book and Manuscript Collection, Perkins Library, Duke University, Durham, NC.

43. "Letters of Itinerant."

44. These statistics were gleaned from: Produce Book, G. W. and S. F. Harper, 1866–1867, vol. 26, Harper Family Account Books, Southern Historical Collection, Wilson Library, University of North Carolina, Chapel Hill; Produce Book, G. W. and S. F. Harper, 1869–1869, vol. 29, Harper Family Account Books; Produce Book, G. W. F. Harper, 1873–1875, vol. 38, Harper Family Account Books; Produce Book, G. W. F. Harper, 1875–1877, vol. 40, Harper Family Account Books; Barter Produce Book, 1869–1870, folder 7, Bernardht-Seagle Co. Records, Southern Historical Collection, Wilson Library, University of North Carolina, Chapel Hill; Produce Book, 1871, folder 8, Bernardht-Seagle Co. Records; Produce Book, 1871–1872, folder 9, Bernardht-Seagle Co. Records; Produce Book, 1872–1873, folder 25, Bernardht-Seagle Co. Records.

45. Carolyn Merchant, *Ecological Revolutions: Nature, Gender, and Science in New England,* 2nd ed. (Chapel Hill: University of North Carolina Press, 2010), 38, 81–82. Other scholars have suggested that a similar division existed among the Cherokee. See Theda Perdue, *Cherokee Women: Gender and Culture Change, 1700–1835* (Lincoln: University of Nebraska Press, 1998), 18–21. That women were the primary conduits through which botanical knowledge was passed down can be seen in Florence Cope Bush, *Dorie: Woman of the Mountains* (Knoxville: University of Tennessee Press, 1992). See also Ronald D. Eller, *Miners, Millhands, and Mountaineers: Industrialization of the Appalachian South, 1880–1930* (Knoxville: University of Tennessee Press, 1982); and Wilma A. Dunaway, *Women, Work, and Family in the Antebellum Mountain South* (Cambridge: Cambridge University Press, 2008).

46. A good source for examining the role of hunting in Appalachian masculine identity is a memoir: Fred M. Burnett, *This Was My Valley* (Ridgecrest, NC: Heritage, 1960).

47. *Carolina Watchman,* 28 July 1862.

48. Quoted in Norman Franke, "Official and Industrial Aspects of Pharmacy in the Confederacy," *Georgia Historical Quarterly* 37, no. 3 (September 1953): 182.

49. "Woman's Work," *Southern Cultivator,* February 1888, 90.

50. Clare Olin Ewing and Ernest Elwood Stanford, "Botanicals of the Blue Ridge," *American Druggist and Pharmaceutical Record*, June 1919.

51. James Lane Allen, *The Blue-Grass Region of Kentucky: And Other Kentucky Articles* (New York: Macmillan, 1907), 232.

52. Michael A. Flannery, *Civil War Pharmacy: A History of Drugs, Drug Supply and Provision, and Therapeutics for the Union and Confederacy*, Pharmaceutical Heritage (New York: Pharmaceutical Products, 2004), 64–70.

53. Julia Morgan, *How It Was: Four Years among the Rebels* (Nashville: Methodist Episcopal Church, 1892), 25.

54. Joseph Jacobs, "Drug Conditions during the War between the States," in *Proceedings of the American Pharmaceutical Association at the Forty-Sixth Annual Meeting, Held at Baltimore, MD, August 1898* (Baltimore: American Pharmaceutical Association, 1898), 192–213.

55. Jacobs, "Drug Conditions during the War between the States."

56. This is based on the fact that more men traded private commodities than commons commodities, and more women traded commons commodities than private commodities. Harper Family Account Books.

57. Taylor and Moore Ledger, W. L. Eury Appalachian Collection, Belk Library, Appalachian State University, Boone, NC.

58. See W. P. Thomas Store Ledger, 1872–1875, Ashe County Historical Museum, Jefferson, NC.

59. Thomas Store Ledger.

60. Store Ledger, 1869–1871, Cathey Family Papers, Special Collections, Hunter Library, Western Carolina University, Cullowhee, NC.

61. John Preston Arthur, *A History of Watauga County, North Carolina: With Sketches of Prominent Families* (Easley, SC: Southern Historical Press, 1976), 190.

62. Arthur, *A History of Watauga County*, 186–93. See also L. B. Love, "Early Pioneer Days in Watauga County," *Watauga Democrat* (Boone, NC), 5 June 1913.

63. H. R. Brinkerhoff, "A Reminiscence," *United Service* 14, no. 2 (August 1895).

64. Quoted in Kristin Johannsen, *Ginseng Dreams: The Secret World of America's Most Valuable Plant* (Lexington: University Press of Kentucky, 2006), 24.

65. "Memoranda of Various Political Arrests—From Reports of Confederate Commissioners," in *The War of the Rebellion: A Compilation of the Official Records of the Union and Confederate Armies*, series 2, vol. 2 (Washington, DC: Government Printing Office, 1897), 1448.

66. "Memoranda of Various Political Arrests," 1448.

67. "Memoranda of Various Political Arrests," 1448.

68. Although the Webster County courthouse was burned in 1888, a newspaper article printed in 1902 included excerpts from the original county court records. That article was reprinted by the Webster County Historical Society in H. Coleman Thurmond, "Webster County and the Foreign Press," *Webster Independent* no. 2 (Fall–Winter 1985–1986): 60.

69. Quoted in Thurmond, "Webster County and the Foreign Press," 60.

70. Roy Bird Cook, "Battle of Droop Mountain," *West Virginia Review,* October 1928, published online by the West Virginia Archives and History, http://www.wvculture.org/history/civilwar/droopmountain01.html.

71. US Bureau of the Census, *Population Schedules of the 8th Census of the United States, 1860, West Virginia, Pocahontas County* (Washington, DC: National Archives and Records Service, 1861); U.S. Bureau of the Census, *Population Schedules of the 9th Census of the United States, 1870, West Virginia, Pocahontas County* (Washington, DC: National Archives and Records Service, 1871).

72. "Webster: A Few Words concerning the 'Independent State,'" *Weston (WV) Democrat,* 14 July 1873.

73. Anna Shue Atkins, "'She Didn't Go Sangin' Alone!'" *Goldenseal* 25, no. 3 (September 1999): 28.

74. It must be noted, however, that the 7 percent total should be taken as the lowest estimate for ginseng's overall economic contribution. As in the case of Cherokee County, it was not uncommon for diggers to contract directly with agents for cash and bypass the store altogether, so some of the cash used by customers likely came from selling ginseng to outside dealers. McNeel himself seems to have sold most of his ginseng to the Boston wholesalers Wilson, Burns & Co. See Ledger, 1871–1874, Isaac McNeel Papers, West Virginia History Center, West Virginia University, Morgantown.

75. Biographical details were established by US Bureau of the Census, *Population Schedules of the 9th Census of the United States, 1870, West Virginia, Pocahontas County;* Compiled Military Service Record, Samuel J. Brown, Pvt. Co. F, 10th West Virginia Infantry, National Archives, Washington, DC; Ledger, 1871–1874, Isaac McNeel Papers.

76. B. Mollohan, "From Webster," *Weston (WV) Democrat,* 21 September 1874. This situation played out across Southern Appalachia as well. While traveling the road from Morganton to Asheville, North Carolina, in 1866, a correspondent for the *Raleigh Sentinel* passed a man with a one-horse wagon heading for the mountains. Asked if he was going over the Blue Ridge, he replied, "Oh, no . . . I'm only hunting 'sang.'" *Raleigh Sentinel,* 13 September 1866.

77. Ronald L. Lewis, *Transforming the Appalachian Countryside: Railroads, Deforestation, and Social Change in West Virginia, 1880–1920* (Chapel Hill: University of North Carolina Press, 1998), 67–77.

78. Harrison Garman, *Ginseng: Its Nature and Culture,* Kentucky Agricultural Experiment Station Bulletin 78 (Lexington: Kentucky Agricultural Experiment Station of the State College of Kentucky, 1898), 128.

79. Garman, *Ginseng,* 128.

80. Maude Chandler, George and Cecilia Brown Life History [interview 4 December 1939], W.P.A. Life Histories, Library of Virginia, Richmond.

81. The two best accounts of this transition remain Eller, *Miners, Millhands, and Mountaineers;* and Lewis, *Transforming the Appalachian Countryside.*

82. Eller, *Miners, Millhands, and Mountaineers*, 226–30.

83. Joann Greer Brassell, correspondence with the author, August 2015.

84. These biographical details were compiled using US Census Bureau, *Seventh Census of the United States, 1850* (Washington, DC: Robert Armstrong, 1853); US Census Bureau, *Eighth Census of the United States, 1860* (Washington, DC: Government Printing Office, 1864); US Census Bureau, *Ninth Census of the United States, 1870* (Washington, DC: Government Printing Office, 1872); US Census Bureau, *Compendium of the Tenth Census of the United States, 1880* (Washington, DC: Government Printing Office, 1883); US Census Bureau, *Compendium of the Eleventh Census of the United States, 1890* (Washington, DC: Government Printing Office, 1892); US Census Bureau, *Twelfth Census of the United States, 1890* (Washington, DC: Government Printing Office, 1902).

85. These biographical details were compiled using: US Census Bureau, *Seventh Census of the United States, 1850;* US Census Bureau, *Eighth Census of the United States, 1860;* US Census Bureau, *Ninth Census of the United States, 1870;* US Census Bureau, *Tenth Census of the United States, 1880;* US Census Bureau, *Eleventh Census of the United States, 1890;* US Census Bureau, *Twelfth Census of the United States, 1890.* The transition from agricultural work to wage work is detailed nicely in Chad Montrie, *Making a Living: Work and Environment in the United States* (Chapel Hill: University of North Carolina Press, 2008), 71–90.

86. "In Highland County," *Richmond Dispatch*, 16 October 1901.

87. Harding, *Ginseng and Other Medicinal Plants*, 155.

88. G. W. Koiner, *Annual Report of the State Board of Agriculture of Virginia* (Richmond: J. H. O'Bannon, Superintendent of Public Printing, 1900), 96.

89. Calvin J. Cowles to Tilden & Co., 25 January 1851, Calvin J. Cowles Papers, Southern Historical Collection, University of North Carolina, Chapel Hill; G. W. F. Harper to Benjamin Gates, 21 September 1870, folder 54, Bernhardt-Seagle Co. Records.

90. Timothy P. Spira, *Wildflowers & Plant Communities of the Southern Appalachian Mountains & Piedmont: A Naturalist's Guide to the Carolinas, Virginia, Tennessee & Georgia*, A Southern Gateways Guide (Chapel Hill: University of North Carolina Press, 2011), 357–58.

91. Henry Kraemer, "The Conservation and Cultivation of Medicinal Plants," *American Journal of Pharmacy*, December 1903.

92. Kraemer, "The Conservation and Cultivation of Medicinal Plants."

93. James Lane Allen, "Through the Cumberland Gap on Horseback," in *The Blue-Grass Region of Kentucky and Other Kentucky Articles* (New York: Harper Brothers, 1892), 250.

94. "Passing of the Sang Digger," *Clinch Valley News*, 25 June 1897.

95. "Wealth Galore: How the Process of Development Is Going on in Remote Parts of the State," *Wheeling Register*, 13 May 1888.

96. James B. McGraw et al., "Ecology and Conservation of Ginseng (*Panax*

Quinquefolius) in a Changing World," *Annals of the New York Academy of Sciences* 1286 (2013): 66.

97. Joanne Braun and Garnett R. Brooks Jr., "Box Turtles (*Terrapene Carolina*) as Potential Agents for Seed Dispersal," *American Midlands Naturalist* 117, no. 2 (April 1987): 312–18.

98. Spira, *Wildflowers & Plant Communities*, 337.

99. Dennis F. Whigham, "Ecology of Woodland Herbs in Temperate Deciduous Forests," *Annual Review of Ecology, Evolution, and Systematics* 35 (2004): 602–3.

100. Thanks to David Hsiung for some of these ideas. Correspondence with the author, January 2019.

6. "Beasts in the Garden"

1. "Ginseng Thief Killed," *Tazewell Republican*, 6 August 1908; "Dead Man Was Robber," *Democratic Banner* (Mt. Vernon, OH), 29 June 1915.

2. Examining the social history of conservation, historians such as Louis Warren, Karl Jacoby, Benjamin Johnson, and others have argued that the movement was a force of modernization that effectively worked to supersede layers of common rights. In their view, outsiders used the power of the state to impose a new resource-use regime on top of the local one. This movement effectively turned fish, game, and private lands into property of the state, which served to benefit urban middle-class sportsmen and hunting clubs at the expense of local users. The movement to conserve ginseng fits into this narrative, but not neatly. Common rights to medicinal plants, as well as fish, game, livestock forage, and other resources, were replaced with a patchwork of laws designed to rationalize the rural landscape and impose "order" on the countryside. Some laws aimed at managing the commons, in part by establishing seasons and bag limits, while others sought to privatize resources. This renegotiation of common rights, however, played out differently in different local contexts. In the case of ginseng in Southern Appalachia, the new regime was not imposed entirely by outside middle-class antagonists. It was largely generated by the demands of rural landowners who, for various reasons, no longer wanted to acquiesce to common rights. For more on the game and fish laws in West Virginia, see Ronald L. Lewis, *Transforming the Appalachian Countryside: Railroads, Deforestation, and Social Change in West Virginia, 1880–1920* (Chapel Hill: University of North Carolina Press, 1998), 278–94. For a discussion on game and fish laws elsewhere in the country, see Karl Jacoby, *Crimes against Nature: Squatters, Poachers, Thieves, and the Hidden History of American Conservation* (Berkeley: University of California Press, 2001); Louis S. Warren, *The Hunter's Game: Poachers and Conservationists in Twentieth-Century America* (New Haven: Yale University Press, 1997); Benjamin H. Johnson, "Conservation, Subsistence, and Class at the Birth of Superior National Forest," *Environmental History* 4, no. 1 (January 1999): 80–99; Scott E.

Giltner, *Hunting and Fishing in the New South: Black Labor and White Leisure after the Civil War,* Johns Hopkins University Studies in Historical and Political Science, 126th ser., 2 (Baltimore: Johns Hopkins University Press, 2008).

3. Maurice G. Kains, *Ginseng: Its Cultivation, Harvesting, Marketing, and Market Value, with a Short Account of Its History and Botany* (New York: Orange Judd, 1903), 13.

4. "Big Profits in Ginseng," *Baltimore Sun,* 17 September 1899.

5. Kains, *Ginseng,* 13.

6. Lewis, *Transforming the Appalachian Countryside,* 3–5, 45–48.

7. John Alexander Williams, *Appalachia: A History* (Chapel Hill: University of North Carolina Press, 2002), 250; Kathryn Newfont, *Blue Ridge Commons: Environmental Activism and Forest History in Western North Carolina,* Environmental History and the American South (Athens: University of Georgia Press, 2012), 42–48.

8. Donald Edward Davis, *Where There Are Mountains: An Environmental History of the Southern Appalachians* (Athens: University of Georgia Press, 2000), 169–72.

9. Quoted in Davis, *Where There Are Mountains,* 168. These changes are noted more broadly for the Southern Appalachian region as a whole in *A Message from the President of the United States, Transmitting a Report of the Secretary of Agriculture in Relation to the Forests, Rivers, and Mountains of the Southern Appalachian Region* (Washington, DC: Government Printing Office, 1902).

10. Dennis F. Whigham, "Ecology of Woodland Herbs in Temperate Deciduous Forests," *Annual Review of Ecology, Evolution, and Systematics* 35 (2004): 583–621; Mary Ann Furedi and James B. McGraw, "White-Tailed Deer: Dispersers or Predators of American Ginseng Seeds?" *American Midland Naturalist* 152, no. 2 (October 2004): 268–76. Studies have shown that these ecological changes had long-term effects on herb populations. See Jennifer Fratterrigo, Monica Turner, and Scott Pearson, "Previous Land Use Alters Plant Allocation and Growth in Forest Herbs," *Journal of Ecology* 94 (2006): 548–57.

11. See Cratis D. Williams, "The Southern Mountaineer in Fact and Fiction" (PhD diss., New York University, 1961), 77. In his recent book, T. R. C. Hutton paints a portrait of "Bloody Breathitt" County, Kentucky, as a community ripped apart at the seams by internal sectionalism rooted in the war experience, generating rounds of political violence that plagued the county for decades. See *Bloody Breathitt: Politics and Violence in the Appalachian South,* New Directions in Southern History (Lexington: University Press of Kentucky, 2013). Another good discussion of the impacts of the war on a community level is Durwood Dunn, *Cades Cove: The Life and Death of a Southern Appalachian Community, 1818–1937* (Knoxville: University of Tennessee Press, 1988).

12. See Ledger, 1871–1874, Isaac McNeel Papers, West Virginia History Center, West Virginia University, Morgantown.

13. "'First of Plants': A Rich West Virginia Product about Which Little is

Known; The Strange Mystery Which Surrounds the Uses to Which Ginseng Is Put by Its Almond-Eyed Consumers—'Man Root,'" *Wheeling Daily Intelligencer,* 8 February 1886.

14. "Hunters After Ginseng," *Bourbon News* (Paris, KY), 19 November 1897.

15. Of a sample of twenty respondents who can be identified in the census, the majority were middle aged, literate (some barely so), white, male farmers of middling status. The group, thus, does not adequately represent the views of nonwhite farmers or of women or of the poorest, illiterate laborers and farmhands. Neither do these respondents represent the views of economic and political elites. They were somewhat typical small landowners. Questionnaire responses are scattered throughout box 13 in the Harrison Garman Papers, University of Kentucky, Lexington.

16. A. M. Weedman to Harrison Garman, 6 November 1898, box 13, Harrison Garman Papers.

17. Elisha Bird to Harrison Garman, 31 October 1898, folder 5, box. 13, Harrison Garman Papers.

18. W. H. R. Markley to Harrison Garman, 25 October 1898, Harrison Garman Papers.

19. H. W. Bens to Harrison Garman, 14 October 1898, Harrison Garman Papers.

20. H. T. Bigley to Harrison Garman, 27 October 1898, Harrison Garman Papers.

21. John Kring to Harrison Garman, n.d., Harrison Garman Papers.

22. S. F. Barrall to Harrison Garman, 22 October 1898, Harrison Garman Papers.

23. Charles Fagan to Harrison Garman, 24 October 1898, Harrison Garman Papers.

24. W. H. Cothringham to Harrison Garman, 15 October 1898, Harrison Garman Papers; P. F. Adams to Harrison Garman, 14 October 1898, Harrison Garman Papers.

25. W. H. C. Johnson to Harrison Garman, 2 November 1898, Harrison Garman Papers.

26. *Public Laws of the State of North Carolina Passed by the General Assembly at the Sessions of 1866–1867* (Raleigh: William E. Pell, State Printer, 1867), 81.

27. *Public Laws of the State of North Carolina,* 81.

28. *Journal of the House of Delegates of the State of West Virginia for the Session Commencing January 18, 1870* (Wheeling: John Frew, 1870), 70, 109.

29. Harrison Garman, *Ginseng: Its Nature and Culture,* Kentucky Agricultural Experiment Station Bulletin 78 (Lexington: Agricultural Experiment Station of the State College of Kentucky, 1898), 127.

30. H.B. 93: "A Bill Prohibiting Persons Digging Ginseng or Other Medical Roots, or Prospecting for the Same on the Land of Another, without the Consent of the Owner, and Prescribing Punishment Thereof," in *Acts of the Legislature of West Virginia at the Eleventh Session, 1872–73* (Charleston: Henry S. Walker, 1873).

31. [Icebound], "Charleston," *Wheeling Daily Intelligencer*, 8 March 1878.

32. Barbara Rasmussen, *Absentee Landowning and Exploitation in West Virginia, 1760–1920* (Lexington: University Press of Kentucky, 1994), 70–89.

33. Reporting on three devastating wildfires tearing through the timber in Western North Carolina, one newspaper, for example, blamed the "root diggers who want the leaves out of their way so the medicinal herbs may have a chance to grow." *Lenoir (NC) Topic*, 17 April 1889.

34. [Henry], "Charleston," *Wheeling Intelligencer*, 28 November 1873.

35. *Journal of the House of Delegates of the State of West Virginia for the Tenth Session, Commencing January 16, 1872* (Charleston: Henry S. Walker, 1872), 128–30.

36. [Alpha], "Charleston Letter," *Wheeling Daily Intelligencer*, 19 February 1873.

37. [Tomahawk], "Charleston," *Wheeling Daily Intelligencer*, 11 November 1873.

38. [Tomahawk], "Charleston."

39. [Henry], "Charleston."

40. *Wheeling Daily Intelligencer*, 9 December 1873.

41. *Journal of the House of Delegates of the State of West Virginia*, 192.

42. Unfortunately, the text of Camden's speech has not survived, but it is referenced in [Henry], "Charleston."

43. Glenn Massay, "The Lost Years: Gideon Draper Camden and the Confederacy," *West Virginia History* 25, no. 3 (April 1964): 194. For more on Camden, see John Edmund Stealey III, "Gideon Draper Camden: A Whig of Western Virginia," *West Virginia History* 26, no. 1 (October 1964): 13–30; Jacob C. Baas Jr., "John Jay Jackson, Jr.: Business, Legal, and Political Activities, 1847–1859," *West Virginia History* 50 (1991): 63–78.

44. *Wheeling Daily Intelligencer*, 19 September 1874.

45. Garman, *Ginseng*, 128.

46. For a good discussion of this wave of fish and game laws, see Lewis, *Transforming the Appalachian Countryside*, 278–83.

47. See chapter 62 of *The Code of West Virginia, 1906, Containing the Declaration of Independence; the Constitution of the United States and Laws Thereof concerning Naturalization and the Election of United States Senators; the Constitution of the State; The Code, as Amended by Legislation to and Including the Year 1906 and Notes to All Prior Laws and Applicable Decisions* (St. Paul: West, 1906), 1122–42.

48. Lewis argues that a legal revolution accompanied the arrival of outside capital that sought to insulate companies from litigation over land use. He detects a change in court decisions beginning in the 1880s that transformed property liability and nuisance law to favor industrial uses of land. Throughout much of the nineteenth century, Virginia and West Virginia high courts upheld a so-called static theory of property rights, in which property was seen as a "natural right" that should not be infringed upon by other property owners. This was used largely to defend agricultural interests against encroachments by industrial

development. By the 1890s, however, the courts adopted a more dynamic theory of property that recognized industrial uses as legitimate economic uses and their side effects (pollution, water diversions, etc.) as sometimes necessary externalities. Thus, the legal revolution involved a weakening of property rights to ease the transition toward an industrial future. The ginseng bill, however, addressed part of the legal culture that Lewis and others have overlooked. Part of this legal revolution, as Woodell's Sang Bill illustrates, was actually the strengthening of property rights to curtail common rights. See Lewis, *Transforming the Appalachian Countryside,* 7–9, 52–55.

49. Anonymous [unsigned] to L. D. Fowler, 15 March 1910, L. D. Fowler Collection, Special Collections Department, James E. Morrow Library, Marshall University, Huntington, WV.

50. Ed Ambrose to L. D. Fowler, 8 November 1909, L. D. Fowler Collection.

51. L. D. Fowler to Whom It May Concern, 27 October 1909, L. D. Fowler Collection.

52. Ira Shockey to Howard K. Sutherland, 13 February 1911, box 9, Howard K. Sutherland Papers, West Virginia State Archives, Charleston.

53. Editorial, "The Cultivation of Medicinal Plants," *American Journal of Pharmacy,* April 1900.

54. [Letter fragment], 2 November 1898, folder 5, box 13, Harrison Garman Papers.

55. Elisha Bird to Harrison Garman, 31 October 1898, folder 5, box 13, Harrison Garman Papers.

56. Essex Spurrier to Harrison Garman, 7 November 1898, folder 5, box 13, Harrison Garman Papers.

57. S. B. Dishman to Harrison Garman, 16 December 1898, folder 5, box 13, Harrison Garman Papers.

58. John Nuttall, *Trees Above with Coal Below* (San Diego: Neyenesch, 1961), 18.

59. Nuttall, *Trees Above with Coal Below,* 18.

60. J. M. Brooks to Harrison Garman, 1 November 1898, in Garman, *Ginseng,* 132–33.

61. Nuttall, *Trees Above with Coal Below,* 19.

62. Nuttall, *Trees Above with Coal Below,* 19.

63. "Ginseng," *Asheville Citizen,* 27 October 1887.

64. Kains, *Ginseng,* 31.

65. J. W. Sears, *The Ginseng Culturist Guide: From Seed to Market, Twenty Years' Practical Experience,* rev. ed. (Somerset, KY: J. W. Sears, 1912), 9.

66. "Some Industries," *Somerset (KY) Semi-Weekly Journal,* 8 January 1904; "American Ginseng Culture," *Somerset (KY) Journal,* 19 October 1900. Both of these clippings can be found in folder 8, box 13, Harrison Garman Papers.

67. J. W. Sears to Harrison Garman, 21 November 1906, Harrison Garman Papers.

68. George Stanton, "Ginseng," *Pharmaceutical Era* 11, no. 6 (March 1894): 254–55.

69. *Documents of the Assembly of the State of New York, One Hundred and Thirty-Fifth Session,* vol. 6, no. 20, part 2 (Albany: Argus, 1912), 842.

70. "The Cultivation of Ginseng," *American Journal of Pharmacy,* August 1894, 399.

71. "The Cultivation of Ginseng," 399.

72. Sears, *The Ginseng Culturist Guide,* 8–9.

73. For a sampling of these pamphlets, see Carlos B. Paseador, *The Crop That's Worth Its Weight in Sterling Silver* (Joplin, MO: Chinese-American Ginseng Co., 1901); M. G. Harrison, *American Ginseng: Its History and Culture* (Centerville, MO: M. G. Harrison, 1897); Arthur Robert Harding, *Ginseng and Other Medicinal Plants: A Book of Valuable Information for Growers as Well as Collectors of Medicinal Roots, Barks, Leaves, etc.* (Columbus, OH: A. R. Harding, 1908); C. M. Root, *What Is Ginseng? An Account of the History and Cultivation of Ginseng* (Omaha: C. M. Root, 1905).

74. "Ginseng Craze Is Spreading," *Lawrence (KS) Daily World,* 6 July 1904.

75. In addition to Sears and Stanton, well-known growers include M. G. Harrison of Redford, Missouri; Harlan P. Kelsey of Boston; A. E. Leavitt of Houston, Missouri; Emmanuel Lewis of Hemlock, Wisconsin; H. S. Seymour of Richland Center, Wisconsin; W. G. Palmer of Boydtown, Wisconsin; G. F. Millard of Houston, Missouri; and W. A. Bates of Cuba, New York.

76. For a good discussion on the growth of cultivated ginseng, see Alvar W. Carlson, "Ginseng: America's Botanical Drug Connection to the Orient," *Economic Botany* 40, no. 2 (April 1986): 233–49.

77. For discussions of the agrarian dimensions of the conservation movement, see Paul Thompson, "Expanding the Conservation Tradition: The Agrarian Vision," in *Reconstructing Conservation: Finding Common Ground,* ed. Ben A. Minteer and Robert E. Manning (Washington, DC: Island, 2003), 77–92; Ben Minteer, "Regional Planning as Pragmatic Conservationism," in Minteer and Manning, 93–114; Richard Judd, "Writing Environmental History from East to West," in Minteer and Manning, 19–32; Sarah T. Phillips, *This Land, This Nation: Conservation, Rural America, and the New Deal* (New York: Cambridge University Press, 2007); Mark D. Hersey, *My Work Is That of Conservation: An Environmental Biography of George Washington Carver,* Environmental History and the American South (Athens: University of Georgia Press, 2011). For a good, thought-provoking article on agrarianism and conservation, see Mart Stewart, "If John Muir Had Been an Agrarian: American Environmental History West and South," in *Environmental History and the American South,* ed. Paul Sutter and Chris Manganiello (Athens: University of Georgia Press, 2009).

78. Allan Carlson, *The New Agrarian Mind: The Movement toward Decentralist Thought in Twentieth-Century America* (New Brunswick, NJ: Transaction, 2000), 7.

79. Scott Peters, "'Every Farmer Should Be Awakened': Liberty Hyde Bailey's Vision of Agricultural Extension Work," *Agricultural History* 80 (2006): 190–219.

80. Kains, *Ginseng,* vi.

81. "Maurice G. Kains, Horticulturist, 77," *New York Times,* 26 February 1946.

82. "Land, Stock, and Crop," *Mount Vernon (KY) Signal,* 11 July 1902.

83. See George C. Butz, *An Experiment in Ginseng Culture,* Pennsylvania State College Experiment Station Bulletin 62 (January 1903); W. M. Munson, "Ginseng," in *Nineteenth Annual Report of the Maine Agricultural Experiment Station,* Orono, Maine, 1903 (Augusta: Kennebec Journal, 1904), 119–20; N. O. Booth, "Ginseng Culture," *Twentieth Annual Report of the Board of Control of the New York Agricultural Experiment Station for the Year 1901* (Albany: J. B. Lyon, 1902), 356–58.

84. "Ginseng," *French Broad Hustler* (Hendersonville, NC), 8 November 1906.

85. "Ginseng," *French Broad Hustler.*

86. A photo shows Elbert Bates's home in rural western Cherokee County with a ginseng garden of about one-eighth of an acre. See Unaka Community Development Club Historic Preservation Committee, *Mountain Heritage: The Story of Western North Carolina's Communities of Unaka, Ogreeta, Bethel, Copper Creek and Upper Beaverdam* (Blairsville, GA: Unaka Community Development Club Historic Preservation Committee, 2011), 218.

87. Horace Kephart, *Our Southern Highlanders: A Narrative of Adventure in the Southern Appalachians and a Study of Life among the Mountaineers* (Knoxville: University of Tennessee Press, 1998), 40.

88. "A Rising Industry," *Charlotte Observer,* 31 May 1908.

89. "Largest Ginseng Farm Is in Swain," *Asheville Citizen-Times,* 12 October 1917.

90. See "Four Ginseng Pictures," *Bulletin of Pharmacy* 22, no. 8 (August 1908): 347–48; "Ginseng Plantation Moved Fifty Miles," *Asheville Citizen-Times,* 24 April 1918; "Making Money out of Ginseng Patch," *Asheville Citizen-Times,* 22 June 1909.

91. "A Rising Industry."

92. Frank S. Woodson, "Money in Ginseng; Wonderful Herb," *Times Dispatch* (Richmond, VA), 7 August 1910.

93. "Ginseng Humbug," *Indianapolis News,* 17 December 1887.

94. "A New Crop—Ginseng," *Southern Planter* 4, no. 58 (April 1897): 177. Although it published numerous articles on ginseng cultivation, the *Progressive Farmer* cautioned its readers that "each one must decide for himself whether or not it is wrong to so impose upon the ignorance of the Chinese." "More about Ginseng," *Progressive Farmer,* 24 January 1899.

95. See *The Pharmacopoeia of the United States of America, Sixth Decennial Revision* (New York: William Wood, 1883), 444.

96. "A New Crop—Ginseng," 177.

97. *Progressive Farmer,* 12 July 1904.

98. C. M. Godspeed, "Ginseng in China," *Special Crops* 4, no. 40 (December 1905): 236.

99. Garman, *Ginseng,* 136.

100. Adolf E. Ibershoff, *Aralia Quinquefolia (Ginseng): An Original Proving by the University of Michigan Society of Drug Provers* (Ann Arbor: University of Michigan, Homoeopathic Department, 1905), 1–8.

101. "Find the Elixir of Life," *Richmond Climax,* 28 December 1904.

102. "Hope Farm Notes," *Rural New Yorker,* 17 December 1904, 895.

103. "Hope Farm Notes," 895.

104. J. R. Pirtle to H. Garman, 15 November 1906, folder 6, box 13, Harrison Garman Papers; J. R. Pirtle to H. Garman, 23 July 1907, folder 6, box 13, Harrison Garman Papers.

105. J. W. Sears to H. Garman, 21 November 1906, folder 6, box 13, Harrison Garman Papers; J. W. Sears to H. Garman, 11 June 1906, folder 6, box 13, Harrison Garman Papers.

106. "Concerning Ginseng," *Biloxi Daily Herald,* 5 September 1900; "Boxers Injuring the Ginseng Trade," *Charlotte Observer,* 26 June 1900.

107. Speyer and Sons to H. Garman, 7 December 1904, folder 8, box 13, Harrison Garman Papers.

108. T. B. Lyon, "Cultivated Ginseng," *Adair County News* (Columbia, KY), 24 May 1905.

109. J. W. Sears to H. Garman, 12 November 1906, folder 6, box 13, Harrison Garman Papers.

110. J. W. Sears to H. Garman, 12 November 1906, folder 6, box 13, Harrison Garman Papers; J. R. Pirtle to H. Garman, 23 July 1907, folder 6, box 13, Harrison Garman Papers. The cause of this particular collapse may have been the result of a Chinese boycott of American goods in response to the United States' regrettable treatment of Chinese immigrants and refusal to repeal the Chinese Exclusion Act. "Boycott," *Eau Claire (WI) Leader,* 29 August 1905.

111. J. S. Lodewick to H. Garman, 1 August 1907, Harrison Garman Papers.

112. Lyon, "Cultivated Ginseng."

113. "The Culture of Ginseng," *Progressive Farmer,* 22 August 1899.

114. "Bear Traps Set in Ginseng Patch," *Asheville Citizen-Times,* 26 May 1909. See also "A Ginseng Patch That Is a Patch," *News Record* (Marshall, NC), 1 August 1913.

115. C. A. Rowley, "Protection for Ginseng," *Special Crops* 4, no. 34 (June 1905): 106–8.

116. Andrew B. Jackson, *Code of Laws of South Carolina, 1912,* vol. 2 (Charlottesville, 1912), 301.

117. Clarence Birdseye, Robert Cumming, and Frank Gilbert, eds., *Annotated Consolidated Laws of the State of New York, as Amended to January 1, 1910,* vol. 3 (New York: Banks Law, 1909), 3812–13; Andrew Howell, *Howell's Annotated Statutes of the State of Michigan, Including the Acts of the Second Extra Session*

of 1912, vol. 2 (Chicago: Callaghan, 1913), 1829; Thomas Womack, Needham Gulley, and William Rodman, eds., *Revisal of 1905 of North Carolina Prepared under Chapter Three Hundred and Fourteen of the Laws of One Thousand Nine Hundred and Three* (Raleigh: E. M. Uzzell, 1905), 1038.

118. *Journal of the Senate of the General Assembly of the State of North Carolina, 1905* (Raleigh: E. M. Uzzell, 1905), 52.

119. "The Garden and the Beast," *Asheville Citizen-Times*, 17 May 1909; US Census Bureau, *Thirteenth Census of the United States, 1910* (Washington, DC: Government Printing Office, 1913).

120. "The Garden and the Beast."

121. US Census Bureau, *Thirteenth Census*.

122. For more on Jobe and the Woolen Mills, see Abraham Jobe, *Mountaineer in Motion: The Memoir of Dr. Abraham Jobe, 1817–1906*, ed. David Hsiung (Knoxville: University of Tennessee Press, 2009), 125–32.

123. "Hunter Gets Fatal Wound," *Asheville Weekly Citizen*, 28 December 1900.

124. "Ginseng Men Are Still at Large," *Asheville Citizen-Times*, 25 May 1909.

125. "Chase Them over Mountains and Down Ravines," *Asheville Weekly Citizen*, 23 July 1909.

126. This fact came from a declaration of Governor Kitchin when he pardoned them. See "Ginseng Pilferers Pardoned from Pen," *Asheville Citizen*, 12 May 1910.

127. "A Growing Nuisance," *Asheville Gazette*, 24 November 1910.

128. "Hodge and Ingle Given Sentences," *Asheville Gazette News*, 7 August 1909.

129. "Bear Traps Set in Ginseng Patch."

130. "Guard Ginseng with Infernal Machines," *Asheville Citizen*, 12 September 1909.

131. "The Garden and the Beast."

132. "Ginseng Pilferers Pardoned from Pen."

7. Progress and Ginseng

1. "Julie, the Huntress," *Baltimore Sun*, 19 November 1888.

2. "Julie, the Huntress."

3. "Julie, the Huntress."

4. The scholarship on Appalachian stereotypes is vast, leading some scholars to call for a shift away from the subject. Yet many scholars have found the topic difficult to overlook. The most important works on Appalachian stereotypes remain Allen Batteau, *The Invention of Appalachia: The Anthropology of Form and Meaning* (Tuscon: University of Arizona Press, 1990); Henry D. Shapiro, *Appalachia on Our Mind: The Southern Mountains and Mountaineers in the American Consciousness, 1870–1920* (Chapel Hill: University of North Carolina Press, 1978); Dwight Billings, Gurney Norman, and Kathryn Ledford, eds., *Confronting Appalachian Stereotypes: Back Talk from an American Region* (Lexington: Univer-

sity Press of Kentucky, 1999); Anthony Harkins, *Hillbilly: A Cultural History of an American Icon* (New York: Oxford University Press, 2004); David Hsiung, *Two Worlds in the Tennessee Mountains: Exploring the Origins of Appalachian Stereotypes* (Lexington: University Press of Kentucky, 1997).

5. See entry for August 15, 1859, on p. 155 in William C. Daily Journal, 1851–1861, Rubenstein Rare Book and Manuscript Library, Duke University, Durham, NC.

6. R. R. Hancock, *Hancock's Diary; or, A History of the Second Tennessee Confederate Cavalry, with Sketches of First and Seventh Battalions* (Nashville: Brandon, 1887), 18, 26–27. The Brown militia of Georgia was apparently also awarded the name. See "Ginseng," *MicMinnville Standard,* 3 October 1885.

7. "Ginseng," *McMinnville Standard.*

8. Ed Thompson, *History of the Orphan Brigade* (Louisville, KY: Lewis Thompson, 1898), 226.

9. In his examination of East Tennessee development during the mid-nineteenth century, historian David Hsiung contends that many of the negative perceptions of mountaineers as lazy, shiftless, and backward were created by members of nearby rural communities with differing views about the issues of railroads and economic modernization. Those with a broad perspective who sought to enhance their economic and social connections to the wider region saw the promise of railroads. These people maintained ties to the region's towns, shared the townspeople's outlook on economic questions, and clashed with their more isolated neighbors, who found themselves increasingly detached from the towns and their influence. Thus, the coming of the railroads brought these two perspectives into conflict. The railroad promoters labeled their opponents in terms of backwardness, and those perceptions, later broadcast to the nation, came to apply to the region as a whole. Hsiung, *Two Worlds in the Tennessee Mountains.*

10. "Ginseng Root Diggers," *Wheeling Register,* 20 September 1883.

11. John McElroy, *Where the Laurel Blooms and Men and Women Live Near Nature's Heart, National Tribune,* 12 August 1897.

12. R. R. Freer, "Ginseng Growers Meet," *New York Times,* 14 September 1902.

13. Reprinted in the *Wheeling Register,* 12 May 1882, 2.

14. "Capitol Notes," *Weekly Register* (Point Pleasant, WV), 28 June 1877.

15. "North Carolina," *New York Herald,* 29 April 1867.

16. "From West Virginia," *Springfield (MA) Republican,* 4 April 1868.

17. "Some Queer Human Beings," *Martinsburg (WV) Statesman,* 14 February 1878.

18. "Some Queer Human Beings."

19. "Some Queer Human Beings."

20. For example, "The Saugers," *Indianapolis Sentinel,* 17 October 1879; *Democratic Advocate* (Westminster, MD), 17 August 1878; *Springfield (MA) Republican,* 8 November 1878.

21. These articles include "The Shy Sang Diggers," *New York Sun,* 30 Decem-

ber 1894; Clifford Smyth, "With the Sang Diggers and Witches of Old Kentucky," *Atlanta Constitution,* 22 February 1903; J. C. Watkins, "Ginseng," *Frank Leslie's Popular Monthly,* May 1890, 614; "Ginseng Root Diggers"; "The Sang Digger," *Coleman's Rural World,* 14 March 1900; "The Sauger," *Indianapolis Sentinel,* 7 October 1879; "With the Sang Diggers," *Louisville Courier-Journal,* 3 September 1899.

22. *Democratic Advocate,* 17 August 1878.

23. "North Carolina," *New York Herald,* 29 April 1867.

24. "The Ginseng Digger," *Cincinnati Commercial Tribune,* 8 March 1889 (reprinted from the *Chicago Times.*)

25. "The Ginseng Digger."

26. *Democratic Advocate,* 17 August 1878; "Some Queer Human Beings."

27. For examples, see "Kentucky Mountaineers," *Morning Oregonian* (Portland), 18 January 1895; "The Hill-Country," *Appleton's Journal of Literature,* 21 December 1872; "Big Profits in Ginseng," *New York Sun,* 17 September 1899.

28. "A Remarkable Discovery," *Weston Democrat,* 23 February 1878.

29. "A Remarkable Discovery."

30. "West Virginia's Ginseng Diggers," *Wheeling Daily Intelligencer,* 20 November 1873.

31. Smyth had gained fame covering the Hatfield-McCoy feud for Joseph Pulitzer's *New York World* and later the Panamanian uprising against Colombia for the *Atlanta Constitution.* See "Clifford Smyth, Writer, 77, Dead," *New York Times,* 2 December 1943.

32. See Clifford Smyth and Hartley Davis, "The Land of Feuds," *Munsey's Magazine,* November 1903.

33. Smyth, "With the Sang Diggers and Witches of Old Kentucky."

34. Charles Randolph, "The Mandragora of the Ancients in Folk-lore and Medicine," *Proceedings of the American Academy of Arts and Sciences* 40, no. 12 (January 1905); H. F. Clark, "The Mandrake Fiend," *Folklore* 73, no. 4 (Winter 1962): 257–69.

35. William Byrd to John Perceval, 20 August 1730, in William Byrd, William Byrd II, and William Byrd III, *The Correspondence of the Three William Byrds of Westover, Virginia, 1684–1776,* ed. Marion Tining (Richmond: Virginia Historical Society, 1977), 436.

36. Smyth's claim is certainly plausible. The mandrake legends proved remarkably durable across time and space, spreading from the Mediterranean region through western Europe over two millennia. When William Byrd first learned about the Chinese regard for American ginseng around 1729, he thought ginseng was "as fabulous as that extraordinary plant mentioned by Theophrastus," referring to mandrake. Byrd remarked that if ginseng "should be the same with Theophrastus's plant, the ladys will cry it down and with very good reason, because it will make their spouses exceedingly troublesome, and introduce a new way of shortening their own lives." See William Byrd to John Perceval, 20 August 1730, in Byrd, Byrd, and Byrd, *Correspondence,* 436.

37. Allen Batteau, *The Invention of Appalachia: The Anthropology of Form and Meaning* (Tucson: University of Arizona Press, 1990), 54–58.

38. James Lane Allen, "Through the Cumberland Gap on Horseback," *Harper's Monthly*, June, 1886, 262.

39. William G. Frost, "Our Southern Highlanders," *Independent*, 4 April 1912.

40. McElroy, *Where the Laurel Blooms*.

41. Historians Tom Lee, Ken Noe, John Inscoe, Gordon McKinney, and Samuel McGuire have thoroughly debunked the myth of Unionist Appalachia, arguing that Civil War loyalties were much more complex and complicated, but the myth was important to contemporaries like McElroy. See John C. Inscoe and Gordon B. McKinney, *The Heart of Confederate Appalachia: Western North Carolina in the Civil War*, Civil War America (Chapel Hill: University of North Carolina Press, 2000); John C. Inscoe and Robert C. Kenzer, eds., *Enemies of the Country: New Perspectives on Unionists in the Civil War South* (Athens: University of Georgia Press, 2001); Samuel B. McGuire, "East Tennessee's Grand Army: Union Veterans Confront Race, Reconciliation, and Civil War Memory, 1884–1913" (PhD diss., University of Georgia, 2016); Tom Lee, "The Lost Cause That Wasn't: East Tennessee and the Myth of Unionist Appalachia," in *Reconstructing Appalachia: The Civil War's Aftermath*, ed. Andrew L. Slap (Lexington: University Press of Kentucky, 2010), 293–322; and Kenneth W. Noe, "Toward the Myth of Unionist Appalachia, 1865–1883," *Journal of the Appalachian Studies Association* 6 (1994): 73–80.

42. Marion G. Rambo, "'The Submerged Tenth' among the Southern Mountaineers," *Methodist Review*, July 1905.

43. Samuel Tyndale Wilson, president of Maryville College and leader of the Presbyterian Synod of Tennessee, published *The Southern Mountaineers* in 1906. Four years later, Samuel H. Thompson published *The Highlanders of the South* on behalf of the Presbyterian Church's Home Missionary Board. Both of these divided mountain society in similar ways.

44. Edward O. Guerrant, "The Galax Gatherers," *Christian Observer*, 8 October 1902.

45. Edward O. Guerrant, *The Galax Gatherers: The Gospel among the Highlanders*, Appalachian Echoes (Knoxville: University of Tennessee Press, 2005).

46. Edgar Tufts, "The Galax Industry," *Christian Observer*, 27 December 1905.

47. Amelie Rives, *Tanis, the Sang-Digger* (New York: Town Topics, 1893).

48. Rives, *Tanis*, 71.

49. *Book Chat*, November 1893, 243.

50. *Book Chat*.

51. "Amelie Rives Chanler's Latest Novel," *Henderson Gold Leaf* (Hendersonville, NC), 19 October 1893.

52. "*Tanis, the Sang Digger*, by Amelie Rives," *Athenaeum*, 2 December 1893.

53. Frederick Jackson Turner, *The Significance of the Frontier in American History* (Madison: State Historical Society of Wisconsin, 1894).

54. Steven Stoll refers to this idea as the "theory of stages." See *Ramp Hollow: The Ordeal of Appalachia* (New York: Hill and Wang, 2017), 37–42.

55. Edmund S. Morgan, *American Slavery, American Freedom: The Ordeal of Colonial Virginia* (New York: Norton, 1975), 78.

56. Benjamin Rush, *An Oration, Delivered February 4, 1774, before the American Philosophical Society, Held at Philadelphia. Containing, an Enquiry into the Natural History of Medicine among the Indians in North-America, and a Comparitive View of Their Diseases and Remedies, with Those of Civilized Nations: Together with an Appendix, Containing, Proofs and Illustrations* (Philadelphia: Joseph Crukshank, 1774), available at Evans Early American Imprints Collection, http://name.umdl.umich.edu/N10722.0001.001.

57. J. Hector St. John de Crèvecoeur, *Letters from an American Farmer* (New York: Fox, Duffield, 1904), 59–60, 63–66. Reprinted from the original edition with a prefatory note by W. P. Trent and an introduction by Ludwig Lewisohn.

58. John R. Finger, *The Eastern Band of Cherokees, 1819–1900* (Knoxville: University of Tennessee Press, 1984), 81.

59. Gail Bederman, *Manliness & Civilization: A Cultural History of Gender and Race in the United States, 1880–1917*, Women in Culture and Society (Chicago: University of Chicago Press, 2000), 26–28.

60. Ellen Churchill Semple, "The Anglo-Saxons of the Kentucky Mountains: A Study in Anthropogeography," *Geographic Journal,* June 1901.

61. "Like a Hog," *Cincinnati Enquirer,* 5 December 1891.

62. Rambo, "'The Submerged Tenth.'"

63. "Chase them over Mountains and down Ravines," *Asheville Weekly Citizen,* 23 July 1909.

64. "Kentucky Mountaineers."

65. "North Carolina."

66. Elizabeth Englehardt has a good analysis of Rives's depictions of Tanis in Elizabeth Sanders Delwiche Engelhardt, *The Tangled Roots of Feminism, Environmentalism, and Appalachian Literature* (Athens: Ohio University Press, 2003), 38–46.

67. Bederman, *Manliness & Civilization,* chapters 1 and 5.

68. Roderick Nash, *Wilderness and the American Mind* (New Haven: Yale University Press, 1969), 135–61. For more discussions of this cultural shift, see Kevin C. Armitage, *The Nature Study Movement: The Forgotten Popularizer of America's Conservation Ethic* (Lawrence: University Press of Kansas, 2009); Richard Slotkin, *Gunfighter Nation: The Myth of the Frontier in Twentieth-Century America* (Norman: University of Oklahoma Press, 1998), chapter 1.

69. Guy LaTourette, "Ginseng and Its Diggers," *Pharmaceutical Journal and Transactions,* vol. 12 (London: J. A. Churchill, 1882), 379–80. LaTourette later

wrote articles for local newspapers recounting the early pioneers of Fayette County. See, for example, "Early Days on Bracken's," *Raleigh Herald,* 17 October 1907.

70. "Tennessee's Herb Diggers Often Reformed Moonshiners," *Springfield Daily Republican,* 22 April 1895.

71. Perhaps the most famous back-to-nature writer to escape his own masculinity crisis and find a home in Appalachia was Horace Kephart. In 1904, Kephart left his family and job as a librarian in St. Louis and lodged himself in the mountains of Swain County, where he took up writing, hunting, and fishing. His *Our Southern Highlanders,* first published in 1913, remains in print. Kephart discusses ginseng cultivation briefly, but he apparently never engaged in digging the plant. He remarked that it was virtually extinct in the wild, suggesting that his arrival in North Carolina was well after the great ginseng boom. Horace Kephart, *Our Southern Highlanders: A Narrative of Adventure in the Southern Appalachians and a Study of Life among the Mountaineers* (Knoxville: University of Tennessee Press, 1998), 39–42.

72. Maurice Thompson, *Stories of the Cherokee Hills* (Boston: Houghton, Mifflin, 1898), 2, http://archive.org/details/storiescherokee00thomgoog.

73. Thompson, *Stories of the Cherokee Hills,* 18.

74. Maurice Thompson, *By-ways and Bird Notes* (New York: John B. Alden, 1885), 96–97.

75. Thompson, *By-ways and Bird Notes,* 104.

76. Harkins, *Hillbilly,* 4–8.

77. Theodore Roosevelt, *The Strenuous Life: Essays and Addresses* (New York: Century, 1900), 2.

78. Perhaps the most relevant passages on this are found in Daniel T. Rodgers, *The Work Ethic in Industrial America, 1850–1920* (Chicago: University of Chicago Press, 1978), 7–29.

79. Allen, "Through the Cumberland Gap on Horseback," 262.

80. For a good discussion on Tennyson's poem as a commentary on epicureanism, see Malcolm MacLaren, "Tennyson's Epicurean Lotos-Eaters," *Classical Journal* 56, no. 6 (March 1961): 259–67.

81. Watkins, "Ginseng," 614.

82. "Julie the Huntress."

83. Gene Stratton-Porter, *The Harvester* (Bloomington: Indiana University Press, 1987).

84. Stratton-Porter, *The Harvester,* 271–72.

85. Stratton-Porter, *The Harvester,* 250.

86. Kevin Armitage, "Gene Stratton Porter's Conservation Aesthetic," *Environmental History* 14, no. 1 (January 2009): 138–45.

87. Cratis D. Williams, "Who Are the Southern Mountaineers?" *Appalachian Journal* 1, no. 1 (Autumn 1972): 48–55; Cratis D. Williams and Martha Pipes,

"The Southern Mountaineer in Fact and Fiction: Part II," *Appalachian Journal* 3, no. 2 (Winter 1976): 100–162.

Epilogue

1. Edward Lansing Cowles, "War Has Stimulated an Old-Time Industry," *Charlotte Observer,* 9 June 1916.
2. "Crude Drug Business Flourishes in This Section," *Lenoir (NC) News-Topic,* 8 October 1920.
3. "Crude Drug Business Flourishes in This Section."
4. Henry C. Fuller, *The Story of Drugs: A Popular Exposition of Their Origin, Preparation, and Commercial Importance* (New York: Century, 1922), 4.
5. Fuller, *The Story of Drugs,* 151.
6. Fuller, *The Story of Drugs,* 151.
7. Patricia Beaver, Sandra Ballard, and Brittany R. Hicks, eds., *Voices from the Headwaters: Stories from Meat Camp, Tamarack (Pottertown) & Sutherland, North Carolina* (Boone, NC: Center for Appalachian Studies, 2013), 198.
8. Leland R. Cooper, *The Pond Mountain Chronicle: Self-Portrait of a Southern Appalachian Community,* Contributions to Southern Appalachian Studies 2 (Jefferson, NC: McFarland, 1998), 22; Leland R. Cooper and Mary Lee Cooper, *The People of the New River: Oral Histories from the Ashe, Alleghany, and Watauga Counties of North Carolina* (Jefferson, NC: McFarland, 2001); Zetta Barker Hamby, *Memoirs of Grassy Creek: Growing Up in the Mountains on the Virginia–North Carolina Line* (Jefferson, NC: McFarland, 1998); Beaver, Ballard, and Hicks, *Voices from the Headwaters.*
9. Beaver, Ballard, and Hicks, *Voices from the Headwaters,* 284.
10. Beaver, Ballard, and Hicks, *Voices from the Headwaters,* 198.
11. Donald L. McCourry, *Us Poor Folks and the Things of Dog Flat Hollow* (Winston-Salem, NC: J. F. Blair, 1975), 113.
12. Varro E. Tyler, "Pharmaceutical Botany in the U.S., 1900–1962: Its Heyday, Decline, and Renascence," *Pharmacy in History* 38, no. 1 (1996): 20–23.
13. Tyler, "Pharmaceutical Botany," 21–22.
14. Benjamin R. Hershenson, "A Botanical Comparison of the United States Pharmacopoeias of 1820 and 1960," *Economic Botany* 18, no. 4 (October–December 1964): 342–56.
15. Tyler, "Pharmaceutical Botany," 21–22.
16. Sherry Joines Wyatt, R. T. Greer and Company Root and Herb Warehouse National Register of Historic Places Nomination, 2003, North Carolina Historic Preservation Office, Raleigh.
17. "Corn Products Merger," *Wall Street Journal,* 21 December 1967.
18. Gary R. Freeze, "Roots, Barks, Berries, and Jews: The Herb Trade in Gilded-Age North Carolina," *Essays in Economic and Business History* 13 (1995): 122.

19. Jackie Greenfield and Jeanine Davis, *Collection to Commerce: Western North Carolina Non-timber Forest Products and Their Markets* (Raleigh: Department of Horticultural Science, North Carolina State University, 2003), 5.

20. Greenfield and Davis, *Collection to Commerce*, 62; Kris Maher, "Demand for Ginseng Boosts Prices, Tempts Poachers," *Wall Street Journal,* 17 September 2014.

21. Greenfield and Davis, *Collection to Commerce*, 62.

22. For more on ginseng regulations by state, see Kim Derek Pritts, *Ginseng: How to Find, Grow, and Use North America's Forest Gold,* 2nd ed. (Mechanicsburg, PA: Stackpole Books, 2010); Scott Persons, *American Ginseng: Green Gold* (Asheville, NC: Bright Mountain Books, 1994).

23. Appalachian Land Ownership Task Force, *Who Owns Appalachia? Landownership and Its Impact* (Lexington: University Press of Kentucky, 2015), 12.

24. Beaver, Ballard, and Hicks, *Voices from the Headwaters,* 50.

25. Cooper, *The Pond Mountain Chronicle,* 188.

26. Beaver, Ballard, and Hicks, *Voices from the Headwaters,* 212.

27. Rhoda H. Halperin, *The Livelihood of Kin: Making Ends Meet "the Kentucky Way"* (Austin: University of Texas Press, 1990), 1–20, 146.

28. Shannon E. McBride, "Political Juxtapositions: Wildcrafting among Herb Diggers in Graham County, North Carolina (1900–2004)" (PhD diss., University of Georgia, 2005).

29. John Jenkins, quoted in McBride, "Political Juxtapositions," 286.

30. Recent books by David Taylor and Kristin Johannsen colorfully document the persistence of ginseng digging. See Taylor, *Ginseng, the Divine Root* (Chapel Hill, NC: Algonquin Books, 2006); Johannsen, *Ginseng Dreams: The Secret World of America's Most Valuable Plant* (Lexington: University Press of Kentucky, 2006).

31. Mary Hufford, "Knowing Ginseng: The Social Life of an Appalachian Root," *Cahiers de littérature orale* 53–54 (2003): 265–92; Eric Edwards, "Stewards of the Forest: An Analysis of Ginseng Harvesters and the Communal Boundaries That Define Their Identity in an Area of Environmental Degradation" (MA thesis, Marshall University, 2011).

32. Greenfield and Davis, *Collection to Commerce*.

33. Appalachian Land Ownership Task Force, *Who Owns Appalachia?* 13–25.

34. Brent Bailey, "Social and Economic Impacts of Wild Harvested Products" (PhD diss., West Virginia University, 1999), 22.

35. Close to 95 percent of the United States' cultivated ginseng crop comes from Wisconsin. See Bailey, "Social and Economic Impacts of Wild Harvested Products," 7; Alvar Carlson, "Ginseng: America's Botanical Drug Connection to the Orient," *Economic Botany* 40, no. 2 (April–June 1986): 233–49.

36. Greenfield and Davis, *Collection to Commerce*, 23, 29, 36, 53.

37. Kathryn Newfont, *Blue Ridge Commons: Environmental Activism and For-*

est History in Western North Carolina, Environmental History and the American South (Athens: University of Georgia Press, 2012).

38. Newfont, *Blue Ridge Commons,* 52–110, 148–50.

39. John Paul Schmidt et al., "Explaining Harvests of Wild-Harvested Herbaceous Plants: American Ginseng as a Case Study," *Biological Conservation* 231 (2019): 139–49.

40. Anna Lowenhaupt Tsing, *The Mushroom at the End of the World: On the Possibility of Life in Capitalist Ruins* (Princeton: Princeton University Press, 2015), 5.

Index

Page numbers in italics refer to illustrations.

Index

Index

"rights-in-the-woods," 7, 34–35
Rives, Amelie, 210–11
R. T. Greer Herb Co., 121, 125–26, 222
Rush, Benjamin, 67, 70–71, 208

salvage capitalism, 6
sang diggers: in census, 155–56; literary "discovery" of, 195–96; as lotos-eaters, 214–15; the myth of, 199–207; romanticization of, 211–16; stigma associated with, 207–10; in West Virginia, 151–53
sassafras (*Sassafras albidum*), 78, 90, 91, *92*, 104, 139, 219, 222
S. B. Penick & Co., 124–25, 222
Schoepf, Johann, 29, 35, 46
Sears, J. W., 176–77, 180, 185
Second Great Awakening, 73–74
Seneca snakeroot (*Polygala senega*), 66, 69, 78, 92, 97–98, 222
Shakers: during the Civil War, 97–98, 111, 260n8; and the origins of pharmaceutical industry, 73, 78–80, 255–56n50
Shortia galacifolia, 86, 87, 118–19
Silva, Robert D., 151–52
Simms, William Gilmore, 102
Smyth, Clifford, 202
Southern nationalism: and medical botany, 101
squatters, 52
Stanton, George, 176–77, 185
Strother Drug Company, 123
"submerged tenth," 204–5

Taylor, Henry, 1–3, 115, 142
therapeutic landscape, 88–89
therapeutic revolutions, 68, 221
Thomas, Wiley P., 142–43
Thomas, William Holland, 55–57, 135, 209
Thompson, Maurice, 212–13
Thomson, Samuel, 72–75
Thomsonianism, 72–74, 89, 91
Tilden & Co, 80–81, 256n54; during the Civil War, 97–98, 111
to'hi, Cherokee concept of, 21–22
Toms, Charles F., 182, 188
"Tragedy of the Commons, The" (Hardin), 9, 236n8. *See also* commons

Valle Crucis, NC, 1–2, 115, 121, 142, 146

Wallace Brothers, 96, 115–21, 126
Waring, James J., 103–4
Webb, Henry, 1–2, 5
Webster County, WV, 147–48, 152–53, 165, 169, 170–71, 272n68
Wheeling, WV, 33–34, 165, 173
Wilcox, Grant, 121, 124–25
Wilcox Drug Company, 222
wild ginger (*Asarum canadense*), 4, 83, 92, 103, *138*, 139, 158
Wilson, James, 183
Woodell, William J., 168
Woodell's Sang Bill, 168–72
World War I: and botanical drug trade, 121–26, 219–20